A History of Public Health

A History of Public Health

Revised Expanded Edition

GEORGE ROSEN

Foreword by
Pascal James Imperato,
MD, MPH&TM

Introduction by
Elizabeth Fee

Biographical Essay &
New Bibliography by
Edward T. Morman

Johns Hopkins University Press
Baltimore

© Copyright 1958 by MD Publications, Inc., New York, New York
© 1993, 2015 Johns Hopkins University Press
Reprinted by permission of Paul P. Rosen, MD
All rights reserved. Published 2015
Printed in the United States of America on acid-free paper
2 4 6 8 9 7 5 3 1

Johns Hopkins University Press
2715 North Charles Street
Baltimore, Maryland 21218-4363
www.press.jhu.edu

Library of Congress Cataloging-in-Publication Data

Rosen, George, 1910–1977, author.
A history of public health / George Rosen ; foreword by Pascal James Imperato ;
introduction by Elizabeth Fee ; biographical essay and new bibliography by
Edward T. Morman. — Revised expanded edition.
p. ; cm.
Includes bibliographical references and indexes.
ISBN 978-1-4214-1601-4 (pbk. : alk. paper) — ISBN 1-4214-1601-8 (pbk. : alk. paper)
— ISBN 978-1-4214-1602-1 (electronic) — ISBN 1-4214-1602-6 (electronic)
I. Title.
[DNLM: 1. Rosen, George, 1910–1977. 2. Public Health—history. WA 11.1]
RA424.R65
614.4—dc23   2014016735

A catalog record for this book is available from the British Library.

*Special discounts are available for bulk purchases of this book. For more information,
please contact Special Sales at 410-516-6936 or specialsales@press.jhu.edu.*

Johns Hopkins University Press uses environmentally friendly
book materials, including recycled text paper that is composed of at least
30 percent post-consumer waste, whenever possible.

WITHDRAWN

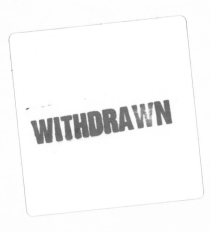

Pascal James Imperato, MD, MPH&TM

FORMER COMMISSIONER OF HEALTH OF NEW YORK CITY

DEAN AND DISTINGUISHED SERVICE PROFESSOR

STATE UNIVERSITY OF NEW YORK

DOWNSTATE MEDICAL CENTER

SCHOOL OF PUBLIC HEALTH

In his preface to the first edition of this volume, George Rosen cogently noted that to understand the present, we must view it "in the light of the past from which it has emerged and of the future which it is bringing forth." He emphasized that advancement into the future required close attention to the past and how it created the possibilities of the present. In setting forth these essential principles that characterize continuity across time, he was in effect saying that the past is never irrelevant. Rather, it informs both the present and the future and helps to shape new ideas and scientific discoveries.

When the first edition of this volume appeared in 1950, the conquest of infectious diseases seemed almost assured. New antibiotics and vaccines held the promise of relegating many of these diseases to archival status. For a time, both medical and public health practitioners witnessed the decline in prevalence of what had once been plagues of both adults and children. As they did so, the focus of attention shifted to chronic diseases.

However, within a short time, antibiotic resistance, the emergence of newer infections, the reemergence of known infections, and the impacts of globalization shifted many public health efforts back to where they had been when Rosen was writing this book. Thus it is that today, infectious diseases are not only in second place globally as the cause of death but also the leading cause of death among those younger than fifty years old.

Several factors have brought about this dramatic return to the past, including world population growth, which in turn has resulted in major population movements. These geographic shifts include encroachment into previously uninhabited environments resulting in exposure to the vectors and reservoirs of diseases previously unknown or little known in humans. At the same time, there has been massive migration to urban environments with weak sanitary infrastructures. Increased transnational and transcontinental population movements have also resulted in the transportation of diseases and insect vectors.

The globalization of the world's food supplies has resulted in the distribution of products contaminated either at the source of production or during various phases of processing. Likewise, global industry and commerce and less than adequate quality production standards have created products that harbor harmful and even deadly chemicals. Human behaviors that alter the environment and bring about climatic changes have directly altered the larger biotope, and thus facilitated the growth of vector and animal reservoir populations. In many resource-poor countries, population growth has outstripped the capacity of public health infrastructures, leading to an expansion of unsanitary environments.

The list of infectious diseases that has emerged over the past forty years is lengthy. It includes HIV/AIDS, Legionnaires' disease, Ebola virus disease, *Cryptosporidium parvum* diarrhea, *Escherichia coli* 0157:H7 hemorrhagic colitis and hemorrhagic uremic syndrome, Lyme disease, severe acute respiratory syndrome (SARS), avian influenza, West Nile virus infection, and many others.

In the absence of a specific vaccine and antiviral agents, the prevention and control of Ebola virus disease uniquely depend on long-established public health interventions discussed in detail by Rosen in this volume. These include patient isolation, concurrent disinfection of everything associated with the patient and his or her environment, identification and surveillance of contacts, and modern versions of quarantine. Enhancing the prevention and control of epidemics and outbreaks of Ebola virus disease, such as those of the late twentieth and early twenty-first centuries, requires the development of effective vaccines and therapeutic agents.

Most of the emerging infections are zoonotic in nature. The reemerging infections, by contrast, are often the result of human behaviors that facilitate transmission. Refusal to have children immunized out of fears that vaccination could cause adverse consequences has resulted in modern outbreaks of measles, pertussis, and poliomyelitis. The prevalence of sexually transmitted diseases such as human papillomavirus infection and herpes virus infections has risen in recent decades because of altered human attitudes and behaviors and individual failure to employ recommended modes of prevention.

The current public health landscape thus includes not only the challenges inherent in the prevention and control of chronic diseases but also those associated with communicable diseases. On the global scene, essential public health infrastructures that provide potable water supplies, sewage disposal, sanitary environments, and safe food and drug supplies are being seriously stressed.

It is clear that a number of public health problems, once a fixture of the distant and not-so-distant past, are largely being addressed with long-established interventions extensively covered in George Rosen's volume. The epidemiology, detection, prevention, and control of most of these emerging and reemerging infections have not appreciably changed over time.

These facts point out the enduring value of Rosen's *A History of Public Health*. For its pages cover not only the public health problems of the past but also some of the public health problems cast against the canvas of a rapidly changing globalized society.

Rosen brought to his writing of this book a unique sense of the intimate relationships between the social and biological determinants of disease and an insightful understanding of the continuity of past, present, and future in the conduct of human affairs. His global account of public health's long and fascinating history benefited from his skills as a historian and from his experiences as a public health practitioner. Although he is best remembered as a medical historian, Rosen also practiced public health. His public health roles practiced in a diversity of venues greatly enriched Rosen's scholarly understanding of the challenges faced across time by those entrusted with protecting and promoting collective well-being.

Initially trained as a clinician at Beth-El Hospital (now Brookdale Hospital) in Brooklyn, New York, he went into private practice for five years. Toward the end of his private practice, he served as a clinic physician in the New York City Department of Health's Bureau of Tuberculosis Control. In this pre-antibiotic era, the prevention, control, and treatment of tuberculosis were daunting, and only the most courageous physicians volunteered for this service. He served as a junior health officer for two years in the health department from 1941 to 1943. Rosen added administrative experiences to the clinical skills he already possessed. During World War II, he served in the Preventive Medicine Service of the Surgeon General's Office and in the European Theater of Operations. After his discharge, he returned to the New York City Department of Health as a district health officer, where he was responsible for overseeing the broad scope of functions and services the department offered. These ranged from maternal and child health clinics to environmental sanitation. Thus, he was responsible for maintaining the public health in a densely populated area of New York City. In so doing, he acquired a vast field-based knowledge of the diverse interventions required to protect the health of the public.

In 1949, Harry S. Mustard, MD, Commissioner of Health of New York City, asked George Rosen to become director of the Bureau of Health Education. Mustard, an academician, had turned to Rosen because he viewed him as someone who could bring new ideas to the bureau. Mustard was also attracted to Rosen because he possessed a PhD in sociology (awarded in 1944 by Columbia University) and a Master of Public Health degree, awarded by Columbia in 1947.

Rosen then served for seven years as director of the Division of Health Education and Preventive Services of the Health Insurance Plan of Greater New

York. He was concurrently professor of public health education at Columbia University's then Faculty of Public Health and Administrative Medicine.

At the time that I joined the New York City Department of Health in 1972, George Rosen was a legendary figure in public health. Within the department, he was remembered for his legacy of important innovations in the Bureau of Health Education. At that time, many of the department's professionals had studied under him at Columbia and greatly admired him as an inspiring teacher. At this stage of his career, he enjoyed an international reputation as a scholar, teacher, and editor. His tenure as editor of the *American Journal of Public Health* (1957–1973) was marked by great improvements in the journal and an expansion of its scope of coverage.

Although my contacts with George Rosen were few, I was always impressed by his warm and welcoming manner and his effortless ability to engage younger public health specialists as respected colleagues. I think that he would be pleased to know that his volume continues to make the exciting history of public health available to younger generations. That audience now includes not only seasoned public health professionals but also an ever-expanding audience of students enrolled in baccalaureate, master's, and doctoral degree programs in public health.

A Shared Social Vision
Elizabeth Fee

George Rosen's *A History of Public Health* is a classic of public health history. An admirably comprehensive synthesis of the development of public health in Europe and North America, it engages the interest of both beginners and specialists. Rosen takes us on a chronological journey from the Greco-Roman ideas of health based on the balance of the four humors, through the plagues and quarantines of the Middle Ages, to the more modern era of political and industrial revolutions, and the health and sanitary reform movements of the nineteenth and twentieth centuries. Throughout, he displays his mastery of public health, his understanding of the social context as well as the biological determinants of disease, and his knowledge of social history, sociology, and political philosophy. Conceived in grand style and incorporating a wealth of detailed knowledge, the *History* is animated by the author's social and scientific optimism and his deep commitment to public health and progressive reform.

At the time of its first publication in 1958, Rosen's *History* filled an absolute vacuum; no book on the history of public health was at once so comprehensive, so accessible, and so informative. It soon became the standard history of the subject; in many ways, it has served to define the content and boundaries of the field ever since. When we consider the purpose, scope, and vision of Rosen's text, we can begin to understand why this book has not been superseded in the intervening decades.

George Rosen's *History* provided the framework and set the agenda for much subsequent research and writing on public health history. Over the past twenty years in particular, historians have paid increasing attention to the history of disease, medicine, and public health. For the most part, they have dealt with specific issues, institutions, personalities, places, and diseases—few have attempted to present a fully comprehensive view across the continents and centuries.[1] A flood of monographs and articles on aspects of public health history has extended Rosen's analysis of specific periods and issues; one purpose of this essay is to provide guidance to this more recent work in the field. Both the notes to this introduction and the new bibliography at the end of the volume thus serve as entry points to the more specialized historical literature. For those new to public health history, Rosen's book provides an excellent starting point and a necessary context for exploring these more specialized studies, but even those familiar with the recent literature will find that Rosen's sweeping synthesis remains useful in relating the diverse aspects of the field and in provoking new questions.

Some of these more recent scholarly studies challenge Rosen's interpretations, and others explore and elaborate them through extensive research in the primary sources. The generation of social historians of health that came of age in the 1960s rejected an older tradition of medical history that seemed to celebrate medical science, glorify the role of physicians, and project a positivist view of scientific progress, while appearing to accept uncritically the existing forms of medical care organization and the underlying structures of social inequality. Instead of a decontextualized story of scientific discoveries, Rosen offered a social history in which he tried to demonstrate the social production of health and disease, to place physicians and public health practitioners within their social context, and to show how their changing ideas and practices related to the larger framework of political and economic conditions. At the same time, he preserved a heroic place in his history for all those struggling to improve health and prevent disease, whether through the development and application of scientific ideas or through social reforms intended to promote the public health. Rosen's *History* thus provided both a model of social criticism and an inspirational tale offering the possibility of (albeit reconceptualized) progress. The first of these themes appeals directly to the critical interests of historians, while the second engages the activist impulses of public health practitioners.

This presentation of the history of public health is especially oriented to the interests of public health practitioners in the United States, the country where he spent most of his life working in public health and medical history. His early years as a medical student in Germany and his long-standing interest in European history, politics, and culture served to broaden his perspective and provided a comparative, and often critical, view. Rosen's medical and sociological training, his social and political concerns, and his almost twenty years of practical and administrative experience—all inform his historical analysis and help make his work relevant to the interests of public health students and practitioners. Most share his social concerns, his essentially optimistic belief in progress and social improvement, and his appreciation for science and positive knowledge.

Rosen showed how the history of public health can capture the attention of practitioners by playing on themes that relate the past to the present. Like his friend and mentor Henry E. Sigerist, he believed that history was an essential discipline in training health professionals; those working in practical and policy positions needed the perspective that could be provided only through knowledge of the past.[2] In his own professional career, Rosen demonstrated the dual interests of the historian and the practitioner. As former editor of the *Journal of the History of Medicine and Allied Sciences* and *Ciba Symposia*, he was familiar with a broad spectrum of research on the history of medicine and public health, and he could draw on his own extensive historical writings as well as on the work of other scholars in the field.[3] As a public health practitioner, administrator, and educator, and as editor of the *American Journal of Public Health*, he was also very much involved in the public health issues and controversies of his day and could speak with authority within the public health community.

Historians often find it difficult to analyze the period in which they live and work, preferring the distant past to the contentious present and welcoming the perspective provided by time's passing. George Rosen, however, sought direct connections between the past and the present—he deliberately used the past as an argument, as a guide, and sometimes as a source of moral lessons for action in the present. Since he believed so firmly in progress, he detected (or perhaps created) a rational progression in the past: a progression in the direction of ever-increasing social concern, social responsibility, equity, and fairness—and he was convinced that history provided precedent and support for continued progress in the future.

Looking Backward: A Later Perspective on Rosen's Politics

Rosen's history ends in the middle of the twentieth century, in the 1950s, and much has changed since then. In the United States, a multiplicity of social protest movements, beginning with the civil rights movement, prompted the expansion of the welfare state through the Great Society programs of the 1960s. The War on Poverty, the Civil Rights Act, and the passage of Medicare and Medicaid are certainly developments of which Rosen would have approved, but the escalation of Vietnam War provoked a large antiwar movement and proved a national as well as an international trauma, marking the end of the United States' assumptions of invincibility. The rise of the decolonialized states and the Non-Aligned Movement also directly challenged the dominance of the United States and European powers. At home, the massive entry of women into the labor market, the flowering of the women's movement, and later of the gay movement, challenged assumptions about gender relations, the family, and sexuality. The occupational health movement and environmental movement created the social consciousness that would lead to the establishment of the Occupational Health and Safety Administration and the Environmental Protection Agency of 1970. Economic stagnation, recession, increased global competition, and the oil crisis were, however, followed by political backlash, attacks on unions and on the political and cultural movements of the 1960s. The

Nixon administration brought the slashing of domestic social expenditures, including public health programs, as again did the Reagan administration in the 1980s. Internationally, the fall of the Berlin Wall and the collapse of the Soviet Union marked the end of superpower rivalries that had structured international relations since World War II. Free-trade policies, international debt crises, economic globalization and growing inequalities among countries and populations were accompanied by the emergence and reemergence of deadly infectious diseases, as Pascal Imperato has explained in his Foreword to this volume. The wars in Iraq and Afghanistan, fears of terrorism and bioterrorism, eruptions in the Middle East, threats of global warming and climate change, and economic expansion collapsing into recession and unemployment have all contributed to making the world a much more threatening and less predictable place than it appeared at the time when George Rosen was writing. In reviewing the history of these more recent decades, it is difficult to see these changes as simply one more chapter in a history already understood: they appear sufficiently discontinuous as to force a more thorough reconsideration of the meaning and scope of contemporary history, including the history of public health.

A progressive, Rosen's political views had been shaped by the experiences and ideas of the 1930s and 1940s, the trade union victories of the Congress of Industrial Organizations (CIO), and the fight against fascism. Progressives and liberals believed firmly in progress, both social and scientific. History offered evidence that human beings, through will and organization, could change their societies for the better. By extrapolation, the future should offer more— more progress, more justice, more equality, and better health. In the future, the benefits from ever-expanding scientific and technological achievements, instead of accruing to a few, would be shared by all.

When Rosen wrote *A History of Public Health* in the 1950s, the Cold War was entrenched and social conflicts that earlier had been overt and obvious were muffled in apparent consensus. A postwar economic boom, widespread prosperity, the retreat to suburbia, and political repression of left-wing ideas had produced a consumer culture of patriotism mixed with complacency. Much of this complacency stemmed from the very gains of the New Deal and the fact that real wages were rising in an expanding economy. Progress, still a pervasive theme in popular culture, was now generally interpreted to mean the acquisition of personal security and material goods. In this context, social conflicts and contradictions were blanketed in silence, as were the politics of gender and sexuality. To be sure, the politics of class and race were being fought out in the factories, in the courts, and in the schools; the civil rights movement, still at its most optimistic, centered on the ideal of racial integration into the mainstream of American life. But for the most part, social and political life seemed untroubled. Rosen's assertion of an alternate vision of progress was a courageous political act as well as a statement of personal conviction.

A few decades later, after the upheavals of the 1960s, 1970s, 1980s, and 1990s, our perceptions of the history of the twentieth century have irrevocably changed. The progressives who triumphed over depression, war, and fascism were able to read the twentieth century as a story of progress. A later generation would find this most basic form of political optimism difficult or impossible. Rosen's very faith in progress and in the continuous steady development of the welfare state, social reform, and public health now gives the final chapters of this book a somewhat old-fashioned air. Today, we tend to be more pessimistic and more cynical. The welfare state is the center of bitter political struggles and can no longer simply be assumed as a measure of social progress and civilization. From immigration to national health insurance, the United States shows deep political divisions and great difficulty moving forward. Other countries around the world are also battling entrenched and, frequently, violent conflicts.

Public Health Issues That Exploded in the 1960s and After

Obviously, it would be unfair to criticize Rosen for not addressing issues that exploded in the 1960s and thereafter, nor can we necessarily fault his reading of progress on the basis of our contemporary skepticism or disillusionment. Anyone writing a history of public health today, for example, would have to pay attention to issues of race; we are incapable of thinking and talking about urban health, poverty, and welfare without dealing with race and racism, particularly as we struggle with differing perceptions and evaluations of the Great Society programs of the 1960s.

By contrast, Rosen's reading of progress led him to frame his discussions of the social context of disease in clear economic terms. Rosen insisted on the importance of class as a factor in public health. This unfashionable emphasis was particularly remarkable in the late 1950s, when the United States and other advanced capitalist countries had supposedly become virtually classless societies. Some readers may still find Rosen's emphasis on class, the impact of class inequalities on health, and the history of occupational health surprising or troubling, as more recent discussions of public health and social policy have often remained blind to the class issues to which Rosen devoted considerable attention. This emphasis on class and on the economic basis of health and illness is, however, all too relevant today, given the falling standard of living of the United States working class, deteriorating occupational health protections, and the return of epidemic tuberculosis and other diseases of poverty, as well as the emergence of devastating new epidemics.[4] We still need histories of public health in which class and race in their domestic and international context are together understood as central ways of shaping social experience and as the twin parameters of social policy in the twentieth and twenty-first centuries. Although sensitive to class issues, Rosen has little to say about gender. He incorporates into his history conventional descriptions of maternal and child health programs but ignores many issues that today convulse discussions of public policy, such as abortion, reproductive rights, and gay marriage. From present perspectives, this volume is curiously silent about such matters as birth control, sex education, and the medicalization of women's health. In the context of the current worldwide pandemic of AIDS, widespread public awareness of sexually transmitted diseases, active contemporary discussions of family violence, battering, and child abuse, and political warfare over abortion rights, it is no longer possible to doubt the relevance to public health of sexuality, sexual behavior, and gender relations.

At his best, Rosen provides interpretations that help us understand the shifting contours of public health in relation to fundamental political and economic changes—mercantilism and cameralism, the Enlightenment, and the philosophic radicalism of the early nineteenth century. In his discussions of the eighteenth and nineteenth centuries, for example, we will see how he draws on elements of Marxist analysis to explore the relationship of public health to the economic and political processes that changed the shape of Europe and North America. At other times, however, when he loses sight of the underlying economic and political processes, his text tends to become a more descriptive listing of efforts and accomplishments—one that is useful, to be sure, but less illuminating and less exciting to read. This is most apparent in Rosen's final sections on public health in the twentieth century, where his inattention to issues of race and gender is also most troubling.

As many readers will note, Rosen pays little attention to the global realities of public health beyond the boundaries he has set by restricting his account to Europe and the United States. There are only a few, fleeting references to Asia, Africa, and South America; these continents appear most frequently as the sources of disease epidemics affecting the more developed world. Rosen gives some indication that he recognizes the need for a larger, more international view of public health problems and interventions, but at the same time, his account is constricted by the implicit conviction—still common today—that all the really important events and activities, at least in modern times, have taken place in Europe and North America. In the preface to his book, he makes explicit reference to an understanding of "development" in which the nations of the Third World are simply lagging several centuries behind their more prosperous neighbors: "For a variety of reasons, a large part of the world—in Asia, in Africa, in the Middle East—stopped developing economically, politically and scientifically around 1400, just about the time that the Western nations entered upon a period of extraordinary growth in these areas. As a result, it is only today that the Asian and African peoples are beginning to effect the far-reaching changes necessary to bridge the gap of centuries." Like most other historians of the period, Rosen's perspective on international health seems innocent of any real comprehension of colonialism, imperial wars, or international political economy, and their impact on the health of the world's populations. Since that time, these subjects have been energetically explored and have generated a considerable literature.[5]

Drawing attention to the issues not covered or minimally discussed by Rosen should not be interpreted as criticism of him for failing to foresee issues that have emerged as present-day concerns, but to point out the ways in which, as health and social policy are reshaped in response to new understandings, so too must their history be revised to reflect a changing universe of meaning. In reading Rosen's *History* from a contemporary perspective, we may observe the subjects he chooses to address and those he omits, notice how his account reflects certain priorities and neglects others, become conscious of the ways in which he guides us and focuses our attention—and at the same time, continue to admire the scope of his accomplishment. With these contemporary concerns and attitudes in mind, we can thus retrace Rosen's history, observing along the way how he has shaped the history of public health in ways that emphasize the moral, political, and social lessons he wished to convey.

Reading Rosen's *History*

We begin as Rosen does, following the traditional outline of European and American history, with the ancient civilizations of Greece and Rome. This framework was certainly the standard when George Rosen was writing, and indeed, it continues to be the dominant framework for much of the history of medicine, science, and public health. There are, however, some indications within the body of Rosen's work that he found the traditional focus on Europe and the United States somewhat constricting. He thus began his *History* with a brief discussion of the sanitary ideas and practices of the ancient civilizations of India, Egypt, and Peru, and he ended with comments on the future of international health.

In his tantalizingly brief introductory chapter on ancient worldwide sanitary practices, Rosen establishes two important points. The first is that the history of public health cannot ultimately be restricted to European civilizations; although his text will be limited mainly to the history of Europe and North America, that history forms but part of a longer and larger history of health and healing throughout the world. The second is that public health includes broad environmental measures and is not restricted to the prevention of specific diseases; Rosen continually emphasizes the idea that such issues as cleanliness, water supplies, and waste removal are more fundamental to health and disease prevention than a sophisticated scientific knowledge of disease causation and transmission.

Turning to the main body of the book, we notice that Rosen devotes the first 40 percent of his text to the history of public health before 1830, the next 20 percent to the nineteenth-century sanitary movement, and the last 40 percent to the bacteriological era and the subsequent developments of the early twentieth century. Some historians would consider this a foreshortened account, but the balance of attention seems appropriate for public health workers, who are likely to be more interested in the relatively recent past than in distant times.

The chapters on the ancient and medieval world are primarily intended to provide a context for discussing the later development of public health in Europe. In these sections, Rosen tries to show how particular ideas of disease causation and prevention fit within their specific social, economic, and political contexts and how they satisfied immediate practical needs. He argues, for example, that the Hippocratic text on *Airs, Waters, and Places* not only represented the first systematic effort to relate environmental factors to disease but also served as a practical guidebook. He explains that the seafaring Greeks needed to understand the relationships of health to climate, soil, water, and nutrition to select the healthiest sites for the establishment of new colonies. Individual Greek physicians, who were essentially wandering craftsmen, also had to understand the geographical distribution of disease; a physician setting up practice in an unfamiliar town could impress potential patients by his familiarity with local diseases and ability to make accurate prognoses.

In a similar way, the Romans, as a great military power, produced public health knowledge and practices compatible with their social and military organization. Although they were dependent on the Greeks for much of their medical knowledge, they were supremely successful as engineers and administrators; their aqueducts, providing water to the cities, were the engineering marvel of the ancient world.[6] Rosen argues that the Roman public baths made personal hygiene and cleanliness possible for all citizens, and he applauds Roman administrative efficiency in the development of public health services, the provision of public hospitals, and the employment of city physicians. Here, he emphasizes themes that will recur in other contexts throughout his *History:* the need for public services, especially for the poor, and the importance of administrative efficiency in providing such services.[7]

Throughout his section on the ancient world, Rosen sets the stage for another key theme—the tension between a broad environmentalist view of disease and one emphasizing the action of specific disease agents. In a global generalization, he argues that the Hippocratic text *Airs, Waters, and Places* served as the basic epidemiological reference for more than two thousand years and that ideas of disease causation did not radically change until the development of bacteriology and immunology in the late nineteenth century. Although he will later provide a glowing account of the achievements of bacteriology, Rosen is clearly sympathetic to the broad, environmentalist perspective.[8]

Rosen's *History* moves rapidly to the monasteries and municipalities of the Middle Ages in Western Europe, referring only briefly to the transmission of Greek and Roman learning by Arab scholars and physicians. As in earlier chapters, he compresses a long and complicated historical development into a few pages, deliberately highlighting themes that show the social context of public health and link historical developments to contemporary concerns. He discusses the sanitary problems of medieval cities, quarantines and the isolation of people with communicable diseases, medical and social assistance to the poor, and the founding of hospitals, hospices, and bathhouses. He concludes that, despite a lack of concrete scientific knowledge, medieval cities were generally able to create "a rational system of public hygiene" for dealing with health problems.[9] Here, he is again trying to counter the scientism of popular culture by showing how much practically useful work can be accomplished in the absence of specific scientific and technological resources.

The Renaissance is associated with the beginnings of modern science and the rise of a new urban middle class, or bourgeoisie, whose wealth was dependent on commerce rather than on land. Their economic activities made possible the development of the national state and, with intellectuals who were often encouraged and directed by royal patronage, helped create a new secular culture, a new science, and the technologies essential for building weapons of war, increasing wealth, and consolidating power.[10]

Rosen argues that the bourgeoisie's growing interest in numerical calculations prompted the gathering of statistical information, first produced in Italian cities during the fourteenth century. Their scientific and quantitative interests also encouraged new approaches to the body: Andreas Vesalius brought a new level of critical observation and precise description to human anatomy, and William Harvey's discovery of the circulation of the blood demonstrated elements of a more functional, experimental, and quantitative approach to physiology. Close clinical observation brought recognizable descriptions of such diseases as whooping cough, typhus fever, and scarlet fever, and studies of disease transmission resulted in what Rosen terms "the first consistent theory of contagious disease," by Girolamo Fracastoro.[11]

In addition to stressing the new importance of scientific observation in the Renaissance, Rosen emphasizes the relationship between new (or newly observed) diseases and the social context in which they developed and were transmitted. Typhus fever traveled with armies and was nourished by constant military campaigns.[12] Scurvy, earlier observed in medieval cities under siege, now became an occupational disease of sailors, sent on voyages of exploration in ships lacking fresh fruits and vegetables.[13] Rickets, a disease born of economic depression, poverty, and malnutrition, was nurtured in dark, overcrowded urban settlements. Deep mines produced the occupational hazards and diseases of mine workers, as recognized by Paracelsus and as discussed comprehensively for the first time in Bernardino Ramazzini's treatise on the diseases of workers.[14]

Rosen also examines how military explorations, trade, and travel generated epidemics by exposing nonimmune populations to new diseases. Around the time of the Columbian voyages, syphilis arrived in Naples and spread from Italy to the rest of Europe.[15] Smallpox, which had smoldered endemically in Europe, proved devastating to Native American populations in the New World. Europeans also brought malaria to the Americas, probably carrying new strains of the parasite from Africa, India, and the Far East. The increasing integration of the world through trade meant the internationalization of disease organisms, which served, all too often, as aids to the armies of conquest.

In examining the early modern period from 1500 to 1750, Rosen shows how new theories of the state and the political and economic doctrines of mercantilism—the new system being built around trade and commerce—integrally involved public health. These theories assumed that no distinction need be made between the welfare of the state and the welfare of society; the interests of the state in building national power and wealth required a large and healthy population. This approach supported public health, albeit of a notably authoritarian form, in the concept of "medical police." The state, wanting to increase the size of the population and the productivity of labor, now began to apply statistical methods to calculations of mortality, life expectancy, and fertility.[16] Statistics thus became more than a matter of curiosity to mathematicians or aristocrats interested in improving their gambling odds; they represented the "book-keeping of the state" or, as William Petty called it, "political arithmetic."

The rulers of the absolutist German states had essentially unlimited powers over their populations. While admiring the spirit of enlightenment and humanitarianism that pervades the monumental work of Johann Peter Frank in the late eighteenth century, Rosen notes that Frank's concept of the "medical police" was based on the political agenda of the absolutist state, which, by the early nineteenth century, was "already outmoded and reactionary."[17] He thus refuses to present Frank as simply a "pioneer" of public health and insists that we read his work in the context of the political struggles between an older concept of the authoritarian state and the more democratic ideals of the French revolution. While rejecting authoritarian power, Rosen also deplores the inefficiency of systems run with purely local controls. He describes without admiration the English system of fragmented, local public health authorities, which lacked any administrative structure linking them to the central government. He praises several sweeping health policy proposals for the provision of national health and medical care—proposals that he admits were, at the time, purely theoretical. For Rosen's purposes, these Utopian proposals provide intellectual precedents within Western culture for the idea that the state should take responsibility for the population's health and welfare.

Rosen presents the Age of Enlightenment (from 1750 to 1830) as pivotal in the evolution of public health. The French philosophers of the Enlightenment had challenged tradition and authority as sources of knowledge and asserted the primacy of reason. In the Enlightenment dream of reason—the belief in the supreme social value of intelligence, the idea that, through reason, man could design and even guarantee social progress, the conviction that education and free institutions could lead to human perfectibility—Rosen found the ultimate justification for even the most mundane efforts to reform social institutions and improve social conditions. From this perspective, the purpose of public health was to translate the ideals of the Enlightenment into practice. Rosen saw the French as intellectuals, the British as administrators: whereas the French philosophers argued the power of human reason and the possibility of progress, the more pragmatic English tried to translate these ideals into legislation and social policy.[18]

In England, Rosen argues, the urban middle class developed a distinctive ethos, based on the values of order, efficiency, and social discipline—but also on the conviction that social conditions must be improved. Theirs was, he says in a wonderful phrase, "a humanitarianism of the successful, tempering sympathy with a firm belief in the sober and practical virtues of efficiency, simplicity, and cheapness." They set about social improvement with campaigns against gin and infant mortality, movements to reform prisons and mental asylums, and efforts to educate poor mothers in child care and to establish maternity hospitals, provincial hospitals, and dispensaries.[19] Rosen emphasizes the social problems of industrialization as motivating the quantitative analysis of health questions, the gathering of vital statistics, the publication of regional health surveys, and the proliferation of health education, advice literature, and home medical guides.[20] Perhaps the single most dramatic and controversial public health measure of the age was smallpox inoculation, followed by Edward Jenner's revolutionary discovery of vaccination.[21]

The chapter on the industrial revolution, the concentration of work and workers inside factories, the explosive growth of cities, and the sanitary reform movement of the nineteenth century stand at the intellectual center of Rosen's book. Following the radical and liberal reformers of this period, he broadly defines public health to include social movements and legislation with clear effects on health, such as efforts to limit the length of the working day, to regulate child labor, to protect pregnant women, and to guarantee employment. A central theme, however, is the continuing debate over theories of disease causation. Rosen discusses the idea, promoted by a minority of mid-nineteenth-century epidemiologists, that specific diseases were caused by specific infections.[22] In recounting the controversies over disease causation, he draws heavily on Erwin Ackerknecht's influential analysis of contagionism and anticontagionism, which suggests that, in an atmosphere of scientific debate and uncertainty, theories of disease were often promoted or opposed for political and economic reasons.[23]

Although Rosen argues that modern public health began as a response to the evils of industrialization, his is not an abstract argument about modernization. He first explains how English sanitary reform was linked to Poor Law reform. The enclosure of common lands had made huge numbers of the rural poor destitute, throwing the existing poor relief system into crisis. At the same time, the factories of the new industrial cities displayed a voracious appetite for laboring bodies. The New Poor Law Act of 1834, drafted by Edwin Chadwick and the economist Nassau Senior, created a national labor market, setting the pool of rural surplus labor "free" to migrate to cities, and supplying factories with a new class of industrial workers. These men, women, and children toiled for long hours of work under dangerous conditions in factories and mines. As they crowded into the towns and cities, speculative builders, interested in maximum profits, constructed back-to-back housing with narrow rooms and tiny back alleys, lacking adequate ventilation, light, or sewerage.[24] The new urban populations were supplied with saloons and bars, but sanitary expenditures were deemed unprofitable.

The spread of cholera and other epidemic diseases drew attention to the disastrous living conditions of the new working class.[25] To Edwin Chadwick, the most influential of the public health reformers, disease was a cause of poverty (and high relief expenditures) while health created wealth. In 1842, Chadwick and his collaborators published their *Report on the Sanitary Condition of the Labouring Population of Great Britain*, which "proved beyond any doubt" that disease stemmed from filthy environmental conditions, polluted water supplies, and the decaying garbage and wastes clogging the streets.[26]

In Rosen's view, and that of the sanitary reformers, unmodified laissez-faire economics was equivalent to a license for exploitation; some degree of public regulation of private property and personal behavior was essential to protect people from unnecessary hazards to their health. Given the deplorable working and living conditions of the new industrial cities, the question was not whether any regulation was necessary, but how much, of what kinds, and for what purposes? At what point should the economic freedom of investors be limited by the demands of public health? English social reformers argued that society had a right to be concerned about disease as an unproductive drain on the economic well-being of the entire community: a sick worker implied the loss of productive labor and each dead male worker added a widow and children to the relief rolls. Where economic rationality reinforced humanitarian feelings, national statistics provided the ammunition for the reformers' campaigns. The new working class, to the extent that it became organized in trade unions and political parties, would help shift the balance of power in favor of developing social and health services.

Examining the public health movements in England, France, and Germany, Rosen shows that fears of the revolutionary movements brewing in Europe in 1848, as much as the dread of cholera, prompted public health reforms. Each nation had intellectuals who pointed out the connections between ill health and poverty and demanded radical or revolutionary change as an answer to the problems of endemic and epidemic diseases. Friedrich Engels in England and Rudolf Virchow in Germany, for example, used public health as a focal point for demonstrating exploitation, dramatizing unhealthy social conditions, and demanding more democratic solutions.[27]

In both England and France, statistical studies of health and disease were becoming an important part of the arsenal of public health reformers.[28] In France, for example, Villermé's statistical study of Paris neighborhoods demonstrated a clear connection between ill-health and poverty.[29] Rudolf Virchow, a leader of the early liberal reform movement in Germany, has gained almost mythic status within public health circles for his social analysis of the causes of disease and his report on the typhus epidemic in Upper Silesia, which recommended economic and political reforms as the solution to the epidemic.[30]

In each of these countries, the reforms eventually enacted fell short of the more ambitious liberal and radical ideas. In England, the Public Health Act of 1848 simply allowed boards of health to appoint medical officers of health and begin dealing with public health problems. The later Public Health Act of 1875 brought a greater centralization of power and more coherence to English public health administration.[31] In France, the legislation of 1848 created a national network of local public health councils (conseils de salubrité) that were merely advisory to local governments.[32] In Germany, the sweeping health and social legislation proposed by liberal and radical reformers was translated, after 1848, into a much more modest set of health and sanitary improvements.[33]

This analysis of Europe sets the stage for Rosen's account of public health in the United States. This essentially begins in the mid-nineteenth century; for the most part, later historians of public health have also tended to focus on the late nineteenth and early twentieth century when public health movements and organizations became more established and visible.[34] Beginning at this point, however, creates a history of public health similar to that of European countries, with many of the particularities of the American colonial situation omitted from the story. There are thus no Native Americans in most American histories of public health,[35] and except for a few recent books on the American South, there are no slaves.[36]

As in England, the early American history of public health consisted of local authorities trying to deal more or less effectively with local sanitary matters and responding at panicked intervals to the threat of epidemics. Rosen sees the massive immigration of the nineteenth century, bringing a population surge to the industrial cities, as equivalent to the migration prompted by poor law reform in England. As in Europe, public health reformers formed committees, undertook sanitary surveys, and wrote impassioned books about the condition of the new urban working class, often modeling their activities on the British and French sanitary movements.[37]

Public health in the latter part of the nineteenth century in Europe and America changes dramatically with the new discoveries in bacteriology.[38] In place of complicated environmentalist theories of disease, germ theory offered apparently simple and scientific explanations for infectious diseases—the microorganisms, made visible in the laboratory, whose life cycles and effects on the human organism could now be investigated and described. Rosen's lively account of Pasteur's pathbreaking work emphasizes its direct relationship to commercial interests in alcohol fermentation and silk production.[39] His largely admiring and uncritical account of the subsequent development of the "golden age" of bacteriology is, however, essentially a descriptive listing of discoveries and accomplishments leading to "the incontrovertible demonstration toward the end of the nineteenth century that specific microscopic creatures rather than vague chemical miasmas produce infectious diseases."[40] Here we find brief accounts of the work of Robert Koch and others in identifying the causative organisms for such diseases as typhoid, leprosy, malaria, tuberculosis, cholera, diphtheria, and tetanus.[41] Rosen describes Pasteur's efforts to produce vaccines by modifying the virulence of bacteria, Joseph Lister's introduction of antiseptic techniques into surgery, William Park's discovery of the carrier state in diphtheria, Ronald Ross's proof that malaria was transmitted by mosquitoes, and Walter Reed's demonstration that the yellow fever virus was similarly transmitted.[42]

Rosen emphasizes the contributions of Americans in developing the practical implications of bacteriological discoveries through the work of diagnostic laboratories and the mass production of diphtheria antitoxin. As the sanitary reform movement generated local health departments, so the bacteriological revolution gave rise to the diagnostic laboratory, the scientific arm of the health department.[43] Bacteriological laboratories allowed many public health procedures to be more efficiently applied, quarantine procedures to be more precisely targeted, and empirical methods and regulations to be enforced with greater discrimination.[44]

Rosen also asks whether the new scientific methods bore any relation to the actual decline of infectious diseases. This question was to be addressed, and answered largely in the negative, in Thomas McKeown's enormously influential book *The Modern Rise of Population* (1976).[45] Writing nearly twenty years earlier, however, Rosen notes that many of the more important infectious diseases began to decline well before the specific causes of these infections were discovered or their transmission clearly understood. He contends that the downward mortality trends reflected, at least in part, the impact of the earlier sanitary reform movement, an argument amplified by Simon Szreter.[46] Rosen maintains that the general reforms of the sanitary era were effective in lowering overall mortality and that the more targeted scientific procedures of the bacteriological era simply accelerated the trend and sharpened the curve in the case of specific diseases. Returning to his broader social and economic theme, he concludes that the success of Europe and North America in lowering infectious disease rates depended on their ability to invest accumulated wealth in the improvement of community health; for much of the world, however, inequalities in health would continue to be directly related to the differential distribution of wealth and poverty.

Much of Rosen's discussion of the early twentieth century is a story of progressive accomplishment in the expanding fields of public health activity and in the organization and financing of medical care. It touches on many topics now more extensively researched by contemporary historians. Rosen first describes the proliferation of child welfare measures in Europe and America through the provision of clean milk, prenatal care, maternal health services, and well-baby clinics, and highlights the establishment of the Children's Bureau in the United States as the first national effort to improve child and maternal health.[47] Assuming the medicalization of childbirth an obvious benefit, Rosen approvingly notes the shift from home births attended by midwives to doctor-assisted hospital births—a transition that has been dealt with much more critically by feminist writers and historians.[48] Responding to a heightened social awareness of the politics of reproduction, contemporary scholars have expanded and sharpened the analysis of birth control, abortion, sexuality, and women's health—themes and issues that Rosen barely mentions.[49] This newer exploration of birth control and population policies clearly links the politics of gender and sexuality to anxiety about class, race, and immigration, as expressed through nativism and eugenics, and ties these concerns to the economic, political, and military interests of countries competing to acquire colonies, define spheres of influence, and secure markets and sources of raw materials.[50]

A History of Public Health devotes much attention to the activities of health departments: school health services, the development of public health nursing,[51] and health education campaigns.[52] Rosen also elaborates on the role of the thousands of voluntary health organizations established to raise money and draw public concern to specific diseases, particular parts of the body, or special population groups.[53] He briefly discusses the work of the United States Public Health Service but is surprisingly silent about the Centers for Disease Control and Prevention (CDC, then the Communicable Disease Center) and the National Institutes of Health (NIH), and mentions schools of public health only in passing.[54] The Communicable Disease Center and the schools of public health were weak and underfunded in the 1950s, and the power of the NIH within the world of biomedical science was perhaps not fully evident.

Rosen displays a particular interest in nutrition, the discovery of vitamins, and efforts to understand deficiency diseases such as scurvy, beriberi, rickets, and pellagra, highlighting Joseph Goldberger and Edgar Sydenstricker's classical studies of the social epidemiology of pellagra in the southern states.[55] He discusses the regulation of food and drugs, the widespread malnutrition following the Depression, the food stamp program inaugurated in 1939, and the distribution of agricultural surpluses through relief programs and school lunches.[56] He concludes that those concerned with community health must address the economic, political, and social problems that create malnutrition and other food-related disorders in both developed and developing countries. Rosen's interest in the relationship between nutrition and health has recently been extended into new areas by other scholars: the history of famine and starvation, the historical relations of class and gender as physically expressed by height and body weight, and the cultural production of bulimia, anorexia nervosa, and obesity.[57]

An extensive discussion of occupational health displays one of Rosen's major interests as a historian. As in the case of much of his twentieth-century survey, however, this section is factual and descriptive, and lacks a clear sense of the changing economic, political, and social context within which research, laws, and regulations were carried out. He says little or nothing about how occupational health policy was affected by war, depression, or the New Deal, about the impact of communism or fascism or, within the United States, about the effects of the McCarthy era or the struggles within trade unions over political and economic policies. The resultant listing of accomplishments is sanguine in tone and lacks much of the tension and drama found in the real-world conflict over this most contested territory of public health.[58]

The section on medical care is more lively; he sketches developments in several European countries, comments very positively on the British National Health Service, and recounts the early efforts to obtain national health insurance in the United States.[59] He also describes the increasing later opposition of insurance companies and the medical profession to the idea of federally funded health care, notes the meager legislative gains to 1950, and discusses the growth of voluntary prepayment plans and private health insurance systems. He highlights the historical contributions of health centers and health districts; these have indeed been followed by more modern incarnations such as neighborhood health centers and community clinics.[60] Subsequent events have, however, countered Rosen's optimistic belief in the continuing steady historical development of state health and welfare services. Recent history has witnessed constant upheavals in policies and funding of both welfare and health services as well as tumultuous battles over the Affordable Care Act.[61]

Rosen suggests that a comprehensive theory of public health administration is needed to address the proper distribution of power and responsibility for health among the federal, state, and local levels; with hindsight, we can see that this political issue is one key to the peculiarities of the American political system. Problems of power, however, are hardly likely to be solved by administrative theory; shifts in political philosophy at the federal level will no doubt continue to determine fiscal and social policy, and state governments will have to cope with the consequences.

The treatment of international issues in the mid-twentieth century focuses on the work of the then newly created World Health Organization and the growth of international cooperative efforts.[62] He briefly, but sharply, criticizes pessimistic reactions to international population growth and disputes the assertion that poverty, malnutrition, and disease necessarily go hand in hand with dense or rapidly increasing populations. The real problem and the real solution, he says, lie with economic development in agriculture and industry, the creation of competent administrative services, and improvements in the educational status of the mass of the population. The international community must help countries solve their health problems by first addressing the larger social and economic issues.

Rosen writes, in terms that are still relevant, about the close relationship between health and economic problems and of the need to provide technical assistance in health within a broader framework of social and economic development. He avoids, however, any direct discussion of the economic relationships between countries, the structure of markets and international debt, and the reasons why much of the developing world remains mired in poverty. Historians since Rosen's time have become much more interested in how colonialism and imperialism have influenced health and medicine from the eighteenth century to the present.[63] The subjects they have examined include the social epidemiology of disease in developing countries, the transmission of disease between countries, and the reasons for the success or failure of international health campaigns.[64]

Rosen ends his *History* with a look toward the future and lists what he antici-
pates will be the public health problems of the next generation. His summary
is a typical one for the 1950s: the aging of the population, chronic diseases, accident prevention, mental health services, environmental health, air pollution,
and radiological health. He mentions the health problems of nuclear radiation
but gives more attention to health and housing, slum clearance, and the building of new suburban developments. Although he refers to an "increasing conservatism in social policy," his conclusion is relentlessly optimistic: "Today,
the community is in a better position than ever before to control its environment and so to preserve health and prevent disease. More and more, man can
consciously plan and organize his campaign for better health because available knowledge and resources make it possible for him in many instances to
act with a clear understanding of what he is doing." He ends by urging public
health workers to preserve and hand on the "noble legacy" of earlier generations
of public health activists.

Current Directions in the History of Public Health

Since the publication of *A History of Public Health* in 1958, there has been an ex-
plosion of scholarship in the field, spurred in no small part by Rosen's work.[65]
As made evident in the accompanying bibliography, new critical books and
monographs have been published on a remarkable diversity of topics. In the
United States, much attention has been devoted to the history of public health
in specific states, cities, and regions.[66] Such studies have the advantage of allowing their authors to explore developments in public health within a particular
social and political context, and thus of relating health issues to the larger politics of the urban environment or to the geography and economy of a particular
region. For the United States, John Duffy's *The Sanitarians* provides a comprehensive view of public health efforts across four centuries, and summarizes or
references many of these more local or specialized studies.[67]

Public health institutions and organizations, both national and regional,
have also received attention. The United States Public Health Service is properly the subject of a number of historical studies; the Centers for Disease Control and Prevention, the National Institutes of Health, the Rockefeller Foundation, and several of the schools of public health have all been variously
applauded, dissected, or criticized by those writing sanctioned or unsanctioned
institutional histories.[68]

Specialized areas of public health, such as maternal and child health, mental
health, popular health education, public health nursing, occupational health,
and environmental health have, and are continuing to develop, a lively historical literature relevant to their specific fields. In some cases, this historical re-

search directly addresses contemporary policy debates; in others, it addresses issues of interpretation within the larger fields of social history, labor history, women's history, and the history of medicine, and is only secondarily, if at all, intended to influence current policies. The directions of historical research and writing do, however, clearly respond to the public health issues considered most critical. Environmental health, for example, has attracted considerable scholarly attention. Similarly, after some years of relative neglect, the history of water, sanitary engineering, and waste disposal have also become issues of interest.[69]

Similarly, the impact of the women's movement and the enormous popular interest in women's health issues has prompted a small industry of research and writing on the history of women's health. Although much of this scholarship is directly related to the history of medicine and nursing, much of it also concerns population issues, public health, social welfare, and health policy.[70] Race and minority health issues, after years of relative neglect, have also received focused attention from a new generation of historians ready to pose questions sharply critical of the medical and public health systems, and more generally, of social practices and public policy. This interest in race and racism extends to the history of eugenics and racial theory, the history of slavery in the United States, the treatment of native and minority populations throughout the Americas, and the application of racial theories in South Africa and Nazi Germany.[71]

One of the richest areas of scholarship continues to be the history of disease, spanning the range from Charles Rosenberg's classic book on cholera and Allan Brandt's lively account of venereal disease, to Richard Evans's impressive *Death in Hamburg* (also on cholera) and Naomi Rogers's engaging study of polio.[72] In between are many significant works on such diseases as yellow fever, hookworm, tuberculosis, syphilis, influenza, anorexia nervosa, and cancer.[73] National and international concern about the AIDS epidemic has certainly stimulated much recent writing about the history of disease, social responses to epidemics, and the contemporary history of AIDS politics and policies.[74] As government agencies and health institutions continue to wrestle with difficult and contested policy options for dealing with the epidemic, the political, ethical, and legal questions posed by HIV and HIV-related diseases have given the history of public health a renewed relevance.

Many of the newer areas of interest have been conceptualized as the history of the body, with the body itself seen as historically constructed through social practices.[75] Our very experience of the body in health and illness—how we perceive ourselves physically, how we eat, move, live, and die—are all part of a history of public health seen as both material and cultural history.[76] Beginning with the experience of the body, the history of food, drugs, sexuality, violence, and disease may all be understood from new perspectives. These allow us to ask different kinds of questions about the history of health and medicine, including those cultural practices considered healthy and those deemed destructive.

When the history of public health is seen as a history of how populations experience health and illness, how social, economic, and political systems structure the possibilities for healthy or unhealthy lives, how societies create the preconditions for the production and transmission of disease, and how people, both as individuals and as social groups, attempt to promote their own health or avoid illness, we find that public health history is not limited to the study of bureaucratic structures and institutions but pervades every aspect of social and cultural life. Hardly surprisingly, these questions direct attention to issues of power, ideology, social control, and popular resistance. These issues may be framed in terms of state intervention versus individual liberties, as the interests of the economically powerful against the relatively powerless, or as the assertion of community rights and interests against the irresponsibility of a few. Such historical concerns engage political philosophy, ideology, ethics, and cultural beliefs and enrich our comprehension of contemporary health policies and politics.[77]

The very variety and multiplicity of themes and interests in the history of public health may help to explain why, with so many excellent studies of specific topics, there have been few attempts at broader, synthetic works.[78] The very proliferation of scholarly research makes the production of any new synthesis, at least one likely to be satisfactory to specialists, a difficult and demanding task. In more than thirty years since the publication of Rosen's *History*, no single text has presented the field in quite such a comprehensive manner.

In part, the fragmentation of public health history reflects the fragmentation of social history in general.[79] Critical scholarship has demolished many of the old assumptions and structures of belief without erecting secure new ones in their place. From a contemporary point of view, for example, the traditional framework of Western civilization, a history that begins with the Greeks and the Romans and ends with twentieth-century America, seems ethnocentric, old-fashioned, and limited. Yet, despite the fact that this framework is no longer persuasive, we do not have a clear alternative. In recent years, scholars have produced a growing body of work on public health in countries other than Western Europe and the United States and have begun the task of preparing new histories of global health.

Busy public health practitioners who do not have the time to keep up with the burgeoning specialist literature may find it easier to ignore history completely. The result is an increasing distance between historians and practitioners, a situation that results in the impoverishment of a public health robbed of historical perspective. Perhaps it is time for historians of public health to be less concerned about addressing each other and more interested in writing for the larger audience of public health professionals.

George Rosen certainly did this; as editor of the *American Journal of Public Health*, he started a historical department in the journal, called "Public Health Then and Now." This has been continued by several editors over time, currently by Elizabeth Fee and Theodore M. Brown. Two additional historical departments have also been added. "Images of Health," as the name suggests, provides a brief discussion of an image (or images) that represent past and continuing public health problems at different times and in different places. "Voices from the Past" provides an extract from words written in the past— whether from a book, speech, or article—where these words offer insights and positions that may since have been forgotten by many, but that are still strikingly relevant today. It would be desirable for public health practitioners to inform themselves more broadly and deeply about the lessons to be learned from a study of the past and, indeed, to contribute to the recovery of significant aspects of their own fields.[80] George Rosen, embedded in the world of public health practice, wrote *A History of Public Health* primarily for practitioners. Strongly influenced by his mentor Henry Sigerist, and sharing Sigerist's social orientation and progressive politics, Rosen wrote history at least in part as a service to the public health profession—a way of giving perspective and informing public health policy and practice. Despite the fact that his book has been superseded in some respects by newer scholarship, it has not been replaced. It still serves in many important ways the functions that Rosen intended and stands as a fine starting point for those in public health who seek a larger historical perspective on their work and who share the idea that public health is not just a set of disciplines, information, and techniques but is, above all, a shared social vision.

NOTES

1. One of the more ambitious books, Dorothy Porter, *Health, Civilization, and the State: A History of Public Health from Ancient to Modern Times* (London: Routledge, 1999) is generally limited to Europe and the United States; John Duffy, *The Sanitarians: A History of American Public Health* (Urbana: University of Illinois Press, 1990), is restricted to the history of public health in the United States and focuses especially on the activities of public health departments. The two volumes by Dona Schneider and David E. Lilienfeld, *Public Health: The Development of a Discipline*, vol. 1, *From the Age of Hippocrates to the Progressive Era* (New Brunswick, NJ: Rutgers University Press, 2008), and *Public Health: The Development of a Discipline, Twentieth Century Challenges* (New Brunswick, NJ: Rutgers University Press, 2011) are selections of classic texts with historical commentaries. Crossing national boundaries, Mark Harrison, *Disease and the Modern World: 1500 to the Present Day* (Cambridge, MA: Polity, 2004), offers a wide-ranging analysis of disease within the context of

the expansion of European colonialism. J. N. Hays, *The Burdens of Disease; Epidemics and Human Response in Western History* (New Brunswick, NJ: Rutgers University Press, 2010), and William H. McNeill, *Plagues and Peoples* (New York: Doubleday/Anchor, 1976), draw on a vast interdisciplinary literature to explore the impact of infectious diseases on human history. Also useful is Robert P. Hudson, *Disease and Its Control: The Shaping of Modern Thought* (Westport, CT: Greenwood Press, 1983). Among the older but still popular texts, Henry E. Sigerist, *Civilization and Disease* (1943; reprint, Chicago: University of Chicago Press, 1962), offers an engaging series of essays on disease and its interpretation; see also Charles-Edward A. Winslow, *The Conquest of Epidemic Disease: A Chapter in the History of Ideas* (New York: Hafner, 1943); and Erwin H. Ackerknecht, *The History and Geography of the Most Important Diseases* (New York: Hafner, 1965). For the twentieth century, Harry Dowling's *Fighting Infection: Conquests of the Twentieth Century* (Cambridge, MA: Harvard University Press, 1977) and Wesley W. Spink, *Infectious Diseases: Prevention and Treatment in the Nineteenth and Twentieth Centuries* (Minneapolis: University of Minnesota Press, 1978) provide general discussions of the history of infectious disease control; much less has been written on the history of chronic diseases.

2. The idea that history was an essential discipline for health professionals prompted several leading historians of medicine of this generation to write textbooks. The preparation of broad, synthetic texts allowed the scholar to present a unified vision of the field and shape the perspective of students and future practitioners. See, for example, Erwin H. Ackerknecht, *A Short History of Medicine* (Baltimore: Johns Hopkins University Press, 1982); Erwin H. Ackerknecht, *Therapeutics from the Primitives to the Twentieth Century* (New York: Hafner, 1973); Henry E. Sigerist, *A History of Medicine* (New York: Oxford University Press), vol. 1, *Primitive and Archaic Medicine* (1951); vol. 2, *Early Greek, Hindu, and Persian Medicine* (1961).

3. For a bibliography of Rosen's writings, see "George Rosen: Bibliography," in *Healing and History: Essays for George Rosen,* ed. Charles E. Rosenberg (New York: Science History Publications, 1979), 252–62.

4. Kevin M. Cahill, ed., *Immanent Peril: Public Health in a Declining Economy* (New York: The Twentieth Century Fund Press, 1991); Vicente Navarro, *Medicine under Capitalism* (New York: Neale Watson, 1976); Barron H. Lerner, "A Case Study of New York City's Tuberculosis Control Efforts: The Historical Limitations of the 'War on Consumption,' " *American Journal of Public Health* 83 (1993): 758–66.

5. For examples of this more recent literature, see Alison Bashford, *Imperial Hygiene: A Critical History of Colonialism, Nationalism and Public Health* (Basingstoke, UK: Palgrave Macmillan, 2004); David Arnold, *Medicine in an Age of Commerce and Empire: Britain and Its Tropical Colonies, 1660–1830* (Oxford: Oxford University Press, 2010); Howard Waitzkin, *Medicine and Public Health at the End of Empire* (Boulder, CO: Paradigm Publishers, 2011); Anne-Emanuelle Birn, Yogan Pillay, and Timothy H. Holtz, *Textbook of International Health: Global Health in a Dynamic World* (New York: Oxford University Press, 2009); Vicente Navarro, ed., *Neoliberalism, Globalization, and Inequalities: Consequences for Health and Quality of Life* (Amityville, NY: Baywood, 2007); Vicente Navarro and Carlos Muntaner, eds., *Political and Economic Determinants of Population Health and Well-Being: Controversies and Developments* (Amityville, NY: Baywood, 2004); Ronald Labonte, Ted Schrecker, David Sanders, and Wilma Meeus, *Fatal Indifference: The G8, Africa, and*

Global Health (Johannesburg: Juta Academic, 2004); Greg Grandin, *Empire's Workshop: Latin America, the United States, and the Rise of the New Imperialism* (New York: Metropolitan Books, 2006); David Sanders and Richard Carver, *The Struggle for Health: Medicine and the Politics of Underdevelopment* (New York: Macmillan, 1991); Ronald Labonte, Ted Schrecker, Corinne Packer, and Vivien Runnels, eds. *Globalization and Health: Pathways, Evidence and Policy* (London: Routledge, 2009); David Arnold, ed. *Warm Climates and Western Medicine* (Amsterdam: Rodopi, 1996); Warwick Anderson, *The Collectors of Lost Souls: Turning Kuru Scientists into Whitemen* (Baltimore: Johns Hopkins University Press, 2008); Warwick Anderson, *Colonial Pathologies* (Durham, NC: Duke University Press, 2006); Meredith Turshen, *The Politics of Public Health* (New Brunswick, NJ: Rutgers University Press, 1989); Paul Farmer, Arthur Kleinman, Jim Yong Kim, and Matthew Basilico, *Reimagining Global Health: An Introduction* (Berkeley: University of California Press, 2013); Joao Biehl and Adriana Petryna, eds., *When People Come First: Critical Studies in Global Health* (Princeton, NJ: Princeton University Press, 2013); David Harvey, *A Brief History of Neoliberalism* (Oxford: Oxford University Press, 2007); Randall Packard, *The Making of a Tropical Disease: A Short History of Malaria* (Baltimore: Johns Hopkins University Press, 2007); Amartya Sen, *Development as Freedom* (Oxford: Oxford University Press, 2001); Amartya Sen and Paul Farmer, *Pathologies of Power: Health, Human Rights, and the New War on the Poor* (Berkeley: University of California Press, 2004); David Arnold, *Warm Climates and Western Medicine: The Emergence of Tropical Medicine, 1500–1900* (Atlanta, GA: Rodopi, 1996); Poonam Bala, *Biomedicine as a Contested Site: Some Revelations in Imperial Contexts* (Lanham, MD: Lexington Books, 2009); Alison Bashford, *Medicine at the Border: Disease, Globalization and Security, 1850 to the Present* (New York: Palgrave Macmillan, 2006); Anne-Emanuelle Birn and Theodore Brown, eds. *Comrades in Health: U.S. Health Internationalists, Abroad and at Home* (New Brunswick, NJ: Rutgers University Press, 2013); Douglas Haynes, *Imperial Medicine: Patrick Manson and the Conquest of Tropical Disease* (Philadelphia: University of Pennsylvania Press, 2001; Ryan Johnson and Amna Khalid, *Public Health in the British Empire: Intermediaries, Subordinates, and the Practice of Public Health, 1850–1960* (New York: Routledge, 2012); Michelle Moran, *Colonizing Leprosy: Imperialism and the Politics of Public Health in the United States* (Chapel Hill: University of North Carolina Press, 2007); Deborah Neill, *Networks in Tropical Medicine: Internationalism, Colonialism, and the Rise of a Medical Specialty,1890–1930* (Stanford, CA: Stanford University Press, 2012; David Arnold, *Warm Climates and Western Medicine: The Emergence of Tropical Medicine, 1500–1900* (Atlanta, GA: Rodopi, 1996); Alison Bashford, *Medicine at the Border: Disease, Globalization and Security, 1850 to the Present* (New York: Palgrave Macmillan, 2006); Douglas Haynes, *Imperial Medicine: Patrick Manson and the Conquest of Tropical Disease* (Philadelphia: University of Pennsylvania Press, 2001; Ryan Johnson and Amna Khalid, *Public Health in the British Empire: Intermediaries, Subordinates, and the Practice of Public Health, 1850–1960* (New York: Routledge, 2012); Michelle Moran, *Colonizing Leprosy: Imperialism and the Politics of Public Health in the United States* (Chapel Hill: University of North Carolina Press, 2007); Deborah Neill, *Networks in Tropical Medicine: Internationalism, Colonialism, and the Rise of a Medical Specialty, 1890–1930* (Stanford, CA: Stanford University Press, 2012; Mark Harrison, *Climates & Constitutions: Health, Race, Environment and British Imperialism in India, 1600–1850* (New Delhi: Oxford University Press, 1999); Pratik Chakrabarti, *Materials and Medicine: Trade, Conquest, and*

Therapeutics in the Eighteenth Century (Manchester: Manchester University Press, 2010); Jack Edward McCallum, *Leonard Wood: Rough Rider, Surgeon, Architect of American Imperialism* (New York: New York University Press, 2006); Sheldon J. Watts, *Epidemics and History: Disease, Power, and Imperialism* (New Haven, CT: Yale University Press, 1997).

6. See Fikret Yegül, *Baths and Bathing in Classical Antiquity* (Cambridge, MA: Architectural History Foundation / MIT Press, 1992).

7. Those interested in public health in the Greco-Roman world are likely to find the following sources helpful: Owsei Temkin, *Hippocrates in a World of Pagans and Christians* (Baltimore: Johns Hopkins University Press, 1991); Geoffrey E. R. Lloyd, ed., *Hippocratic Writings* (New York: Penguin, 1978); Wesley D. Smith, *The Hippocratic Tradition* (Ithaca, NY: Cornell University Press, 1979); Owsei Temkin, *Galenism: Rise and Decline of a Medical Philosophy* (Ithaca, NY: Cornell University Press, 1973); Heinrich von Staden, *Herophilus: The Art of Medicine in Early Alexandria* (New York: Cambridge University Press, 1989); "The Dietetics of Antiquity," and other essays by Ludwig Edelstein in *Ancient Medicine: Selected Papers of Ludwig Edelstein*, ed. Owsei Temkin and C. Lilian Temkin (Baltimore: Johns Hopkins Press, 1967); Robert Parker, *Miasma: Pollution and Purification in Early Greek Religion* (Oxford: Clarendon Press, 1983); Guido Majno, *The Healing Hand: Man and Wound in the Ancient World* (Cambridge, MA: Harvard University Press, 1975); John Scarborough, "Roman Medicine and Public Health," in *Public Health*, ed. Teizo Ogawa (Tokyo: Taniguchi Foundation, 1981), 33–74; the chapter on hygiene in Ralph Jackson, *Doctors and Diseases in the Roman Empire* (Norman: University of Oklahoma Press, 1988); Vivian Nutton, "The Seeds of Disease: An Explanation of Contagion and Infection from the Greeks to the Renaissance," *Medical History* 27 (1983, supp. 1): 1–34; Owsei Temkin, "The Scientific Approach to Disease: Specific Entity and Individual Sickness" (and other essays) in *The Double Face of Janus* (Baltimore: Johns Hopkins University Press, 1977), 442–48; Mirko D. Grmek, *Diseases in the Ancient Greek World* (Baltimore: Johns Hopkins University Press, 1989); Vivian Nutton, "Continuity or Rediscovery? The City Physician in Classical Antiquity and Medieval Italy," in *The Town and State Physician in Europe from the Middle Ages to the Enlightenment*, ed. Andrew Russell (Wolffenbutel: Herzog August Bibliothek, 1981), 9–46.

8. In many areas of domestic public health, environmental health policy, and international health, we continue to debate the relative importance and effectiveness of categorical programs targeted at the prevention of specific diseases versus those oriented to broader social, economic, and environmental reform. See, for example, N. Krieger, *Epidemiology and the People's Health: Theory and Context* (New York: Oxford University Press, 2011),

9. For a general discussion of medieval hygiene and epidemics, see the relevant chapters in C. H. Talbot, *Medicine in Medieval England* (London: Oldbourne, 1967), 144–69. Useful discussions may also be found in more general histories of the medieval period: see, for example, David Herlihy, *Cities and Societies in Medieval Italy* (London: Variorum Reprints, 1980); David Herlihy, ed., *The Medieval City* (New Haven, CT: Yale University Press, 1977); and Josiah C. Russell, *Medieval Regions and Their Cities* (Bloomington: Indiana University Press, 1972). Epidemic diseases, while not the only issues of medieval public health, mark times of particular drama. The Black Death, the catastrophic bubonic plague epidemic of the fourteenth century, has especially gripped the popular historical imagination; Philip Ziegler's *The Black Death* (New York: Harper & Row, 1969) and Barbara Tuchman's *A Dis-*

tant Mirror: The Calamitous Fourteenth Century (New York: Knopf, 1978) are two lively accounts. Like other more popular works, these may not be considered fully reliable by experts in the field. Faye Marie Getz has a witty review of the extensive and growing scholarly literature on the Black Death in "Black Death and the Silver Lining: Meaning, Continuity, and Revolutionary Change in Histories of the Medieval Plague," *Journal of the History of Biology* 24 (1991): 265–89; see also Nancy Siraisi's introduction to *The Black Death: The Impact of the Fourteenth Century Plague,* ed. Daniel Williman (Binghamton, NY: Center for Medieval and Early Renaissance Studies, 1982), 9–22. Anna M. Campbell, *The Black Death and Men of Learning* (New York: AMS Press, 1966), is an early but well-regarded work for those interested in serious explorations of the subject. Leprosy, characteristic of the early Middle Ages, seems to have received less attention; see, however, Saul N. Brody, *The Disease of the Soul: Leprosy in Medieval Literature* (Ithaca, CT: Cornell University Press, 1974), and Peter Richards, *The Medieval Leper and His Northern Heirs* (Totowa, NJ: Rowman & Littlefield, 1977). Those interested in more contemporary views of leprosy should consult Zachary Gussow, *Leprosy, Racism, and Public Health: Social Policy in Chronic Disease Control* (Boulder, CO: Westview, 1989).

10. Considerable work has been done in recent years on public health in the Renaissance. See Katherine Park, *Doctors and Medicine in Early Renaissance Florence* (Princeton, NJ: Princeton University Press, 1985); Ann G. Carmichael, *Plague and the Poor in Renaissance Florence* (Cambridge: Cambridge University Press, 1986); and Carlo M. Cipolla, *Public Health and the Medical Profession in the Renaissance* (Cambridge: Cambridge University Press, 1976). Nancy Siraisi, *Medieval and Early Renaissance Medicine: An Introduction to Knowledge and Practice* (Chicago: University of Chicago Press, 1990), provides a very useful introduction to the larger context of medical thought and practice, although she does not focus on public health. On early modern Europe, see also the essays in Charles Webster, ed., *Health, Medicine, and Mortality in the Sixteenth Century* (Cambridge: Cambridge University Press, 1979). Several of Carlo Cipolla's books on the plague are as lively and interesting as novels; see, for example, *Christofano and the Plague: A Study in the History of Public Health in the Age of Galileo* (Berkeley: University of California Press, 1973); *Faith, Reason, and the Plague in Seventeenth-Century Tuscany* (Ithaca, NY: Cornell University Press, 1979); and *Fighting the Plague in Seventeenth-Century Italy* (Madison: University of Wisconsin Press, 1981). For accounts of the plague in countries other than Italy, see J. F. Shrewsbury, *A History of Bubonic Plague in the British Isles* (Cambridge: Cambridge University Press, 1970); Paul Slack, *The Impact of Plague in Tudor and Stuart England* (London: Routledge & Kegan Paul, 1985); J. T. Alexander, *Bubonic Plague in Early Modern Russia: A Public Health and Urban Disaster* (Baltimore: Johns Hopkins University Press, 1980); and M. W. Dols, *The Black Death in the Middle East* (Princeton, NJ: Princeton University Press, 1977).

11. Fracastoro, in the sixteenth century, argued that epidemic diseases were caused by minute infective agents that were transmissible, self-propagating, and disease specific. These seeds of disease could be spread by direct contact from person to person, through intermediate agents, or at a distance, through the air. In the seventeenth century, after Anthony van Leeuwenhoek described the microscopic organisms, or "little animals," he had found in rainwater, soil, and human excretions, several observers suggested that these "little animals" could be the cause of contagious diseases. Various confusing and conflict-

ing reports, however, led to a reaction against this early "germ" theory of disease, which would only be revived, in a different form, in the nineteenth century. See especially Nancy Tomes, *The Gospel of Germs: Men, Women, and the Microbe in American Life* (Cambridge, MA: Harvard University Press, 1999).

12. As an introduction to the history of typhus fever, Hans Zinsser's *Rats, Lice and History* (1935; reprint, New York: Bantam Books, 1965) may be read with some caution and great enjoyment.

13. On scurvy, see especially Kenneth J. Carpenter, *The History of Scurvy and Vitamin C* (New York: Cambridge University Press, 1986).

14. The best introduction to occupational health in this period is still George Rosen, *The History of Miners' Diseases: A Medical and Social Interpretation* (New York: Schuman's, 1943).

15. The transmission of disease is controversial, especially the still-debated origins and spread of syphilis. Several interesting and well-written books trace the histories of syphilis, smallpox, and malaria over a broad time frame: Claude Quetel, *History of Syphilis* (Baltimore: Johns Hopkins University Press, 1990); Donald R. Hopkins, *Princes and Peasants: Smallpox in History* (Chicago: University of Chicago Press, 1983); Gordon Harrison, *Mosquitoes, Malaria, and Man: A History of Hostilities since 1880* (New York: Dutton, 1978). For discussion of the importance of geographical patterns of disease transmission, see William H. McNeill, *Plagues and Peoples* (New York: Anchor, 1976); Alfred W. Crosby, *Ecological Imperialism: The Biological Expansion of Europe, 900–1900* (Cambridge: Cambridge University Press, 1986); Alfred W. Crosby, *The Columbian Exchange: Biological and Cultural Consequences of 1492* (Westport, CT: Greenwood Press, 1972); and, for a contemporary virologist's view, Stephen S. Morse, "AIDS and Beyond: Defining the Rules for Viral Traffic," in *AIDS: The Making of a Chronic Disease*, ed. Elizabeth Fee and Daniel M. Fox (Berkeley: University of California Press, 1992), 23–48. Giovanni Berlinguer provides a thoughtful framework for discussing the consequences for public health of the Columbian voyages in "The Interchange of Disease and Health in the Old and New Worlds," *American Journal of Public Health* 82 (1992): 1407–13.

16. Lorraine Daston, *Classical Probability in the Enlightenment* (Princeton, NJ: Princeton University Press, 1988); Theodore M. Porter, *The Rise of Statistical Thinking, 1820–1900* (Princeton, NJ: Princeton University Press, 1986); Andrea Rusnock, "The Quantification of Things Human: Medicine and Political Arithmetic in Enlightenment England and France," PhD dissertation, Princeton University, 1990.

17. For the concept of medical police, see Erna Lesky's introduction to Johann Peter Frank, *A System of Complete Medical Police*, ed. Erna Lesky (Baltimore: Johns Hopkins University Press, 1976); George Rosen, "Cameralism and the Concept of Medical Police" (and other essays), in his *From Medical Police to Social Medicine: Essays on the History of Health Care* (New York: Science History Publications, 1974), 120–41; and Ludmilla Jordanova, "Policing Public Health in France, 1780–1815," in *Public Health*, ed. Teizo Ogawa (Tokyo: Taniguchi Foundation, 1981). For a helpful general introduction to the Enlightenment, see Guenter B. Risse, "Medicine in the Age of Enlightenment," in *Medicine in Society: Historical Essays*, ed. Andrew Wear (Cambridge: Cambridge University Press, 1992): 149–95.

18. The history of public health in France is, however, more than the ideas and theories of the Encyclopedists and Ideologues. For the medical context, see Matthew Ramsey, *Professional and Popular Medicine in France, 1170–1830* (Cambridge: Cambridge Univer-

sity Press, 1988). On the handling of epidemics in eighteenth-century France, see Caroline C. Hannaway, "The Société Royale de Médecine and Epidemics in the Ancien Régime," *Bulletin of the History of Medicine* 46 (1972): 254–73. See also George D. Sussman, *Selling Mothers' Milk: The Wet-Nursing Business in France, 1715–1914* (Urbana: University of Illinois Press, 1982).

19. Rosen is somewhat critical of the ideology of the utilitarians, while praising many of their practical accomplishments. Since then, Michel Foucault has offered a more damning critique of utilitarian reforms, especially in relation to prisons and mental hospitals. See, for example, his *Madness and Civilization: A History of Insanity in the Age of Reason* (New York: Pantheon Books, 1965); *Discipline and Punish: The Birth of the Prison* (New York: Pantheon Books, 1977); and *The Birth of the Clinic: An Archaeology of Medical Perception* (New York: Pantheon Books, 1973).

20. For fascinating accounts of the experience and meaning of sickness and popular ideas about health, as reflected in personal accounts such as diaries and letters, see Roy Porter and Dorothy Porter, *In Sickness and in Health: The British Experience, 1650–1850* (New York: Blackwell, 1988); Mary E. Fissell, *Vernacular Bodies: The Politics of Reproduction in Early Modern England* (Oxford: Oxford University Press, 2004). See also Charles E. Rosenberg, "Medical Text and Social Context: Explaining William Buchan's *Domestic Medicine*," *Bulletin of the History of Medicine* 57 (1983): 22–42; Charles E. Rosenberg, *Right Living: An Anglo-American Tradition of Self-Help Medicine* (Baltimore: Johns Hopkins University Press, 2003); and Antoinette Emch-Dériaz, "Towards a Social Conception of Health in the Second Half of the Eighteenth Century: Tissot (1728–1787) and the New Preoccupation with Health and Well-Being," PhD dissertation, University of Rochester, 1984.

21. The controversies over smallpox inoculation are discussed in much detail in Genevieve Miller, *The Adoption of Inoculation for Smallpox in England and France* (Philadelphia: University of Pennsylvania Press, 1957); see also John B. Blake, *Benjamin Waterhouse and the Introduction of Vaccination: A Reappraisal* (Philadelphia: University of Pennsylvania Press, 1957). For a worldwide history of smallpox, see Donald R. Hopkins, *Princes and Peasants: Smallpox in History* (Chicago: University of Chicago Press, 1983). For the story of the final eradication of smallpox, see F. Fenner, D. A. Henderson, I. Arita, Z. Jezek, and I. D. Ladnyi, *Smallpox and Its Eradication* (Geneva: World Health Organization, 1988), or, for a much shorter version, D. A. Henderson, "The History of Smallpox Eradication," in *Times, Places, and Persons: Aspects of the History of Epidemiology*, ed. Abraham M. Lilienfeld (Baltimore: Johns Hopkins University Press, 1980), 99–108.

22. Peter Ludwig Panum, *Observations during the Epidemic of Measles on the Faroe Islands in the Year 1846*, with a biographical memoir by Julius Jacob Petersen (New York: Delta Omega Society; distributed by American Public Health Association, 1940); John Snow, *Snow on Cholera*, a reprint of two papers by John Snow, together with a biographical memoir by B. W. Richardson, MD, and an introduction by Wade Hampton Frost, MD (New York: Commonwealth Fund, 1936); William Budd, *Typhoid Fever, Its Nature, Mode of Spreading, and Prevention* (London: Longmans, 1873; reprint, New York: Arno Press, 1977).

23. Erwin Ackerknecht, "Anticontagionism between 1821 and 1867," *Bulletin of the History of Medicine* 22 (1948): 562–93. Margaret Pelling has recently criticized and modified Ackerknecht's thesis and presented a rather more complex view of nineteenth-century debates over disease etiology; see Margaret Pelling, *Cholera, Fever and English Medicine, 1825–1865* (Oxford: Oxford University Press, 1978); William Coleman, *Yellow Fever in the North:*

The Methods of Early Epidemiology (Madison: University of Wisconsin Press, 1987); John M. Eyler, *Victorian Social Medicine: The Ideas and Methods of William Farr* (Baltimore: Johns Hopkins University Press, 1979); Roger Cooter, "Anticontagionism and History's Medical Record," in *The Problem of Medical Knowledge: Examining the Social Construction of Medicine*, ed. P. Wright and A. Treacher (Edinburgh: Edinburgh University Press, 1982), 87–108; Abraham M. Lilienfeld and David E. Lilienfeld, "Epidemiology and the Public Health Movement: A Historical Perspective," *Journal of Public Health Policy* 3 (1982): 140–49; Abraham M. Lilienfeld, ed., *Times, Places, and Persons: Aspects of the History of Epidemiology* (Baltimore: Johns Hopkins University Press, 1980); V. P. Vandenbroucke, H. M. Eelkman Rooda, and H. Beukers, "Who Made John Snow a Hero?," *American Journal of Epidemiology* 133 (1991): 967–73; Mervyn Susser, "Epidemiology in the United States after World War II: The Evolution of Technique," *Epidemiological Reviews* 7 (1985): 147–77; Abraham M. Lilienfeld and David E. Lilienfeld, "A Century of Case Control Studies: Progress?," *Journal of Chronic Diseases* 32 (1979): 5–13.

24. A number of public health histories provide graphic descriptions of living conditions. See especially Anthony S. Wohl, *Endangered Lives: Public Health in Victorian Britain* (Cambridge, MA: Harvard University Press, 1983).

25. The several cholera epidemics of the nineteenth century were socially traumatic and generated a considerable literature. Some of the best work in the history of public health takes the cholera epidemics as a focal point for analyzing the social, political, and cultural context of disease and for exploring the variety of social responses to epidemics. See especially the classic account by Charles E. Rosenberg, *The Cholera Years: The United States in 1832, 1849, and 1866* (Chicago: University of Chicago Press, 1962), and more recently, Richard J. Evans, *Death in Hamburg: Society and Politics in the Cholera Years, 1830–1910* (Oxford: Oxford University Press, 1987). See also François Delaporte, *Disease and Civilization: The Cholera in Paris, 1832*, trans. Arthur Goldhammer (Cambridge, MA: MIT Press, 1986); Roderick E. McGrew, *Russia and the Cholera, 1823–1832* (Madison: University of Wisconsin Press, 1965); R. J. Morris, *Cholera 1832: The Social Response to an Epidemic* (New York: Holmes & Meier, 1976); Michael Durey, *The Return of the Plague: British Society and the Cholera, 1831–2* (Atlantic Highlands, NJ: Gill & Macmillan, 1980); Charles E. Rosenberg, "Cholera in Nineteenth-Century Europe: A Tool for Social and Economic Analysis," *Comparative Studies in Society and History* 8 (1966): 452–63; Richard J. Evans, "Epidemics and Revolutions: Cholera in Nineteenth-Century Europe," *Past and Present* 120 (1988): 123–46.

26. Rosen makes good use of Chadwick to show the relationship of public health to a larger social and political agenda. See also M. W. Flinn's introduction to *Report on the Sanitary Condition of the Labouring Population of Great Britain* [1842], ed. M. W. Flinn (Edinburgh: Edinburgh University Press, 1965), 1–73; S. E. Finer, *The Life and Times of Sir Edwin Chadwick* (London: Methuen, 1952); R. A. Lewis, *Edwin Chadwick and the Public Health Movement, 1832–1854* (London: Longmans & Green, 1952); John Eyler, *Victorian Social Medicine* (Baltimore: Johns Hopkins University Press, 1979); F. B. Smith, *The Peoples Health* (London: Croom Helm, 1979); Dorothy E. Watkins, "The English Revolution in Social Medicine, 1880–1911," PhD dissertation, University of London, 1984; Royston Lambert, *Sir John Simon 1816–1904 and English Social Administration* (London: MacGibbon & Kee, 1963); Margaret Pelling, *Cholera, Fever and English Medicine, 1825–1865* (Oxford: Oxford University Press, 1978).

27. Friedrich Engels, *The Condition of the Working Class in England* (Leipzig, 1845; reprint, New York: Oxford University Press, 1993); Erwin H. Ackerknecht, *Rudolf Virchow. Doctor, Statesman, Anthropologist* (Madison: University of Wisconsin, 1953).

28. For public health in France in the early nineteenth century, see William Coleman, *Death Is a Social Disease: Public Health and Political Economy in Early Industrial France* (Madison: University of Wisconsin Press, 1982); Ann F. La Berge, "Public Health in France and the French Public Health Movement, 1815–1848," PhD dissertation, University of Tennessee, 1974; and Erwin H. Ackerknecht, *Medicine at the Paris Hospital, 1794–1848* (Baltimore: Johns Hopkins Press, 1967).

29. For Villermé's work, see Coleman, *Death Is a Social Disease.*

30. Erwin H. Ackerknecht, *Rudolf Virchow: Doctor, Statesman, Anthropologist* (Madison: University of Wisconsin Press, 1953; Rudolf Carl Virchow, "Report on the Typhus Epidemic in Upper Silesia." Reprint excerpt, *American Journal of Public Health* 96(2006): 2102–5; Theodore M. Brown and Elizabeth Fee, *"Rudolf Carl Virchow," American Journal of Public Health* 96 (2006): 2104–2105. Rosen helped enshrine Virchow's reputation as a forerunner of social medicine. See George Rosen, "What Is Social Medicine?" *Bulletin of the History of Medicine* 21 (1947): 674–733.

31. On the subsequent history of public health in Britain, see Jeanne L. Brand, *Doctors and the State: The British Medical Profession and Government Action in Public Health, 1870–1912* (Baltimore: Johns Hopkins Press, 1965); Virginia Berridge: *Health and Society in Britain since 1939* (New York: Cambridge University Press, 1999); Jane Lewis, *What Price Community Medicine?: The Philosophy, Practice and Politics of Public Health Since 1919* (Brighton: Wheatsheaf, 1986); the essays by Dorothy Porter, Elizabeth Fee, and Jane Lewis in *A History of Education in Public Health: Health That Mocks the Doctors' Rules,* ed. Elizabeth Fee and Roy M. Acheson (Oxford: Oxford University Press, 1991), 195–229; Frank Honigsbaum, *The Struggle for the Ministry of Health, 1914–1919* (London: G. Bell, 1971); Charles Webster, "Health, Welfare and Unemployment During the Depression," *Past and Present* 109 (1985): 204–30; Frank Honigsbaum, *Health, Happiness, and Security: The Creation of the National Health Service* (London: Routledge, 1989). See also Greta Jones, *Social Hygiene in Twentieth-Century Britain* (London: Croom Helm, 1986); Pauline M. H. Mazumdar, *Eugenics, Human Genetics and Human Failings: The Eugenics Society, Its Source and Its Critics in England* (New York: Routledge, 1992); Jane Lewis, *The Politics of Motherhood: Child and Maternal Welfare in England, 1900–1939* (London: Croom Helm, 1980); and Deborah Dwork, *War Is Good for Babies and Other Young Children* (London: Tavistock, 1987).

32. Ann F. La Berge, "The Early Nineteenth-Century French Public Health Movement: The Disciplinary Development and Institutionalization of *Hygiene Publique,*" *Bulletin of the History of Medicine* 58 (1984): 363–79; Evelyn B. Ackerman, *Health Care in the Parisian Countryside, 1800–1914* (New Brunswick, NJ: Rutgers University Press, 1990); Martha L. Hildreth, *Doctors, Bureaucrats, and Public Health in France, 1888–1902* (New York: Garland, 1987).

33. Richard J. Evans, *Death in Hamburg: Society and Politics in the Cholera Years, 1830–1910* (Oxford: Oxford University Press, 1987); Paul Weindling, *Health, Race, and German Politics between National Unification and Nazism, 1810–1945* (New York: Cambridge University Press, 1989).

34. Some major exceptions to this observation are John Duffy, *Epidemics in Colonial*

America (Baton Rouge: Louisiana State University Press, 1953); John Blake, *Public Health in the Town of Boston, 1630–1822* (Cambridge, MA: Harvard University Press, 1959); and James H. Cassedy, *Demography in Early America: Beginnings of the Statistical Mind, 1600–1800* (Cambridge, MA: Harvard University Press, 1969). See also Roslyn Stone Wolman, "Some Aspects of Community Health in Colonial Philadelphia," PhD dissertation, University of Pennsylvania, 1974, and David T. Courtwright, "Disease, Death, and Disorder on the American Frontier," *Journal of the History of Medicine and Allied Sciences* 46 (1991): 467–92.

35. Some important recent books, however, do focus on this neglected topic: Calvin Martin, *Keepers of the Game: Indian-Animal Relationships and the Fur Trade* (Berkeley: University of California Press, 1978); Stephen J. Kunitz, *Disease, Change, and the Role of Medicine: The Navaho Experience* (Berkeley: University of California Press, 1983); Russell Thornton, *American Indian Holocaust and Survival: A Population History Since 1492* (Norman: University of Oklahoma Press, 1987); and Alfred W. Crosby, *The Columbian Exchange.*

36. Among the exceptions are Todd L. Savitt, *Medicine and Slavery: The Diseases and Health Care of Blacks in Antebellum Virginia* (Urbana: University of Illinois Press, 1978); Edward H. Beardsley, *A History of Neglect: Health Care for Blacks and Mill Workers in the Twentieth-Century South* (Knoxville: University of Tennessee Press, 1987); Todd L. Savitt and James Harvey Young, eds., *Disease and Distinctiveness in the American South* (Knoxville: University of Tennessee Press, 1988); William Stanton, *The Leopards Spots: Scientific Attitudes toward Race in America, 1815–1859* (Chicago: University of Chicago Press, 1960); Nancy Krieger, "Shades of Difference: Theoretical Underpinnings of the Medical Controversy on Black/White Differences in the United States, 1830–1870," *International Journal of Health Services* 17 (1987): 259–73.

37. Gert H. Brieger, "Sanitary Reform in New York City: Stephen Smith and the Passage of the Metropolitan Health Bill," *Bulletin of the History of Medicine* 40 (1966): 407–29; Charles E. Rosenberg and Carroll Smith-Rosenberg, "Pietism and the Origins of the American Public Health Movement: A Note on John H. Griscom and Robert M. Hartley," *Journal of the History of Medicine and Allied Sciences* 23 (1968): 16–35; Barbara Gutmann Rosenkrantz, *Public Health and the State: Changing Views in Massachusetts, 1842–1936* (Cambridge, MA: Harvard University Press, 1972); John Duffy, *A History of Public Health in New York City* (New York: Russell Sage Foundation, 1968–1974).

38. Rosen's story turns on the scientific pivot of bacteriology. Although he mentions epidemiology and statistics, these are subsidiary sciences in his account. A history of public health written by a contemporary practitioner would surely give equal weight to epidemiology as a central discipline of public health. Milton Terris, "The Epidemiologic Tradition: The Wade Hampton Frost Lecture," *Public Health Reports* 94 (1979): 203–9; F. H. Top, ed., *The History of American Epidemiology* (St. Louis, MO: C. V. Mosby, 1952); Abraham M. Lilienfeld, ed., *Times, Places, Persons: Aspects of the History of Epidemiology* (Baltimore: Johns Hopkins University Press, 1980); John M. Eyler, *Victorian Social Medicine: The Ideas and Methods of William Farr* (Baltimore: Johns Hopkins University Press, 1979); William Coleman, *Yellow Fever in the North: The Methods of Early Epidemiology* (Madison: University of Wisconsin Press, 1987); Carol Buck et al., eds., *The Challenge of Epidemiology: Issues and Selected Readings* (Washington, DC: PAHO/WHO, 1988); Mervyn Susser, "Epidemiology in the United States after World War II: The Evolution of Technique," *Epidemiological Reviews* 7 (1985): 147–77. On the early history of statistics in America, see James H.

Cassedy, *Demography in Early America: Beginnings of the Statistical Mind, 1600–1800* (Cambridge, MA: Harvard University Press, 1969); and James H. Cassedy, *American Medicine and Statistical Thinking, 1800–1860* (Cambridge, MA: Harvard University Press, 1984).

39. While Rosen's summary of Pasteur's scientific career is useful, it may be contrasted with the more critical view of Gerald L. Geison, *The Private Science of Louis Pasteur* (Princeton, NJ: Princeton University Press, 1995); and Bruno Latour, *The Pasteurization of France*, trans. Alan Sheridan and John Law (Cambridge, MA: Harvard University Press, 1988). For older accounts, see René Dubos, *Louis Pasteur: Free Lance of Science* (London: Gollancz, 1951); and René J. Dubos and Thomas D. Brock, *Pasteur and Modern Science* (1960; reprint, Madison, WI: Science Tech Publishers, 1988).

40. Much has been written about the social construction of science and laboratory research, countering the sometimes uncritical perspective offered by Rosen and many earlier historians. See, for example, Bruno Latour and Steve Woolgar, *Laboratory Life: The Construction of Scientific Facts* (Princeton, NJ: Princeton University Press, 1986); Bruno Latour, *Science in Action: How to Follow Scientists and Engineers through Society* (Cambridge, MA: Harvard University Press, 1987); Daniel P. Todes, *Pavlov's Physiology Factory: Experiment, Interpretation, Laboratory Enterprise* (Baltimore: Johns Hopkins University Press, 2001).

41. Thomas D. Brock, *Robert Koch: A Life in Medicine and Bacteriology* (Madison, WI: Science Tech Publishers, 1988); Patricia Gossel, "The Emergence of American Bacteriology, 1875–1900," PhD dissertation, Johns Hopkins University, 1989; William Coleman, "Koch's Comma Bacillus: The First Year," *Bulletin of the History of Medicine* 61 (1987): 315–42.

42. These are all heroic stories in the annals of public health and have been told many times in different versions. A standard source is William Bulloch, *The History of Bacteriology* (London: Oxford University Press, 1938; reprint, 1960); see also Harry F. Dowling, *Fighting Infection: Conquests of the Twentieth Century* (Cambridge, MA: Harvard University Press, 1977). On surgery, see Gert H. Brieger, "American Surgery and the Germ Theory of Disease," *Bulletin of the History of Medicine* 40 (1966): 135–45. The yellow fever story has been given an entirely new reading in François Delaporte, *The History of Yellow Fever: An Essay on the Birth of Tropical Medicine* (Cambridge, MA: MIT Press, 1991). For recent work on the history of immunology, see Arthur Silverstein, *A History of Immunology* (San Diego, CA: Academic Press, 1989); and Pauline Mazumdar, *Immunology, 1930–1980: Essays on the History of Immunology* (Toronto: Wail and Thompson, 1989).

43. David Blancher, "Workshops of the Bacteriological Revolution: A History of the Laboratories of the New York Department of Health," PhD dissertation, City University of New York, 1979; Evelynn Hammonds, *Childhood's Deadly Scourge: The Campaign to Control Diphtheria in New York City, 1880–1930* (Baltimore: Johns Hopkins University Press, 1999); John Duffy, *A History of Public Health in New York City*, 2 vols. (New York: Russell Sage Foundation, 1968–74).

44. See James H. Cassedy, *Charles V. Chapin and the Public Health Movement* (Cambridge, MA: Harvard University Press, 1972).

45. Thomas McKeown, *The Modern Rise of Population* (New York: Academic Press, 1976). See also Thomas McKeown, *Medicine: Dream, Mirage, or Nemesis?* (Princeton, NJ: Princeton University Press, 1979); and Thomas McKeown and R. G. Record, "Reasons for the Decline in Mortality in England and Wales during the Nineteenth Century," *Population Studies* 16 (1962): 94–122.

46. Simon Szreter, "The Importance of Social Intervention in Britain's Mortality De-

cline, c. 1850–1914: A Reinterpretation of the Role of Public Health," *Social History of Medicine* 1 (1988): 1–37.

47. Maternal and child health has recently received considerable attention from public health historians and feminist scholars. See Molly Ladd-Taylor, ed., *Raising a Baby the Government Way: Mothers' Letters to the Children's Bureau, 1915–1932* (New Brunswick, NJ: Rutgers University Press, 1986); Richard A. Meckel, *Save the Babies: American Public Health Reform and the Prevention of Infant Mortality, 1850–1920* (Baltimore: Johns Hopkins University Press, 1990); Rima D. Apple, *Mothers and Medicine: A Social History of Infant Feeding, 1890–1950* (Madison: University of Wisconsin Press, 1987); Jane Lewis, *The Politics of Motherhood: Child and Maternal Welfare in England, 1900–1939* (Montreal: McGill-Queen's University Press, 1980); and Alisa Klaus, "Babies All the Rage: The Movement to Prevent Infant Mortality in the United States and France, 1890–1920," PhD dissertation, University of Pennsylvania, 1986.

48. Feminist writers and historians of medicine have generally challenged the older automatic assumptions that physicians were safer than midwives and hospital deliveries superior to home births. See, for example, Jean Donnison, *Midwives and Medical Men: A History of Inter-Professional Rivalry and Women's Rights* (New York: Schocken, 1977). On women and the social context of childbirth, Judith W. Leavitt, *Brought to Bed: Childbearing in America, 1750–1950* (New York: Oxford University Press, 1986), and Laura Thatcher Ulrich, *A Midwife's Tale: The Life of Martha Ballard, Based on Her Diary, 1785–1812* (New York: Knopf, 1990), are both excellent.

49. Andrea Tone, *Devices and Desires: A History of Contraceptives in America* (New York: Hill and Wang, 2002); Ellen Chesler, *Woman of Valor: Margaret Sanger and the American Birth Control Movement in America* (New York: Simon & Schuster, 1992); Linda Gordon, *Woman's Body, Woman's Right: A Social History of Birth Control in America* (New York: Grossman, 1976; revised edition, New York: Penguin, 1990); James Reed, *From Private Vice to Public Virtue: The Birth Control Movement and American Society since 1830* (New York: Basic Books, 1978); Leslie J. Reagan, *When Abortion Was a Crime: Women, Medicine, and Law in the United States, 1867–1973* (Berkeley: University of California Press, 1997); James C. Mohr, *Abortion in America: The Origins and Evolution of National Policy, 1800–1900* (New York: Oxford University Press, 1978); Carroll Smith-Rosenberg, *Disorderly Conduct: Visions of Gender in Victorian America* (New York: Knopf, 1985); Rosalind P. Petchesky, *Abortion and Woman's Choice: The State, Sexuality, and Reproductive Freedom* (Boston: Northeastern University Press, 1985); Rima D. Apple, ed., *Women, Health, and Medicine in America: A Historical Handbook* (New York: Garland, 1990).

50. In this context, a perceived decline in the numbers of births, especially to middle-class women, and the discovery that many young men were physically unfit for military service stimulated public health and child welfare efforts as well as nativism and the eugenics movement. See Daniel J. Kevles, *In the Name of Eugenics: Genetics and the Uses of Human Heredity* (New York: Knopf, 1985). For an interesting discussion of the intersections of sexuality and power, see Alain Corbin, *Women for Hire: Prostitution and Sexuality in France after 1850* (Cambridge, MA: Harvard University Press, 1990).

51. For public health nursing, see especially Karen Buhler-Wilkerson, *False Dawn: The Rise and Decline of Public Health Nursing, 1900–1930* (New York: Garland, 1989). Also interesting is Mary Breckinridge, *Wide Neighborhoods: A Story of the Frontier Nursing Service* (New York: Harper, 1952; reprint, Lexington: University Press of Kentucky, 1981).

52. Rosen asserts, with Charles-Edward A. Winslow, that health education had been as important as the germ theory to public health. See Winslow's *The Evolution and Significance of the Modern Public Health Campaign* (New Haven, CT: Yale University Press, 1923); Richard K. Means, *A History of Health Education in the United States* (Philadelphia: Lea & Febiger, 1962); and, for a different and provocative perspective, John C. Burnham, *How Superstition Won and Science Lost: Popularizing Science and Health in the United States* (New Brunswick, NJ: Rutgers University Press, 1987). On the related issues of health, fitness, and health reform, see Harvey Green, *Fit for America: Health, Fitness, Sport, and American Society* (New York: Pantheon Books, 1986); James C. Whorton, *Crusaders for Fitness: The History of American Health Reformers* (Princeton, NJ: Princeton University Press, 1982); and Martha H. Verbrugge, *Able-Bodied Womanhood: Personal Health and Social Change in Nineteenth-Century Boston* (New York: Oxford University Press, 1988).

53. On tuberculosis, the first of the voluntary health organizations, see Michael E. Teller, *The Tuberculosis Movement: A Public Health Campaign in the Progressive Era* (New York: Greenwood Press, 1988); Richard H. Shryock, *National Tuberculosis Association, 1904–1954: A Study of the Voluntary Health Movement in the United States* (New York: National Tuberculosis Association, 1957). More broadly, the history of voluntary organizations includes the public perception of disease hazards and the politics of funding. See, for example, Richard A. Rettig, *Cancer Crusade: The Story of the National Cancer Act of 1971* (Princeton, NJ: Princeton University Press, 1977); James T. Patterson, *The Dread Disease: Cancer and Modern American Culture* (Cambridge, MA: Harvard University Press, 1977); and Stephen P. Strickland, *Politics, Science, and Dread Disease: A History of United States Medical Research Policy* (Cambridge, MA: Harvard University Press, 1972).

54. These institutions have received more attention in recent years. On the CDC, see Elizabeth W. Etheridge, *Sentinel for Health: A History of the Centers for Disease Control* (Berkeley: University of California Press, 1992); on the NIH, see Victoria Harden, *Inventing the NIH: Federal Biomedical Research Policy, 1887–1937* (Baltimore: Johns Hopkins University Press, 1986); on schools of public health, see Elizabeth Fee, *Disease and Discovery: A History of the Johns Hopkins School of Hygiene and Public Health, 1916–1939* (Baltimore: Johns Hopkins University Press, 1987); Robert R. Korstad, *Dreaming of a Time: The School of Public Health; The University of North Carolina at Chapel Hill, 1939–1989* (Chapel Hill: University of North Carolina, 1990); Elizabeth Fee and Roy M. Acheson, eds., *A History of Education in Public Health: Health That Mocks the Doctors' Rules* (Oxford: Oxford University Press, 1991). A recent book complements the older histories of the United States Public Health Service: Fitzhugh Mullan, *Plagues and Politics: The Story of the United States Public Health Service* (New York: Basic Books, 1989).

55. On pellagra, see Elizabeth W. Etheridge, *The Butterfly Caste* (Westport, CT: Greenwood Press, 1972); Daphne A. Roe, *A Plague of Corn: The Social History of Pellagra* (Ithaca, NY: Cornell University Press, 1973); and Milton Terris, ed., *Goldberger on Pellagra* (Baton Rouge: Louisiana State University Press, 1964).

56. On food regulation, see James Harvey Young, *Pure Food: Securing the Federal Food and Drugs Act of 1906* (Princeton, NY: Princeton University Press, 1989); on food relief, see Jan Poppendieck, *Breadlines Knee-Deep in Wheat: Food Assistance in the Great Depression* (New Brunswick, NJ: Rutgers University Press, 1986). For an introduction to the world of illegal and street drugs and efforts to control their use, see David F. Musto, *The American Disease: Origins of Narcotic Control* (New York: Oxford University Press, 1987).

57. Joan Jacobs Brumberg, *Fasting Girls: The Emergence of Anorexia Nervosa as a Modern Disease* (Cambridge, MA: Harvard University Press, 1988); Lucile F. Newman et al., eds., *Hunger in History: Food Shortage, Poverty and Deprivation* (Cambridge, MA: Basil Blackwell, 1990); Roderick Floud, Kenneth Wachter, and Gregory Annabel, *Height, Health and History: Nutritional Status in the United Kingdom, 1750–1980* (New York: Cambridge University Press, 1990); David Arnold, ed., *Famine, Social Crisis and Historical Change* (Oxford: Basil Blackwell, 1988).

58. The history of occupational health has received considerable attention in the United States. Some important recent books include David Rosner and Gerald E. Markowitz, *Deadly Dust: Silicosis and the Politics of Occupational Disease in Twentieth-Century America* (Princeton, NJ: Princeton University Press, 1991); Gerald Markowitz and David Rosner, *Deceit and Denial: The Deadly Politics of Industrial Pollution* (Berkeley: University of California Press: 2013); David Rosner and Gerald E. Markowitz, eds., *Dying for Work: Workers' Safety and Health in Twentieth-Century America* (Bloomington: Indiana University Press, 1987); Alan Derickson, *Workers' Health, Workers' Democracy: The Western Miners' Struggle, 1891–1925* (Ithaca, NY: Cornell University Press, 1989); Alan Derickson, *Black Lung: Anatomy of a Public Health Disaster* (Ithaca, NY: Cornell University Press, 1998); Claudia Clark, *Radium Girls: Women and Industrial Health Reform, 1910–1935* (Berkeley: University of California Press, 1997); Paul Weindling, ed., *The Social History of Occupational Health* (London: Dover, 1986); Edward H. Beardsley, *A History of Neglect: Health Care for Blacks and Mill Workers in the Twentieth-Century South* (Knoxville: University of Tennessee Press, 1987); Barbara Sicherman, *Alice Hamilton: A Life in Letters* (Cambridge, MA: Harvard University Press, 1984); Ronald Bayer, ed., *The Health and Safety of Workers: Case Studies in the Politics of Professional Responsibility* (New York: Oxford University Press, 1988). On child labor, see Alan Derickson, "Making Human Junk: Child Labor as a Health Issue in the Progressive Era," *American Journal of Public Health* 82 (1992): 1280–90. Related literature on the history of environmental health includes James Whorton, *Before Silent Spring: Pesticides and Public Health in Pre-DDT America* (Princeton, NJ: Princeton University Press, 1974); Samuel P. Hays, *Beauty, Health, and Permanence: Environmental Politics in the United States, 1955–1985* (New York: Cambridge University Press, 1987); and Catherine Caulfield, *Multiple Exposures: Chronicles of the Radiation Age* (London: Seeker & Warburg, 1989). See also Samuel S. Epstein's controversial book, *The Politics of Cancer* (Garden City, NY: Anchor Press, 1979). Especially important in linking public health and the environmental movement is Robert Gottlieb, *Forcing the Spring: The Transformation of the American Environmental Movement* (Washington, DC: Island Press, 1993).

59. On the British National Health Service, see Charles Webster, *Peacetime History: The Health Services since the War*, vol. 1, *Problems of Health Care: The National Health Service before 1957* (London: H.M.S.O., 1988); Frank Honigsbaum, *Health, Happiness, and Security: The Creation of the National Health Service* (London: Routledge, 1989); and Daniel M. Fox, *Health Policies, Health Politics: The British and American Experience, 1911–1965* (Princeton, NJ: Princeton University Press, 1986). Ronald Numbers has elaborated on Rosen's brief account of the early efforts to gain national health insurance in the United States; see Ronald L. Numbers, *Almost Persuaded: American Physicians and Compulsory Health Insurance, 1912–1920* (Baltimore: Johns Hopkins University Press, 1978). There is an extensive literature on the subsequent struggles around national health insurance; see, for example, Ronald Numbers, ed., *Compulsory Health Insurance: The Continuing American Debate* (West-

port, CT: Greenwood Press, 1982); Monty Poen, *Harry S. Truman versus the Medical Lobby* (Columbia: University of Missouri Press, 1979); Richard Harris, *A Sacred Trust* (Baltimore: Penguin, 1966); Paul Starr, *The Social Transformation of American Medicine* (New York: Basic Books, 1982), and *Remedy and Reaction: The Peculiar American Struggle over Health Care Reform* (New Haven, CT: Yale University Press, 2011); Beatrix Hoffman, *Health Care for Some: Rights and Rationing in the United States since 1930* (Chapel Hill: University of North Carolina Press, 2012). Georges C. Benjamin, Theodore M. Brown, Susan Ladwig, and Elyse Berkman, *The Quest for Health Reform: A Satirical History* (Washington, DC: American Public Health Association, 2013). Anne-Emanuelle Birn, Theodore M. Brown, Elizabeth Fee, and Walter J. Lear, "Struggles for National Health Reform in the United States," *American Journal of Public Health* 93(2003): 86–91.

60. See George Rosen's influential article about early community health centers, "The First Neighborhood Health Center Movement: Its Rise and Fall," in *From Medical Police to Social Medicine: Essays in the History of Health Care* (New York: Science History Publications, 1974), 304–27. See also Alice Sardell, *The U.S. Experiment in Social Medicine: The Community Health Center Program, 1965–1986* (Pittsburgh: University of Pittsburgh Press, 1988).

61. Robert B. Stevens and Rosemary Stevens, *Welfare Medicine in America: A Case Study of Medicaid* (New York: Free Press, 1974); Paul Starr, *The Social Transformation of American Medicine* (New York: Basic Books, 1982); Vicente Navarro, *Crisis, Health, and Medicine: A Social Critique* (New York: Tavistock, 1986); J. Rogers Hollingshead, *A Political Economy of Medicine: Great Britain and the United States* (Baltimore: Johns Hopkins University Press, 1986); Vicente Navarro, "Why Some Countries Have National Health Insurance, Others Have National Health Services, and the United States Has Neither," *Social Science and Medicine* 28 (1989): 383–404.

62. We still lack a good one-volume history of the World Health Organization. Some of the earliest international cooperative efforts are included in Norman Howard-Jones, *The Scientific Background of the International Sanitary Conferences* (Geneva: World Health Organization, 1975). The series of volumes produced by the Taniguchi Foundation include a number of interesting essays on international health issues. See, for example, Teizo Ogawa, ed., *Public Health* (Tokyo: Taniguchi Foundation, 1981); see also the many references on international health and tropical medicine in the bibliography to this volume.

63. See, for example, John Farley, *Bilharzia: A History of Imperial Tropical Medicine* (New York: Cambridge University Press, 1991); Randall M. Packard, *White Plague, Black Labor: Tuberculosis and the Political Economy of Health and Disease in South Africa* (Berkeley: University of California Press, 1989); Philip D. Curtin, *Death by Migration: Europe's Encounter with the Tropical World in the Nineteenth Century* (Cambridge: Cambridge University Press, 1989); Gerald W. Hartwig and K. David Patterson, eds., *Disease in African History: An Introductory Survey and Case Studies* (Durham, NC: Duke University Press, 1978); David Arnold, ed., *Imperial Medicine and Indigenous Societies* (Manchester: Manchester University Press, 1988); Roy McLeod and Milton Lewis, eds., *Disease, Medicine and Empire: Perspectives on Western Medicine and the Experience of European Expansion* (London: Routledge, 1988); Teresa Meade and Mark Walker, *Science, Medicine, and Cultural Imperialism* (New York: St. Martin's Press, 1991).

64. For example, Philip D. Curtin, *Death by Migration: Europe's Encounter with the Tropical World in the Nineteenth Century*; K. David Patterson, *Pandemic Influenza, 1700–*

1900: A Study in Historical Epidemiology (Totowa, NJ: Rowman & Littlefield, 1986); Dennis Carlson, *African Fever: A Study of British Science, Technology, and Politics in West Africa, 1787–1864* (New York: Science History, 1984); Maryinez Lyons, *The Colonial Disease: A Social History of Sleeping Sickness in Northern Zaire, 1900–1940* (New York: Cambridge University Press, 1992); Armando Solórzano, "The Rockefeller Foundation in Mexico: Nationalism, Public Health, and Yellow Fever (1911–1924)," PhD dissertation, University of Wisconsin, 1990.

65. For historiographical discussions relevant to the history of public health, see Charles Rosenberg, "The History of Disease: Now and in the Future," in Lloyd Stevenson, ed., *A Celebration of Medical History* (Baltimore: Johns Hopkins University Press, 1982); Gerald Grob, "The Social History of Medicine and Disease in America: Problems and Possibilities," *Journal of Social History* 10 (1977): 391–409; Judith W. Leavitt, "Medicine in Context: A Review Essay of the History of Medicine," *American Historical Review* 95 (1990): 1471–84; Ronald L. Numbers, "The History of American Medicine: A Field in Ferment," *Reviews in American History* 10 (1982): 245–63; Edwin Clarke, *Modern Methods in the History of Medicine* (London: Athlone Press, 1977). Useful collections of articles in the field include Charles Rosenberg, ed., *Healing and History* (New York: Neale Watson, 1979); Judith Walzer Leavitt and Ronald L. Numbers, eds., *Sickness and Health in America* (Madison: University of Wisconsin Press, 1985); Elizabeth Fee and Daniel M. Fox, eds., *AIDS: The Burdens of History* (Berkeley: University of California Press, 1988); Charles E. Rosenberg and Janet Golden, eds., *Framing Disease: Studies in Cultural History* (New Brunswick, NJ: Rutgers University Press, 1992); Andrew Wear, ed., *Medicine in Society: Historical Essays* (Cambridge: Cambridge University Press, 1992).

66. See, for example, Barbara G. Rosenkrantz, *Public Health and the State: Changing Views in Massachusetts, 1842–1936* (Cambridge, MA: Harvard University Press, 1972); Judith Walzer Leavitt, *The Healthiest City: Milwaukee and the Politics of Health Reform* (Princeton, NJ: Princeton University Press, 1982); Stuart Galishoff, *Newark: The Nation's Unhealthiest City, 1832–1895* (New Brunswick, NJ: Rutgers University Press, 1988); Stuart Galishoff, *Safeguarding the Public Health: Newark, 1895–1918* (Westport, CT: Greenwood Press, 1975); James H. Cassedy, *Charles V. Chapin and the Public Health Movement* (Cambridge, MA: Harvard University Press, 1962); John Duffy, *Sword of Pestilence: The New Orleans Yellow Fever Epidemic of 1853* (Baton Rouge: Louisiana State University Press, 1966); John Duffy, *A History of Public Health in New York City*, 2 vols. (New York: Russell Sage Foundation, 1968–74); Philip D. Jordan, *The People's Health: A History of Public Health in Minnesota to 1948* (St. Paul: Minnesota Historical Society, 1953); Jacqueline K. Corn, *Environment and Health in Nineteenth Century America: Two Case Studies* (New York: Peter Lang, 1989); J. W. Estes and David M. Goodman, *The Changing Humors of Portsmouth: The Medical Biography of an American Town, 1623–1983* (Boston: Countway Library, 1986); Michael P. McCarthy, *Typhoid and the Politics of Public Health in Nineteenth-Century Philadelphia* (Philadelphia: American Philosophical Society, 1987); Edward T. Morman, "Scientific Medicine Comes to Philadelphia: Public Health Transformed, 1854–1899," PhD dissertation, University of Pennsylvania, 1986. See also Heather MacDougall, *Activists and Advocates: Toronto's Health Department, 1883–1983* (Toronto: Dundern Press, 1990).

67. John Duffy, *The Sanitarians: A History of American Public Health* (Urbana: University of Illinois Press, 1990).

68. Fitzhugh Mullan, *Plagues and Politics: The Story of the United States Public Health*

Service (New York: Basic Books, 1989); Elizabeth W. Etheridge, *Sentinel for Health: A History of the Centers for Disease Control* (Berkeley: University of California Press, 1992); Victoria Harden, *Inventing the NIH: Federal Biomedical Research Policy, 1887–1931* (Baltimore: Johns Hopkins University Press, 1986); E. Richard Brown, *Rockefeller Medicine Men: Medicine and Capitalism in America* (Berkeley: University of California Press, 1979); John Ettling, *The Germ of Laziness: Rockefeller Philanthropy and Public Health in the New South* (Cambridge, MA: Harvard University Press, 1981); Elizabeth Fee, *Disease and Discovery: A History of the Johns Hopkins School of Hygiene and Public Health, 1916–1939* (Baltimore: Johns Hopkins University Press, 1987); Robert R. Korstad, *Dreaming of a Time: The School of Public Health; The University of North Carolina at Chapel Hill, 1939–1989* (Chapel Hill: University of North Carolina, 1990); Paul A. Bator with Andrew J. Rhodes, *Within Reach of Everyone: A History of the University of Toronto School of Hygiene and the Connaught Laboratories* (Ottawa: Canadian Public Health Association, 1990); Elizabeth Fee and Roy M. Acheson, eds., *A History of Education in Public Health: Health That Mocks the Doctors' Rules* (Oxford: Oxford University Press, 1991), especially the essay by Arthur J. Viseltear, "The Emergence of Pioneering Public Health Education Programmes in the United States," 114–54.

69. See, for example, Christopher Sellers, *Crabgrass Crucible: Suburban Nature and the Rise of Environmentalism in the Twentieth Century* (Chapel Hill: University of North Carolina Press, 2012); Gerald Markowitz and David Rosner, *Lead Wars and the Fate of America's Children* (Berkeley: University of California Press, 2013); Robert Gottlieb, *Forcing the Spring: The Transformation of the American Environmental Movement* (Washington, DC: Island Press, 1993); J. C. Wharton, *Before Silent Spring: Pesticides and Public Health in Pre-DDT America* (Princeton, NJ: Princeton University Press, 1974); Jean-Pierre Goubert, *The Conquest of Water: The Advent of Health in the Industrial Age*, trans. Andrew Wilson (Princeton, NJ: Princeton University Press, 1989); Christopher Hamlin, *A Science of Impurity: Water Analysis in Nineteenth Century Britain* (Berkeley: University of California Press, 1990); Louis P. Cain, *Sanitary Strategy for a Lakefront Metropolis: The Case of Chicago* (DeKalb: Northern Illinois University Press, 1978); Georges Vigarello, *Concepts of Cleanliness: Changing Attitudes in France since the Middle Ages* (Cambridge: University of Cambridge Press, 1988); Martin V. Melosi, *Garbage in the Cities: Refuse, Reform, and the Environment, 1880–1980* (College Station: Texas A&M University Press, 1981); Martin V. Melosi, ed., *Pollution and Reform in American Cities, 1870–1930* (Austin: University of Texas Press, 1980); Elizabeth Fee, *Garbage: The History and Politics of Trash in New York City* (New York: New York Public Library, 1994). A fascinating book dealing with ideas of disease, health, and the environment is Alain Corbin, *The Foul and the Fragrant: Odor and the French Social Imagination*, trans., Miriam Kochan (Cambridge, MA: Harvard University Press, 1986). Joel A. Tarr has written a number of important articles on waste management and environmental history, including Joel A. Tarr, Terry Yosie, and James McCurley III, "Disputes over Water Quality Policy: Professional Cultures in Conflict, 1900–1917," *American Journal of Public Health* 70 (1980): 427–35; Joel A. Tarr, "Industrial Wastes and Public Health: Some Historical Notes, Part I, 1876–1932," *American Journal of Public Health* 75 (1985): 1059–67; Joel A. Tarr, "The Search for the Ultimate Sink: Urban Air, Land, and Water Pollution in Historical Perspective," *Records of the Columbia Historical Society of Washington, D.C.* 51 (1984): 1–29; Joel A. Tarr and Charles Jacobson, "Environmental Risk in Historical Perspective," in *The Social and Cultural Construction of Risk: Essays on Risk Selection and Perception,*

ed. Branden B. Johnson and Vincent T. Covello (Dordrecht: D. Reidel, 1987), 317–44. See also an earlier study, Nelson M. Blake, *Water for the Cities: A History of the Urban Water Supply Problem in the United States* (Syracuse, NY: Syracuse University Press, 1956).

70. For an excellent guide to this voluminous literature, see Rima Apple, ed., *Women, Health, and Medicine in America: A Historical Handbook* (New York: Garland, 1990). Judith Walzer Leavitt, ed., *Women and Health in America: Historical Readings* (Madison: University of Wisconsin Press, 1984), is a fine collection of articles in the field. On public policy, see especially Linda Gordon, ed., *Women, the State, and Welfare* (Madison: University of Wisconsin Press, 1990). On domestic hygiene, see Nancy Tomes, "The Private Side of Public Health: Sanitary Science, Domestic Hygiene, and the Germ Theory, 1870–1900," *Bulletin of the History of Medicine* 64 (1990): 467–80; see also Marilyn T. Williams, *Washing "The Great Unwashed": Public Baths in Urban America, 1840–1920* (Columbus: Ohio State University Press, 1991).

71. Keith Wailoo, *Dying in the City of the Blues: Sickle Cell Anemia and the Politics of Race and Health* (Chapel Hill: University of North Carolina Press, 2000); Keith Wailoo, *How Cancer Crossed the Color Line* (New York: Oxford University Press, 2011); Susan L. Smith, *Sick and Tired of Being Sick and Tired: Black Women's Health Activism in America, 1890–1950* (Philadelphia: University of Pennsylvania Press, 1995); Dorothy Roberts, *Killing the Black Body: Race, Reproduction, and the Meaning of Liberty* (New York: Vintage, 1998); Vanessa N. Gamble, *The Black Community Hospital: An Historical Perspective* (New York: Garland, 1989); Vanessa N. Gamble, ed., *Germs Have No Color Lines: Blacks and American Medicine, 1900–1945* (New York: Garland, 1989); David McBride, *Integrating the City of Medicine: Blacks in Philadelphia Health Care, 1910–1965* (Philadelphia: Temple University Press, 1989); David McBride, *From TB to AIDS: Epidemics among Urban Blacks Since 1900* (Albany: State University of New York Press, 1991); Todd L. Savitt, *Medicine and Slavery: The Diseases and Health Care of Blacks in Antebellum Virginia* (Urbana: University of Illinois Press, 1978); Edward H. Beardsley, *A History of Neglect: Health Care for Blacks and Mill Workers in the Twentieth-Century South* (Knoxville: University of Tennessee Press, 1987); Todd L. Savitt and James Harvey Young, eds., *Disease and Distinctiveness in the American South* (Knoxville: University of Tennessee Press, 1988); Stephen J. Kunitz, *Disease Change and the Role of Medicine: The Navajo Experience* (Berkeley: University of California Press, 1983); Russell Thornton, *American Indian Holocaust and Survival: A Population History since 1492* (Norman: University of Oklahoma Press, 1987); Randall M. Packard, *White Plague, Black Labor: Tuberculosis and the Political Economy of Health and Disease in South Africa* (Berkeley: University of California Press, 1989); Paul Weindling, *Health, Race, and German Politics between National Unification and Nazism, 1870–1945* (New York: Cambridge University Press, 1989); Angus McLaren, *Our Own Master Race: Eugenics in Canada, 1885–1945* (Toronto: McClelland & Stewart, 1990); Mark B. Adams, ed., *The Wellborn Science: Eugenics in Germany, France, Brazil, and Russia* (New York: Oxford University Press, 1990).

72. Charles E. Rosenberg, *The Cholera Years: The United States in 1832, 1849, and 1866* (Chicago: University of Chicago Press, 1962); Richard J. Evans, *Death in Hamburg: Society and Politics in the Cholera Years, 1830–1910* (Oxford: Oxford University Press, 1987); Allan M. Brandt, *No Magic Bullet: A Social History of Venereal Disease in the United States since 1880* (New York: Oxford University Press, 1985); Naomi Rogers, *Dirt and Disease: Polio before FDR* (New Brunswick, NJ: Rutgers University Press, 1992).

73. François Delaporte, *The History of Yellow Fever: An Essay on the Birth of Tropical*

Medicine (Cambridge, MA: MIT Press, 1991); John Ettling, *The Germ of Laziness: Rocke-feller Philanthropy and Public Health in the New South* (Cambridge, MA: Harvard University Press, 1981); Barbara Bates, *Bargaining for Life: A Social History of Tuberculosis, 1816–1938* (Philadelphia: University of Pennsylvania Press, 1992); Linda Bryder, *Below the Magic Mountain: A Social History of Tuberculosis in Twentieth Century Britain* (New York: Oxford University Press, 1988); F. B. Smith, *The Retreat of Tuberculosis, 1850–1950* (New York: Croom Helm, 1988); Claude Quetel, *History of Syphilis* (Baltimore: Johns Hopkins University Press, 1990); K. David Patterson, *Pandemic Influenza, 1700–1900: A Study in Historical Epidemiology* (Totowa, NJ: Rowman & Littlefield, 1986); Alfred W. Crosby, *Epidemic and Peace, 1918* (Westport, CT: Greenwood Press, 1976): Joan Jacobs Brumberg, *Fasting Girls: The Emergence of Anorexia Nervosa as a Modern Disease* (Cambridge, MA: Harvard University Press, 1988); James T. Patterson, *The Dread Disease: Cancer and Modern American Culture* (Cambridge, MA: Harvard University Press, 1987). See also the essays in Charles E. Rosenberg and Janet Golden, eds., *Framing Disease* (New Brunswick, NJ: Rutgers University Press, 1992).

74. Mirko D. Grmek, *History of AIDS: Emergence and Origin of a Modern Pandemic* (Princeton, NJ: Princeton University Press, 1990); Elizabeth Fee and Daniel M. Fox, eds., *AIDS: The Burdens of History* (Berkeley: University of California Press, 1988); Ronald Bayer, *Private Acts, Social Consequences: AIDS and the Politics of Public Health* (New York: Free Press, 1989); Elizabeth Fee and Daniel M. Fox, eds., *AIDS: The Making of a Chronic Disease* (Berkeley: University of California Press, 1992); Peter Arno and Karen L. Felden, *Against the Odds: The Story of AIDS Drug Development, Politics, and Profits* (New York: Harper-Collins, 1992); David L. Kirp and Ronald Bayer, eds., *AIDS in the Industrialized Democracies: Passions, Politics, and Policies* (New Brunswick, NJ: Rutgers University Press, 1992).

75. Thomas Laqueur, *Making Sex: Body and Gender from the Greeks to Freud* (Cambridge, MA: Harvard University Press, 1990); Emily Martin, *The Woman in the Body: A Cultural Analysis of Reproduction* (Boston: Beacon Press, 1987); Barbara Duden, *The Woman beneath the Skin: A Doctor's Patients in Eighteenth-Century Germany* (Cambridge, MA: Harvard University Press, 1991); Michel Feher, with Ramona Naddaff and Nadia Tazi, eds., *Fragments for a History of the Human Body* (Cambridge: MIT Press, 1989); Roger Cooter, "The Power of the Body: The Early Nineteenth Century," *Natural Order*, ed. Barry Barnes and Steven Shapin (Beverly Hills, CA: Sage Publications, 1979).

76. Roy Porter, *Patients and Practitioners: Lay Perceptions of Medicine in Pre-industrial Society* (Cambridge: Cambridge University Press, 1985); Roy Porter and Dorothy Porter, *In Sickness and in Health: The British Experience, 1650–1850* (London: Fourth Estate, 1988); Andrew Wear, ed., *Medicine in Society: Historical Essays* (Cambridge: Cambridge University Press, 1992); Mary Fissell, *Patients, Power, and the Poor in Eighteenth-Century Bristol* (New York: Cambridge University Press, 1991); John Woodward and David Richards, eds., *Health Care and Popular Medicine in Nineteenth Century England: Essays in the Social History of Medicine* (New York: Holmes & Meier, 1977).

77. See, for example, Barbara G. Rosenkrantz, *Public Health and the State: Changing Views in Massachusetts, 1842–1936* (Cambridge, MA: Harvard University Press, 1972); Allan M. Brandt, *No Magic Bullet: A Social History of Venereal Disease in the United States since 1880* (New York: Oxford University Press, 1985); Ronald Bayer, *Private Acts, Social Consequences: AIDS and the Politics of Public Health* (New Brunswick, NJ: Rutgers University Press, 1991).

78. For some steps in this direction, see the two volumes by Dona Schneider and David E. Lilienfeld, *Public Health: The Development of a Discipline, from the Age of Hippocrates to the Progressive Era* (New Brunswick, NJ: Rutgers University Press, 2008), and *Public Health: The Development of a Discipline, Twentieth Century Challenges* (New Brunswick, NJ: Rutgers University Press, 2011); Mark Harrison, *Disease and the Modern World: 1500 to the Present Day* (Boston: Polity, 2004); J. N. Hays, *The Burdens of Disease: Epidemics and Human Response in Western History* (New Brunswick, NJ: Rutgers University Press, 2010).

79. Oliver Zunz has complained about the fragmentation of social history, the proliferation of specialized monographs, and the reluctance to attempt a higher level of generalization. See Oliver Zunz, "The Synthesis of Social Change: Reflections on American Social History," in *Reliving the Past: The Worlds of Social History* (Chapel Hill: University of North Carolina Press, 1985), 53–114. See also Thomas Bender, "Wholes and Parts: The Need for Synthesis in Social History," *Journal of American History* 73 (1986): 120–36; Allan Megill, "Fragmentation and the Future of Historiography," *American Historical Review* 96 (1991): 693–98.

80. Jay Glasser in organizing the American Public Health Association's History Project asked for contributions from every area of public health, so there are openings for those interested in preserving the past; the *American Journal of Public Health* is interested in similar submissions.

Edward T. Morman

When this book first appeared in 1958, George Rosen was professor of health education at Columbia University and editor of the *American Journal of Public Health*. A public health worker and educator with more than fifteen years' experience, he was also the author of dozens of articles and several books on the history of medicine. He had been pursuing scholarly work in history since medical school, and his interest in a public health career developed only when he recognized that he had little chance of gaining a position in medical history while still a young man.

Rosen had a passion for history, driven by an insatiable curiosity about all human activity; but as a physician, he also had a practical motive for his historical interests. For him disease was a social phenomenon and medicine a social endeavor, and study in the history of medicine, done correctly, would demonstrate these truths. Rosen cultivated the *social* history of medicine—the history of patients, of medical institutions, of the physician's role in society, of public health—because he saw social history as indispensable for an understanding of present-day health care.[1]

During and immediately after World War II, Rosen involved himself in the social medicine movement. "Social medicine" meant something different to each of its advocates, but at its core was a critical approach to health care that stressed the social determinants of disease.[2] Rosen planned a book that would trace the history of the idea and propose means for implementing it. By thus appropriating the role of historian of social medicine, Rosen hoped to be able to specify its intellectual lineage and thereby define its content.

As a preliminary exercise, Rosen published an essay in 1947 on the history of social medicine, and his continuing research in this area yielded some important detailed empirical studies.[3] But he never completed a book-length treatment of the subject—perhaps because the phrase "social medicine" sounded very much like "socialized medicine," and the concept incorporated the politically suspect idea of a national health system. By the early 1950s, advocacy of programs that were to the left of the New Deal had become dangerous, and the

American social medicine movement lost its momentum during the red scare of the McCarthy era.

Without an existing social medicine movement, Rosen had no motivation for publishing a book on its history; but there did exist an audience for a book on public health history—an audience that could be taught many of the same lessons that would have been conveyed by a history of social medicine. A comparison of his earlier writings with the content of *A History of Public Health* demonstrates the impact of his interest in social medicine on this book.

A History of Public Health is an important work that for good reason remains the standard text on the subject. As this new edition is published, though, George Rosen's treatise is almost sixty years old. So that we may understand it better both as a textbook and as a piece of historical source material, a review of Rosen's life, scholarship, and political philosophy is in order.

I

George Rosen was born in Brooklyn, New York, on June 23, 1910. His parents were immigrant Jews who spoke Yiddish at home, and it was not until he entered the New York City public schools that Rosen himself learned English. Years later, to motivate his own children, Rosen would claim that a teacher had once told him that he "would never amount to anything." His father, a presser in a laundry, was an ardent trade unionist who sometimes took George to union functions. His younger brother Jack, neither as motivated nor as scholarly as George, eventually became a lawyer. His mother kept house for the family of four.[4]

In high school, Rosen was known to devour books on almost any subject, and a required drafting course led to a lifetime hobby of drawing and painting. He did his undergraduate work at the College of the City of New York, which was, for bright young men (especially Jews) of the city's working class, simultaneously a gateway to upward mobility and a center of radical politics. At college Rosen devoted himself to schoolwork, his post office job as an armed security guard, and his voracious reading. He joined the City College swim team, but the pressure of his other obligations forced him to quit after a few months. Though sympathetic to the trade union movement, he showed little interest in politics.

Following an uncle's example, Rosen took the premedical course at CCNY— only to find himself the victim of the *numerus clausus*, which restricted the number of Jewish students in American medical colleges. At first he hoped that his uncle could help him gain admission into an American school the following year, but when a friend suggested going immediately to Germany (where there was no such barrier to medical education), Rosen agreed. When he arrived in Berlin in September 1930, Rosen joined several dozen young Americans (all Jews except for one African American) who had gone abroad for the type of high-quality medical education denied them at home. Much about Weimar Germany impressed Rosen, especially the national health insurance system; and he never confused the crimes of the Nazis with the general legacy of German culture.[5] Throughout his career—and especially in his work on social medicine—Rosen's writings reflected the attention he had paid, during his four and a half years in Berlin, to German liberal and socialist traditions.

The experiences of the American medical students in Berlin were paradoxical. As citizens of the United States, they enjoyed the cultural amenities of a European capital even after the Nazi seizure of power, but they were also well aware of the increasingly precarious status of the Jews of Germany. This was brought home to Rosen as he became involved with Beate Caspari, a German Jewish medical student to whom he proposed marriage after knowing her for only a few weeks. Rosen was not unique in marrying a classmate (women accounted for about one-quarter of the medical school class in Berlin, a proportion that surprised the all-male American contingent); but whether or not they had established intimate ties with particular families, many of the Americans made themselves available to protect Jewish households in Berlin. Rosen personally disposed of the family's unused pistol on a night when the Casparis feared that their apartment would be searched.

Beate's father, a successful physician, was an "old German democrat," and the Caspari household was simultaneously religious and worldly. While observing the traditions of Orthodox Judaism, Beate also belonged to a socialist youth group. The kosher food customs of the Caspari home would have been quite familiar to Rosen, but the presence of a servant and the atmosphere of genteel culture were a far cry from his parents' proletarian apartment in the Bronx. In his father-in-law, George Rosen found a model of a compassionate physician who maintained a Jewish identity within a comfortable household, while also participating in the broader secular culture.

Though he was a nonbeliever, indifferent to Zionism, and an aspiring cosmopolite, Rosen always acknowledged his Jewish roots.[6] More significantly for both his historical and public health work, as a middle-class intellectual Rosen continued to associate with health issues important to the labor movement.

II

The University of Berlin required each candidate for the MD degree to write a dissertation, and in the fall of 1933, Rosen asked Paul Diepgen, professor of the history of medicine, to serve as his thesis adviser. Rosen hoped to develop a topic in the history of American medicine that he could pursue using local library resources. Diepgen agreed to work with him, but because he was no expert in American medicine, he urged Rosen to contact Henry Sigerist for further advice.

Sigerist, who had come to the United States a year earlier from the University of Leipzig, was then director of the Institute of the History of Medicine at Johns Hopkins. A Swiss citizen, literate in a dozen languages and fluent in four, the forty-two-year-old Sigerist was regarded as perhaps the world's leading historian of medicine. Sigerist was a political liberal on a leftward trajectory who was excited by the dynamism and openness he had seen on an earlier lecture tour of the United States. He therefore had been happy to leave Germany and the specter of Nazism to take on the task of professionalizing the history of medicine in North America. By the time Rosen first wrote to him, Sigerist had established a program of courses as well as a monthly journal, the *Bulletin of the History of Medicine*. Within the next few years, he would make the Johns Hopkins Institute a vital center for all who were interested in the history of medicine and the future of medical care.

Sigerist proposed a thesis topic for Rosen and began corresponding with the younger man. Once the thesis was completed, both he and Diepgen praised it highly.[7] Sigerist would have liked to have more American students, but in 1935 Johns Hopkins did not have many resources to put into medical history. Rosen, with his capacity for distinguished independent work and his expected ability to earn a living in medical practice, was just the sort of informal student Sigerist wanted.

Rosen began an internship in New York City soon after returning from Berlin in May 1935, and within a few months, he began submitting articles to Sigerist's journal. The two men shared interests in social history and the organization of medical care, and over the next several years, they developed a warm student-teacher relationship.[8] At one point Rosen informed Sigerist that he was prepared to pursue a topic big enough for a book; when Sigerist proposed a history of miners' diseases, Rosen proceeded to do fundamental work in the history of occupational medicine.[9] Between 1936 and 1947, Rosen published no fewer than twenty articles in Sigerist's *Bulletin*, aided by Beate's library research, often at the New York Academy of Medicine. He was a perfectionist in this work, writing in ink on lined yellow paper. When he wanted to make a correction, he tore the offending sheet from the pad and rewrote the entire page. Until he became a university professor and had a secretary to do this work, Beate typed all of his manuscripts from the handwritten yellow sheets.

While establishing himself as a historian of medicine, Rosen completed his internship, opened a medical practice, and became a fanatical book collector. This, however, was a difficult time in his life. While his intelligence and hard work permitted him to pursue two careers simultaneously, he was not temperamentally suited for clinical practice. As a result, he was dissatisfied with his circumstances, and his income suffered (a problem worsened by his constant purchase of books). To relieve the financial strain, Rosen took a part-time job in the tuberculosis service of the New York City Department of Health. Meanwhile, Sigerist recommended him to the publisher Alfred A. Knopf as a translator, and to the Ciba-Geigy drug firm as editor of their new magazine, *Ciba Symposia.*

It was relatively easy for someone as well connected as Sigerist to find lucrative part-time jobs for a protégé as capable as Rosen, but it was impossible for Sigerist to help him achieve his main ambition—a professorial position in medical history. Rosen therefore eventually developed an alternative strategy. He would give up medical practice in favor of public health work and complete a PhD in a field allied with medical history. Then he would supplement his practical work in public health with an MPH degree. Rosen hoped that on completing this program he would be able to find a faculty position in a school of medicine or public health where his historical work would be appreciated.

In the fall of 1939, Rosen began taking courses in the Sociology Department at Columbia University, and within six months, he was at work on his PhD thesis. At Columbia he developed close ties with several prominent faculty members, including Robert K. Merton and Robert Lynd. He became a full-time health officer for the New York City Department of Health in 1942, and soon qualified for a fellowship-in-training that would involve one year of practical work followed by a year of study. Rosen began the fellowship that fall and hoped to use the academic year 1943–44 to work on an MPH—possibly at the Johns Hopkins School of Hygiene, just across the street from Henry Sigerist's institute.

In the meantime, his wife, Beate, qualified to practice medicine in the United States, undertook additional training at the New York Eye and Ear Infirmary, and began part-time work as one of the few female ophthalmologists in New York City—all the while assisting Rosen in his research, writing, and editing. Beate saw patients at an office in the Rosens' apartment on Riverside Drive and worked in the clinics of the New York City Health Department and the International Ladies' Garment Workers' Union. With the invaluable help of her own mother, Flora Caspari—who had left Germany after the elder Dr. Caspari's death and became responsible for daily supervision of the children, grocery shopping, and preparing meals for the family—Beate took on the role of primary parent to the two Rosen children, who were born in 1938 and 1941.

George Rosen earned his PhD in 1944 (with a dissertation that remains a standard work on the history of medical specialization),[10] but World War II postponed his formal public health training. He joined the army in the spring of 1943 and spent the following two years working at the global epidemiology program in Washington, DC. He regretted being separated from Beate and the children but enjoyed his work and took advantage of being a short train ride away from Sigerist. In Washington Rosen also made contact with a circle of Sigerist protégés who were interested primarily in health policy and only secondarily in history. Toward the end of the war, Rosen was transferred to London, where he interviewed captured German military doctors and uncovered some of the abuses of Nazi experimentation on humans. Although he also used this time to make contacts with British medical historians, he was not interested in his work and was anxious to return to a new project in New York. While George was in London, Beate took up the work of editing *Ciba Symposia*, working closely with the noted medical illustrator Frank Netter.

Shortly after his arrival in England, Rosen had learned that the rare book dealer Henry Schuman was planning to publish a scholarly periodical and that Schuman wanted him to serve as editor. Rosen began working on the *Journal of the History of Medicine and Allied Sciences* while still overseas, and in February 1946 the first issue appeared. Unlike *Ciba Symposia*, the *Journal* was not a mere supplement to his income but rather an unpaid labor of love. Sigerist's *Bulletin* had been the only English-language scholarly periodical in the field for the past several years. Now editor of a comparable publication, the thirty-five-year-old Rosen had arrived as a major medical historian.

After his discharge in April 1946, Rosen returned to the New York City Health Department to prepare its *Manual of District Health Administration*—all the while writing medical history articles and editing the new journal. Again an employee of the health department, he was able to take advantage of the second year of his fellowship, and in September 1946 he enrolled as an MPH student at Columbia University. Meanwhile he and Beate began co-editing *400 Years of a Doctor's Life*, a popular work of collective biography, published by Henry Schuman in 1948. Beate was responsible for most of the research for this book, which was largely based on excerpts from the writings of the eighty-two physicians whose lives and careers are covered.

In the winter of 1946–47, just months away from completing his third graduate degree, Rosen learned that Sigerist had decided to retire from Hopkins at the end of the academic year. At first Rosen was hopeful that he would succeed Sigerist, but by the time he finished the MPH program, he knew that this was not likely. The most honest appraisal of his chances was provided by Erwin Ackerknecht, another young historian of medicine who had become Rosen's friend while working at the institute during the war. "This holy institution," Ackerknecht warned Rosen about Hopkins, "has not yet had a Jewish chair holder."[11] Rosen was once more confronted with institutional anti-Semitism. Moreover, the administration and trustees of Hopkins had had enough of Sigerist's vocal advocacy of socialized medicine and friendliness toward the

Soviet Union. As a close associate of Sigerist, Rosen—although sharply opposed to Russian communism and never a political activist—was tarred with the same brush.

With the Hopkins job closed to him and no other positions likely to open in history of medicine, Rosen resolved to continue his historical scholarship on his own time, while earning his living in public health. In 1949 he became director of health education for New York City, where he developed techniques for exhibits, radio broadcasts, and publications and coordinated health education activities. He left city government in 1950 to found the Department of Health Education and Preventive Services at the Health Insurance Plan of Greater New York (HIP).

HIP, a medical care program for families of moderate income, had begun operations in 1947. It consisted of about thirty semiautonomous medical partnerships, compensated by capitation payments derived from enrollees' premiums and coordinated through a central office. In some ways HIP resembles the HMOs that have developed since the 1970s, but many of its early administrators regarded HIP as a small-scale, privately organized model for a government-based national health system.[12] Not only was medical care at HIP based on principles of prepayment and group practice, but care for the sick was only a part of HIP's broader mission of disease prevention and health promotion. For example, while with HIP, Rosen played an important role in implementing the innovative program that introduced mammographic screening for breast carcinoma to the United States. At HIP Rosen had achieved a major position in the world of public health—a position in which he could apply aspects of his theory of social medicine.[13] Nonetheless, his passion remained history, and his goal was still a faculty position.

At this time Rosen also became increasingly active in the American Public Health Association. He was invited to join the editorial board of its *American Journal of Public Health* in 1948, and he regularly contributed to the *AJPH* and participated at APHA meetings. He was appointed editor in 1957 and presided over the *AJPH* until 1973, a period during which expanding federal programs challenged lagging state and local health agencies. As public health work in America became increasingly fragmented, Rosen struggled against narrow specialization and tried to forge a broad vision of the field. His editorials made good use of his understanding of history in support of points of social and political significance. While editor, Rosen also inaugurated and regularly contributed to the feature "Public Health: Then and Now," a series intended to cultivate a sense of shared heritage among public health workers.[14]

In 1951 Rosen reaped the first fruits of his career strategy, when he was appointed to a part-time faculty position at the Columbia University School of Public Health and Administrative Medicine. His position was made full time in 1957, allowing him to leave HIP and concentrate on his scholarship and editorial duties. At Columbia he taught courses in health education, education theory, community health, the sociology of mental illness, and, of course, history. Finally, in 1969, after turning down several offers from universities farther from New York City, Rosen became professor of the history of medicine and of public health at Yale University, where, as at Columbia, he was highly regarded by his students. He died in Oxford in August 1977, while touring Great Britain on his way to give the keynote address at an international history of science conference in Edinburgh.

Through the end of his life Rosen remained a leading innovator in social history of medicine. Always universal in scope—writing about Britain, continental Europe, and America, and comfortably covering conditions from the seventeenth century through his own day—in his later work, Rosen turned toward the history of mental illness,[15] while reserving some of his most insightful analysis for the history of urban health.[16] A man of broad culture, whose interests extended from New Orleans jazz to medieval architecture, he was remembered at a memorial service with a reading of a Dylan Thomas poem and performance of a Mozart string quartet.

III

Rosen's most significant works have a definite political content, and it would be a mistake to approach his historical writings without acknowledging this. Because he was a man of principle and integrity, concerned about meeting scholarly norms of objectivity and evidence, Rosen recognized that all historians approach their subjects with certain presuppositions. In an early essay he made his own preferences clear.[17]

At different times in his life, Rosen might have characterized himself as a democratic socialist or a left liberal. In any case, he was consistently a man of the moderate left, with a commitment to social reform on behalf of the poor and the working class. By temperament, though, he was not an activist, and he never joined any political organization. He had strong views about many of the issues of his day, but he restricted his public utterances to questions of health and medical care. In his *AJPH* editorials, he was a spokesman for the public health profession and health advocacy was his job. As a historian, he felt that it was also his duty, and he viewed his historical scholarship as a means to influence health policy—by demonstrating that health and disease were social matters and that the best health professionals had always recognized this. For George Rosen, scholarship was a form of activism.

Two distinct strains merged in Rosen's politics. A child of the working class and a victim of discrimination, he sympathized with the poor and sought to reform society. But his burning desire to systematize knowledge also influenced his politics and his historical scholarship. Once he mastered the language for the purposes of medical education, he immersed himself in the traditions of German intellectual culture. He began using Hegelian philosophy and other strains of German idealism as tools for historical analysis and read works in the Marxist tradition. His early writings particularly reflect the prominent role of Marxist ideas, and these ideas remained important throughout his life, even after he absorbed many of the lessons of American functionalist sociology at Columbia. Rosen took Marxism seriously enough in the early 1940s to prepare two essays on Marx's view of history. In these pieces, Rosen argued that, while Marx saw economic factors as basic, he did not regard them as the sole determinants of historical development. Rosen submitted the articles to *Science and Society,* a leading left-wing scholarly journal, but they were rejected "because of dire lack of space" and remain unpublished.[18]

Rosen's early articles in the *Bulletin of the History of Medicine* also demonstrate his debt to German theoretical works. Setting the tone for one piece, the twenty-six-year-old Rosen used the ideas of Hegel, Marx, and the German sociologist Karl Mannheim to explain intellectual history in economic and political terms. He insisted that a new, social, history of medicine must be dialectical, and discussed historical development as a series of contradictions where thesis and antithesis create synthesis.[19] In his theoretical discussion of occupational health, Rosen demanded that the historian recognize the centrality of economic structure and incorporate the activities of the working class into medical history. The history of occupational health was pivotal to Rosen because occupational diseases were so evidently caused by social circumstances.[20]

Like Sigerist, Rosen put the patient first in the patient-disease-physician triad, but he added the insight that a patient is also a person with a social role. He stressed that diseases are not immutable entities and are intelligible only within their biological *and* social contexts,[21] and he suggested that history of medicine had been deficient in viewing the patient as "only an accident in the history of the disease."[22] Rosen claimed to have learned from Marx and Engels that human beings were "central actors on the stage of history"; until the very end of his career he protested against a "biologism" in history that devalued human action in relationship to disease and other natural forces.[23]

Rosen made this argument to demonstrate to doctors that their endeavor was necessarily social. He wanted to show that the most astute physicians were those who understood the social etiology of disease and that the most successful healers were those who acted on this understanding.[24] But there was one further lesson that Rosen proposed for doctors who granted this point. This was to recognize "the necessity of becoming a social critic."[25] Through his early work on occupational medicine and the role of the physician, Rosen was germinating the conception of social medicine that he articulated in the years immediately following World War II.

Just as Rosen denied that Marx was a strict economic determinist, he also looked to other cultural elements in explaining the development of health care. In his efforts to demonstrate that medicine could not be understood outside of a broad social context, Rosen was willing to invoke the power of ideas as much as the means of production. In a highly regarded article, Rosen demonstrated how a philosophical outlook influenced the subsequent history of both medical knowledge and the organization of medical care. In another essay, he stressed the importance of "the mental struggles, the ideological and philosophical conflicts that preceded action."[26]

IV

Rosen's political views were formed in the 1920s, 1930s, and 1940s, and his thinking thereafter reflected the dominant ideas of that period. For Rosen, progressive politics was democratic, class based, and trade union oriented. Therefore, while sympathetic to radical political movements that developed in the 1960s and 1970s, Rosen was wary of what he regarded as their excesses.

Although he was not drawn to scholarship about the health of blacks or the role of blacks in health care, Rosen was interested in African American culture and history and had no tolerance for prejudice based on race. His sensitivity to racism is attested to by a letter he received from a black public health worker who had been his student at Columbia. Coming from the South in the mid-1960s, this man was severely disappointed by the racism he encountered at a leading northern university. Sometime after leaving New York, he made a point of writing to Rosen, to commend him for a decency, sensitivity, and goodwill that were almost unique among the northern white academics whom he had met.[27]

Rosen similarly viewed women's liberation as a basic question of democratic rights and opposed all institutional and formal barriers to civil equality for women.[28] Late in his career he wrote two articles on women in public health,[29] and he prepared an exhibit for the Yale Medical Historical Library on women as healers. Gender, however, like race, did not greatly interest him as a dimension of social history. When asked to review the manuscripts of two books of feminist scholarship on American medical history, he strongly recommended their publication but expressed somewhat pedantic reservations about terminology. He was uncomfortable with neologisms like "chairperson," and he objected to what he viewed as mythmaking in the service of ideology.[30]

Rosen opposed the war in Vietnam much as he had supported the Spanish

Republic in the late thirties (although in neither case did he take a vocal stand outside his circle of friends and family). He was therefore sympathetic to the antiwar movement of the 1960s, but he was wary of scholarship that was explicitly anti-imperialist and he distrusted what he considered the irrational side of the youth revolt.[31]

Most important for understanding *A History of Public Health* is Rosen's response to the radical health movement of the 1960s and 1970s. As a former health educator and advocate of social medicine, Rosen thought it essential to involve people in their own health care and to give them the information necessary for informed decisions. His perspective, however, was always that of the health administrator working for a large centralized organization; and just as he opposed individualistic notions of responsibility for health and disease, he was wary of voluntarism and too much decentralization.[32] Coming from an older socialist and public health tradition, Rosen focused on global, grand strategic planning. In a sense, he was a typical midcentury rationalizer who believed that enlightened public leaders (most often liberal Democrats) could solve social problems using efficiently organized government bureaucracies. Ultimately, for Rosen, it was the state that must guarantee health: through health education, housing reform, occupational medicine, food inspection, medical care, and so on.

V

George Rosen completed *A History of Public Health* while in the midst of numerous other projects. It is neither his most elegant nor his most scholarly work, but it is infused both with the findings of his earlier research and with the passions that motivated his scholarship. In this book, Rosen makes clear his belief that a turning point in history occurred in the early nineteenth century, when "a new social class, the industrial workers, was beginning to express itself politically and socially." "Furthermore," he adds, "the new class of industrial workers, taking seriously the democratic implications of liberalism in terms of human rights and human dignity . . ., organized themselves . . ., refused to compete against one another, and took action to secure . . . social services."

Rosen was particularly sympathetic to a current in progressive thought that looked to events and thinkers of the eighteenth century as its source. In both France and Britain, the legacy of the Enlightenment included the theoretical underpinnings of the nineteenth-century public health movement—the organizational achievements of which remained in place in Rosen's own day. Rosen was a subtle and critical thinker, but what frequently showed itself in his writings—and perhaps most of all in *A History of Public Health*—was his attachment to the optimism and rationalism of the Age of Revolution.

NOTES

The author wishes to acknowledge the following people for their encouragement and for the information they provided through interviews and personal communications: Dr. Beate Caspari-Rosen, Dr. Paul Peter Rosen, Prof. Susan Koslow (aka Susan Rosen-Olejarz), Dr. Louis Schneider, Dr. Thomas Patrick, Prof. Saul Benison, Prof. Arnold Koslow, and Mr. Erich Meyerhoff.

1. See "What Medical History Should Be Taught to Medical Students?," in *Education in the History of Medicine,* ed. John B. Blake (New York: Hafner, 1968), 19–27.

2. For more on the social medicine movement and its relationship to public health (especially in Great Britain), see Dorothy Porter and Roy Porter, "What Was Social Medicine? An Historiographical Essay," *Journal of Historical Sociology* 1 (1989): 90–106.

3. "What Is Social Medicine? A Genetic Analysis of the Concept," *Bulletin of the History of Medicine* 21 (1947): 674–733. For a nearly complete list of Rosen's publications that includes all of his major articles on the history of social medicine, see the bibliography in *Healing and History: Essays for George Rosen* (New York: Science History, 1979), 252–62.

4. Unless otherwise noted, information on Rosen's life throughout this essay was abstracted from a series of interviews with his relatives, friends, and associates.

5. See "Medicine under Hitler," *Bulletin of the New York Academy of Medicine* 25 (1949): 125–29.

6. See his introduction to the reprint edition of Harry Friedenwald's *The Jews and Medicine: Essays* (New York: Ktav, 1967).

7. Rosen later translated the thesis and published it as *The Reception of William Beaumont's Discovery in Europe* (New York: Schuman's, 1942). Beaumont's work on gastric physiology during the 1820s and 1830s was probably the earliest significant contribution to basic biomedical science by a doctor in the United States.

8. The entire Rosen-Sigerist correspondence through June 1947 is preserved in the papers of the Institute of the History of Medicine at the Alan Mason Chesney Medical Archives of the Johns Hopkins Medical Institution (hereinafter IHMP). Unless otherwise noted, all discussion of Rosen's activities through 1947 is based on this correspondence.

9. *The History of Miners' Diseases: A Medical and Social Interpretation* (New York: Schuman's, 1943).

10. *The Specialization of Medicine with Particular Reference to Ophthalmology* (New York: Froben Press, 1944).

11. Ackerknecht to Rosen, 7 March 1947 (George Rosen papers, Yale University Archives, MS group 862 [hereinafter GRP], Addition of 4 June 1979, Box 2). Ackerknecht, who was not Jewish but had been a political refugee from Nazi Germany, admired Rosen's continuing self-identification as a Jew. See Ackerknecht, "George Rosen as I Knew Him," *Journal of the History of Medicine and Allied Sciences* 33 (1978): 254–55.

12. See John Z. Bowers, "Remarks at George Rosen Memorial Service, 14 October 1977, Yale University," *Journal of the History of Medicine and Allied Sciences* 33 (1978): 256.

13. A good source on the early history of HIP is Louis L. Feldman, "Organization of a Medical Group Practice Prepayment Program in New York City" (New York: Health Insurance Plan of Greater New York, 1953), mimeographed. For Rosen's view of health education, see "Health Education and Preventive Medicine—'New Horizons in Medical Care,'" *American Journal of Public Health* 42 (1952): 687–93.

14. See Alfred Yankauer, "The American Journal of Public Health 1957–73," in *Healing and History: Essays for George Rosen* (New York: Science History Publications, 1979), 229–41; and Milton Terris, "George Rosen and the American Public Health Tradition," *American Journal of Public Health* 69 (1979): 173–76. "Public Health: Then and Now" continues as a regular feature in the *AJPH* and is currently edited by Elizabeth Fee and Theodore M. Brown.

15. His most significant essays in this area were collected as *Madness in Society: Chapters in the Historical Sociology of Mental Illness* (Chicago: University of Chicago Press, 1968). For a detailed analysis of Rosen's work in psychiatric history, see Edward T. Morman, "George Rosen and the History of Mental Illness," in *Discovering the History of Psychiatry*, ed. Roy Porter and Mark S. Micale (New York: Oxford University Press, 1993).

16. See, for example, "Disease, Debility and Death," in *The Victorian City: Images and Reality*, ed. H. J. Dyos and Michael Wolff (London: Routledge & Kegan Paul, 1973), 625–67.

17. See "A Theory of Medical Historiography," *Bulletin of the History of Medicine* 8 (1940): 655–65.

18. "Some Pre-suppositions of Marxian Socialism" and "An Analysis of Certain Sections of Marx's *Kritik der Hegelschen Rechtsphilosophie*" (GRP, Addition of 15 June 1979, Box 1); Bernhard Stern to Rosen, 23 July 1942 (GRP, Addition of 26 October 1978).

19. "Social Aspects of Jacob Henle's Medical Thought," *Bulletin of the History of Medicine* 5 (1937): 509–37.

20. "On the Historical Investigation of Occupational Diseases: An Aperçu," *Bulletin of the History of Medicine* 5 (1937): 941–46.

21. "A Theory of Medical Historiography."

22. "Disease and Social Criticism: A Contribution to a Theory of Medical History," *Bulletin of the History of Medicine* 10 (1941): 5–15.

23. See "Some Pre-suppositions of Marxian Socialism," and "The Biological Element in Human History," *Medical History* 1 (1957): 150–59.

24. See, for example, the discussion of Lind and Blane in "Occupational Diseases of English Seamen during the Seventeenth and Eighteenth Centuries," *Bulletin of the History of Medicine* 7 (1939): 751–58.

25. "Disease and Social Criticism," 14.

26. "The Philosophy of Ideology and the Emergence of Modern Medicine in France," *Bulletin of the History of Medicine* 20 (1946): 328–39; "Medicine in Utopia," *Ciba Symposia* 7 (1945): 188–200.

27. Kenneth L. Howard to Rosen, 26 June 1974 (GRP, Addition of 28 August 1978, Box 1).

28. When he visited New York with his wife soon after moving to New Haven, Rosen was incensed to learn that women were not allowed to enter the Yale Club of New York through the front door. He resigned from the club after vocally complaining to the management. Rosen to William Milo Barnum, 20 December 1971, 21 January 1972 (GRP, Addition of 28 August 1978, Box 1). Rosen was also sensitive to the social dimensions of homosexuality. See "Homosexuality in Primitive Societies," *Ciba Symposia* 2 (1940): 495.

29. "Sara Josephine Baker," in *Dictionary of American Biography: Supplement Three, 1941–1945* (New York: Scribner's, 1973), 27–29; and "Ellen H. Richards (1842–1911), Sanitary Chemist and Pioneer of Professional Equality for Women in Health Science," *American Journal of Public Health* 64 (1974): 816–19.

30. "Referee's report [on two manuscripts on the history of American midwifery]" (GRP, Addition of 28 August 1978, Box 5).

31. See "The Revolt of Youth: Some Historical Comparisons," in *The Psychopathology of Adolescence,* ed. J. Zubin and A. M. Freedman (New York: Grune & Stratton, 1970), 1–14.

32. "The First Neighborhood Health Center Movement—Its Rise and Fall," *American Journal of Public Health* 61 (1971): 1620–37.

Man's the reality that mak's / A'things possible, even himsel'.
Hugh M'Diarmid

The protection and promotion of the health and welfare of its citizens is considered to be one of the most important functions of the modern state. This
function is the embodiment of a public policy based on political, economic,
social, and ethical considerations. But whence this concern for the health of
the group? And how does it relate to the individual citizen? For answers to
these questions we must turn to the history of the community and its health
problems.

History performs a social task. It may be regarded as the collective memory
of the human group and for good or evil helps to mold its collective consciousness. It creates an awareness of oneself in relation to the world around one, including both our yesterdays and our tomorrows. A meaningful understanding
of the present requires that it be seen in the light of the past from which it has
emerged and of the future which it is bringing forth. Every situation that man
has faced and every problem that he has had to solve have been the product of
historical developments. Furthermore, the way in which we act in a given situation is, in large measure, determined by the mental image of the past that
we have. To understand the problems of our own society and to be capable of
playing an intelligent role in shaping our civilization, we must have a sense of
continuity in time, an awareness that one cannot advance intelligently into
the future without a willingness to look attentively at the past, we must have
knowledge of the past and how it brought the present into being.

History illuminates the public concern with health. Man is a social being. It
is characteristic of human beings to associate with each other for mutual protection and advantage. Throughout known history, men living in communities
have had to take account in one way or another of health problems that derive
from the biological needs and attributes of their fellows. Out of the need for
dealing with these problems of social life, there has developed with increasing
clarity a recognition of the signal importance of community action in the promotion of health and the prevention and treatment of disease. This recognition
is summed up in the concept of public health.

The aim of this book is to tell the story of community health action, from its beginnings in the earliest civilizations to the state of development achieved at present in the economically and technologically advanced countries of the world. For this reason, the narrative, especially for the modern period, relates chiefly to those lands which have been the major centers of modern public health—especially Great Britain, France, Germany, and the United States. Where there have been developments of special interest in other countries, reference is made to them. For a variety of reasons, a large part of the world—in Asia, in Africa, in the Middle East—stopped developing economically, politically, and scientifically around 1400, just about the time that the Western nations entered upon a period of extraordinary growth in these areas. As a result, it is only today that the Asian and African peoples are beginning to effect the far-reaching changes necessary to bridge the gap of centuries, and the importance of this development for public health is considered in its implications for the future.

The story of community health action is written for a wide range of potential readers and is designed to be read by interested laymen as well as professional health workers. Various strands have contributed and are continuing to add to the growing fabric that is community action in the interest of health. To trace this process, however, is not an end in itself. Ultimately, the value of such an analysis and interpretation resides in the light thrown upon the formation of policy and the application of knowledge. The dynamic and changing character of community health action requires both professional and layman to be aware of the significant trends and issues involved. If this book contributes to an increased awareness of the nature of the factors involved in dealing with community health problems, its aim will have been achieved. For in the field of health, we may echo the ancient Roman,

Salus publica suprema lex.

George Rosen, MD

A History of Public Health

-I-
The Origins of Public Health

Throughout human history, the major problems of health that men have faced have been concerned with community life, for instance, the control of transmissible disease, the control and improvement of the physical environment (sanitation), the provision of water and food of good quality and in sufficient supply, the provision of medical care, and the relief of disability and destitution. The relative emphasis placed on each of these problems has varied from time to time, but they are all closely related, and from them has come public health as we know it today.

SANITATION AND HOUSING. Evidence of activity connected with community health has been found in the very earliest civilizations. Some four thousand years ago, a people of whom little is known developed a great urban civilization in the north of India. Sites excavated at Mohenjo-Daro in the Indus valley and at Harappa in the Punjab indicate that these ancient Indian cities were consciously planned in rectangular blocks, apparently in accordance with building laws. Bathrooms and drains are common in the excavated buildings. The streets were broad, paved, and drained by covered sewers. These drains were laid some two feet or less below the level of the street, and they consisted for the most part of molded bricks, cemented with a mortar of mud. Within the houses better materials were used, and in at least one instance there is a report of drain pipes made of pottery and embedded in gypsum plaster against the possibility of leakage.

Finds dating from the Middle Kingdom (2100–1700 B.C.) give some idea of conditions in Egypt. The archeologist Flinders Petrie discovered the ruins of the city of Kahun, which had been built at the royal command according to a unified plan. Care was taken to drain off water by means of a stone masonry gutter in the center of the street. The ruins of Tel-el-Amarna, dating from the fourteenth century B.C., are essentially like those of Kahun. One detail, however, deserves mention. The remains of a bathroom were found in one of the smaller houses.

Two thousand years before the Christian era, the problem of procuring an adequate supply of drinking water for larger communities had in considerable measure already been solved. For example, the Cretan-Mycenean culture had large conduits. Excavations have also revealed that Troy had a very ingenious water supply system. Just as in any place where drinking water supply systems were accepted facts, the disposal of wastes was likewise regulated and the sewer age system was well developed. In palaces, such as that of Knossos on Crete, which dates from the second pre-Christian millenium, there were not only magnificent bathing facilities, but also water flushing arrangements for the toilets. Water pipes in private houses, the remains of which are still clearly evident at present among the ruins of Priene in Asia Minor, were probably installed at an early date, even though in many places, water was usually drawn from public wells.

Impressive ruins of sewerage systems and baths testify to the achievements of the Incas in public health engineering. They established well-drained cities that were adequately supplied with water, thus providing a good basis for the health of the community. The Incas were also aware that other elements of the physical environment could have an effect upon health. Thus, they recognized the connection between acclimatization and ill-health. Troops from the highlands served in the hot valleys under a rotation system, remaining there only for a few months at a time.

CLEANLINESS AND GODLINESS. Cleanliness and personal hygiene are to be found among present-day primitives and were unquestionably practiced by prehistoric and early historic men. Primitive peoples generally dispose of their excretions in a sanitary manner, but their reasons for this behavior are not necessarily identical with ours. Throughout large periods of human history, cleanliness has been next to godliness because of religious beliefs and practices. People kept clean so as to be pure in the eyes of the gods and not for hygienic reasons. Cleanliness and hygiene were emphasized on such grounds among the the Egyptians, the Mesopotamians, the Hebrews, and other peoples.

An interesting example of the connection between cleanliness and religion is the Inca feast, Citua. Every year, in September, at the beginning of the rainy season, which was associated with disease, the people led by the Inca carried out the health ceremony. In addition to prayer, propitiatory offerings to the gods, and other religious practices, all homes were thoroughly cleaned.

DISEASE AND THE COMMUNITY. As long as man has lived on earth, disease has plagued him. Sickness is associated with life, and man everywhere endeavors to deal with it as best he can. Studies in paleopathology have shown not only the antiquity of disease, but also that it has always occurred in the same basic forms, such as infection, inflammation, disturbances of development and metabolism, traumatism, and tumors. For example, schistosomiasis, prevalent in Egypt today, has been found in kidneys 3000 years old, and tuberculosis of the spine has been diagnosed in the skeletal remains of pre-Columbian Indians. Furthermore, pictorial evidence from Egypt suggests the existence of poliomyelitis and achondroplastic dwarfism. However, while the basic types have not changed, the incidence and prevalence of illness have varied from time to time and from place to place. Knowledge of such changes in the occurrence of disease is essential for an understanding of the health problems faced by communities in the course of human history and of the thoughts and actions of those who dealt with them.

Faced with problems of endemic or epidemic disease, communities and individuals have acted in terms of some prevailing concept of the nature of illness. On the primitive level of knowledge, this action is generally couched in super natural terms. Modern medicine, on the other hand, seeks to understand and to manage illness by studying normal and morbid structures and processes in the body. Modern medicine identifies and differentiates many distinct diseases, defining the disease as clearly as possible in terms of its symptoms, location, and cause. This concept of distinct disease entities is, however, of comparatively recent origin.

Ancient and medieval physicians did not generally distinguish different diseases as such, but they were concerned rather with various groups of symptoms exhibited by sick people. Such evidences of disordered health were explained by theories about the abnormal mixture of the body fluids (humoralism) or about the constricted and relaxed states in the solid parts of the body (solidism). As long as such conceptions of disease prevailed, physicians could not, in the nature of the case, concentrate on specific seats of disease.

However, the transmissibility of certain diseases was noted long before their causes were known, and certain communicable diseases have been recognized for many centuries. There is not any doubt that the ancient world was repeatedly visited by epidemics. The possible existence of smallpox in Egypt around 1000 B.C. was suggested by M. A. Ruffer. He examined a mummy of the Twentieth Dynasty, in which the skin was "the seat of a peculiar vesicular or bulbous eruption which in form and general distribution bore a striking resemblance to that of smallpox." In the *Iliad* we read of Apollo with his darts inflicting epidemic illness on the army before Troy; and in the *Old Testament* of the Bible in the book of I Samuel we are told that the hand of the Lord was against the Philistines who were smitten so that "emerods broke out upon them."

For thousands of years, epidemics were looked upon mainly as divine judgments on the wickedness of mankind, and it was believed that these punishments were to be avoided by appeasing the wrathful gods. In Egypt, for instance, Sekhmet, goddess of pestilence, produced epidemics when aroused and abated them when she was mollified. This theurgical theory of disease lasted for several millennia, but alongside it there gradually developed the idea that pestilence is due to natural causes involving especially climate and the physical environment. This great liberation of thought took place in Greece and culminated during the fifth and fourth centuries B.C. in the first attempts at a rational, scientific theory of disease causation. This is not to say that Greek medical thought was completely devoid of religious aspects, but more and more the great physicians and thinkers of Greece oriented themselves in terms of this world.

- II -
Health and the Community in the
Greco-Roman World

Greece

PROBLEMS OF DISEASE. The first clear-cut accounts of acute communicable diseases occur in the literature of classical Greece. Thucydides has a vivid account of the epidemic that broke out at Athens in the second year of the Peloponnesian War. Curiously enough, however, there is an apparent absence of most communicable diseases in the writings of the Hippocratic collection. There is no mention of smallpox or measles, nor is there any certain reference to diphtheria, chicken pox, or scarlet fever. The great plague of Athens does not appear in the Hippocratic writings. Yet there is an unmistakable clinical description of mumps in the book known as *Epidemics I*. Attention is centered chiefly on endemic disease in the Hippocratic works; included are such conditions as colds, pneumonia, malarial fevers, inflammations of the eyes, as well as various unidentified illnesses.

DIPHTHERIA. Classical medical literature contains numerous references to severe sore throats often ending in death. Owing to the ambiguity of the terms employed, however, it is difficult to say with certainty what diseases were involved. The Greek word *kynanche* (cynanche) was applied to various forms of acute inflammatory disease of the throat and the larynx, characterized by difficulty in swallowing and in breathing to the point of suffocation. The equivalent term in Latin was *angina*. While we are unable to draw any firm conclusion from the symptoms described, it seems likely that diphtheria was included.

Several Hippocratic treatises contain tantalizing statements suggestive of diphtheria and its sequelae. In *Epidemics II* the writer mentions certain complications of cynanche, among them a nasal voice, difficulty in swallowing, escape of fluid through the nostrils when drinking, and inability to stand upright. Similarly, in the aphoristic collection *On Dentition*, two statements seem to suggest diphtheria. The one states that "in cases of ulcerated tonsils, the formation of a membrane like a spider's web is not a good sign" (XXIV). According to the other, "Ulcers on the tonsils that spread over the uvula alter the voice of those who recover" (XXXI). These comments may refer to diphtheria and the nasal voice of diphtheritic paralysis.

While there may be some doubt whether the Hippocratic writings deal with diphtheria, the clinical picture of the Egyptian or Syrian ulcer described by Aretaeus the Cappadocian in the second century A.D. may be identified as diphtheria with greater certainty. He gives a clear description of a severe inflammatory disease of the throat, attacking children particularly, and accompanied by the formation of a whitish or discolored membrane covering the throat, which might extend into the mouth or descend into the windpipe, causing difficulty in breathing or suffocation. Aretaeus goes on to say that the disease was engendered in Egypt and Syria, particularly in Coelesyria, hence the name Egyptian and Syrian ulcer. He also noted that in extremely severe cases of the disease, before death occurred, food and drink were regurgitated through the nostrils, hoarseness and loss of speech supervened, and there was great difficulty in breathing. Finally, such patients were released by death.

There would seem to be small doubt that this author had observed cases of diphtheria and had noted various post-diphtheritic sequelae. Furthermore, from an epidemiological viewpoint, the disease appears to have been endemic in the Mediterranean area, occurring in Italy, Greece, Syria, and Egypt, and it may have been especially prevalent around the eastern and southeastern shores of the Mediterranean.

MALARIA. The Greek physicians of the fifth century B.C. were very familiar with malaria. References to malarial fevers abound in the Hippocratic writings. The Hippocratic authors knew of the periodicity of these fevers. They spoke of tertians and quartans and referred to the benign character of the latter. Notable is the observation that children are the main sufferers in endemic areas. The Hippocratic writers observed and noted the seasonal character of the disease as well as the detrimental consequences of wet springs and dry summers. They also associated marshes and malarial fevers, even though they misunderstood the relationship and thought the fevers were caused by drinking swamp water. How early the Greeks established a rational association between malaria and swamps is indicated by the story told of the philosopher Empedocles of Agrigentum (c. 504–443 B.C.). According to the tradition, as reported by Diogenes Laertius, he delivered the people of Selinus in Sicily from an epidemic by turning two rivers into its marshes so as to prevent stagnation and to sweeten the waters.

THE NATURE OF DISEASE. The great physicians of Greece were likewise natural philosophers, whose aim was not only to deal with health problems but also to fathom the nature of the universe and to understand the interrelations of man and nature. Based on philosophic reasoning as well as on observations like those already described, and in response to practical needs, the Greeks developed a naturalistic concept and explanation of disease. They realized that health and disease resulted from natural processes. Thus, the author of the Hippocratic work on *The Sacred Disease* (believed to be epilepsy) says at the outset: "It is not, in my opinion, any more divine or more sacred than any other diseases, but has a natural cause. . . ." Ill-health developed when there was an imbalance between man and his environment.

AIRS, WATERS, AND PLACES. The belief in the balance between man and his environment is most clearly evident in the Hippocratic book on *Airs, Waters and Places*. The importance of this work cannot be overestimated. It constitutes the first known systematic endeavor to present the causal relations between environmental factors and disease. For more than 2000 years, it was the basic epidemiological text and provided the theoretical underpinning for an understanding of endemic and epidemic disease. No fundamental change occurred in this respect until late in the nineteenth century when the new sciences of bacteriology and immunology made their appearance.

The writer of *Airs, Waters and Places* recognized that there were diseases that were always present in a population. These he called *endemic*, a term we still use. He was further aware that other diseases, which were not always present, at certain times became excessively frequent, and these he called *epidemic*, a term that is likewise still current. The book endeavors to give an answer to the question: "What are the factors of local endemicity?" The eight introductory paragraphs present and summarize the essential factors. These are climate, soil, water, mode of life, and nutrition.

COLONIZATION AND MEDICAL CARE. *Airs, Waters and Places*, however, is not only a theoretical treatise. It also had a very practical purpose, and thus throws light on the way in which Greek communities dealt with certain problems of health. Extensive movements of colonization are a characteristic feature of ancient Greek history. From some time about 1000 B.C., the Greeks expanded eastward and westward beyond Greece proper and the coasts of the Aegean. Colonies were planted on the shores of Thrace and the Black Sea, in Italy and Sicily, even in Spain and Gaul. In establishing a new community, it was necessary to make sure that the site would not only satisfy religious and military requirements, but also that it would be salubrious. *Airs, Waters and Places* is intended to provide guidance in this matter. Thus, the author advises that before a place is colonized physicians should be questioned and the character of the soil should be subjected to detailed investigation. Marshy lowlands and swamp regions are said to be harmful. It is best to erect houses on elevated areas warmed by the sun, so that they would have contact only with salubrious winds.

Another practical purpose was to help the physician about to set up practice in an unfamiliar town. This purpose is intimately linked to the way in which a Greek community provided medical care for its members and to the peculiar conditions of medical practice in the fifth century B.C.

Like other arts and crafts, medicine in ancient Greece was an itinerant vocation. The number of physicians was small, and like other craftsmen, such as the shoemaker or the artist, the Hippocratic physician practiced his craft while wandering. In smaller towns, medical service was provided exclusively by these itinerant practitioners. When the physician came to town, he would knock at the doors offering his services, and where he found enough work, he opened a shop (the *iatreion*) and settled down for a while. Larger communities had permanent municipal physicians. About 600 B.C., individual cities began to appoint such physicians. When a community wanted a doctor to settle there, it offered him an annual salary, for which the money was raised through a special tax. By the end of the fifth century, this arrangement became general throughout the Greek cities. The physician was not prevented from accepting fees, but he was guaranteed an income even when there was not much work. To a large extent, the community doctor served the needy. During the Hellenistic period, this practice was to be found wherever Greek culture prevailed.

That many of these physicians proved eminently satisfactory to their communities is evident from the numerous decrees of thanks passed to them. The municipal doctors were not a wealthy lot; the one salary known is about $180.00 a year. Nevertheless, many were like Damiades of Sparta of whom it is reported that he "made no difference between rich and poor, free and slaves." There was a high standard of devotion to duty among these men, and often they forwent their salaries during epidemics. Apollonius of Miletus fought the plague in the islands without reward; and when all the Coan doctors were down with an epidemic, Xenotimus voluntarily came to the city's assistance.

However, since physicians were not licensed, how could one distinguish a competent physician from a charlatan? Furthermore, how could the physician gain the confidence of the public? Some doctors were known to a town because they had already established a reputation for themselves. Others were new to the community and had to gain the confidence of their patients rapidly by predicting the future course of the illness. If the physician could do this and if events proved him correct, his reputation was established. The social situation of the Greek physician in the fifth century explains why he placed such emphasis on prognosis. *Airs, Waters and Places* is intended to aid the physician entering an unfamiliar city by indicating how he might cope with local diseases and make successful prognoses.

HYGIENE AND HEALTH EDUCATION. Throughout its history, Greek medicine was never exclusively curative medicine. From the very beginning, the preservation of health seemed the more important task and a great deal of thought was given to problems of hygiene. An old Attic drinking song declared that "Health is the first good lent to men." The poet Ariphron in a paean praised "Health, eldest of Gods" with whom he wanted to dwell for the rest of his life.

Health to the Greek physician was a condition in which the various forces or elements constituting the human body were perfectly balanced. Disturbed equilibrium resulted in disease. It was important therefore to maintain a mode of life in which such disturbances might be reduced to a minimum. Since the balance could easily be upset by external elements, a great deal of attention was paid to the influence of physical and nutritional factors on the human body. The ideal mode of life, according to the physicians, was one in which nutrition and excretion, exercise and rest were perfectly balanced. In addition, for each individual, account had to be taken of age, sex, constitution, and the seasons. In essence, one's whole life had to be organized for this purpose.

Very few people, however, could afford to lead such a life. This was a regimen for a small upper class leading a life of leisure, a class supported by a slave economy. It was an aristocratic hygiene. The mass of the people, said the writer of the Hippocratic book, *On Diet*, "by necessity must lead a haphazard life and . . . neglecting all, cannot take care of their health."

OCCUPATIONAL HEALTH. The emphasis on an aristocratic hygiene is reflected as well in the lack of attention paid to the occupational health problems of those who had to work for a living. Allusions to such matters are infrequent in the medical literature of classical Greece. Nevertheless, occupational diseases did occur. For example, there are pictures of flute players wearing a mouthband of leather like a halter around their cheeks and lips. Its purpose, apparently, was to prevent excessive puffing of the cheeks in order to avoid eventual relaxation of the muscles. The Greeks worked their mines with slaves and convicts, who toiled for long hours in narrow, poorly ventilated galleries. Yet only one reference in the Hippocratic writing can be interpreted as relating to a miner. This reference may refer to a case of lead poisoning or to a case of pneumonia. Not until the Roman period do we find more frequent references to occupational health.

PUBLIC HEALTH ADMINISTRATION. The public services, which the Greek cities provided for their inhabitants, varied both in scope and in magnitude according to their size and wealth. The municipal services, which we today associate with public health, are not mentioned very frequently in antiquity. Nevertheless, there were specific officials, *astynomi*, who were responsible for such matters as drainage and water supply. The Athenians, for example, had ten *astynomi* (five for Athens and five for Piraeus). In the cities of the Hellenistic period the administration became more complex and was generally uniform with Roman practice.

Rome

THE LEGACY OF GREECE. When Rome conquered the Mediterranean world and took over the legacy of Greek culture, she also accepted the medicine and ideas on health of the Greeks. However, in taking over from Greece her teeming ideas, Rome stamped them with her own character and formed them to her own purposes. As clinicians, the Romans were hardly more than imitators of the Greeks, but as engineers and administrators, as builders of sewerage systems and baths, and as providers of water supplies and other health facilities, they set the world a great example and left their mark in history.

WATER SUPPLY AND SANITATION. According to Strabo, because springs and streams of pure water were abundant, the Greeks did little to bring water supplies from a distance to their cities, and it was left to the Romans to introduce a system of aqueducts and organized water supply. This statement is not entirely correct and requires qualification. The Romans possibly learned from the Etruscans, who knew how to transport water and exploit this resource. Nevertheless, taking into account levels of technological development as well as the achievements of their predecessors, the Roman system of water supply is unparalleled in history.

All ancient cities relied to some extent on wells and rainwater cisterns for their water supply. At an early date, a number of Greek cities undertook to supplement these supplies from outside sources. Sometime in the sixth century B.C., water was brought into Athens from hills outside to augment the city supplies. Excavations at Olynthus dating from the fifth century B.C. have revealed an elaborate water-supply system in which the water was brought from a mountain 10 miles away and piped to bathrooms and a public fountain within the city. Even closer to the Roman practice was the system developed by the city of Pergamon in Asia Minor about 200 B.C. In this instance, an aqueduct was installed on true hydraulic principles. The source of supply was a high-level reservoir at a height of about 1220 feet on Mount Hagios Georgios, whence the water was carried over intervening lower ground to a cistern 369 feet above sea level. Other Greek cities also developed systems of this type. However, even when these achievements are accorded due recognition, there is no doubt that the Romans far outstripped their forerunners.

For our knowledge of the water supply of Rome, we are indebted to the very comprehensive account prepared by Sextus Julius Frontinus (c. 40–104 A.D.). After having served as consul in 73 and 74, and then as governor of Britain, Frontinus was appointed water commissioner of Rome in 97 under the Emperor Nerva. He served in this capacity until his death in 103 or 104, and during his tenure, he prepared the book *De aquis urbis Romae* (*The Aqueducts of Rome*). This work is primarily a source of information about the water supply of Rome. But it is much more than that. It is the first full account that we have of an important branch of public health administration. Futhermore, it depicts the motives and ideals, the springs of conduct of a zealous and conscientious public servant who could proudly boast that by his labors he had not only made Rome cleaner and its air purer but also removed the causes of disease, which previously had given the city a bad reputation.

According to Frontinus, for 441 years after the founding of Rome, the inhabitants obtained water from the Tiber and from private wells. In 312 B.C., however, the censor Appius Claudius Crassus, who built the first of the great Roman roads, the Appian Way, was responsible for bringing a supply of water to Rome by means of an aqueduct. This first venture in the provision of a public water supply was followed by a succession of others, until at the time of Frontinus nine aqueducts were bringing water into the city. Later four others were built to bring water into Rome.

The total capacity of these aqueducts cannot be stated with certainty. Various estimates have been made but these differ widely. Ashby has deduced from the figures of Frontinus that the total system was capable of delivering no less than 222 million gallons in 24 hours. According to another estimate by F. W. Robins, the 11 principal aqueducts (presumably in the third century A.D.) probably delivered about 40 million gallons a day. At the height of the Empire, the population of Rome numbered a million, which means that the total consumption was at least 40 gallons per head per day, and possibly more. This compares favorably with modern conditions. Recent figures for a group of American cities showed variations from a minimum of 45 gallons to a maximum of 357 gallons, with the larger cities varying between 100 and 150 gallons per person.

Attention was paid to the purity of the water. At specified points along the aqueduct, generally near the middle and the end, there were settling basins (*piscinae*) in which sediment might be deposited. At Rome, the water was received in large reservoirs (*castella*) whence it flowed into smaller reservoirs from which it was then piped off for use. Because of its purity, water from some aqueducts was reserved for drinking purposes, while the supply from others, owing to its pollution, was employed to water gardens.

At first, the maintenance of the aqueducts and the distribution of water was the responsibility of the censors and the aediles. Under Augustus, a board was appointed consising of a *curator* of consular rank and two assistants of senatorial rank. Under Claudius, the position of *procurator aquarum* was created, and the person occupying this post probably did most of the administrative work. The board had at its disposal a permanent staff consisting at first of 240 skilled slaves bequeathed by Augustus. To these Claudius added 460 slaves. Among these workers were masons, pavers, *castellarii* to attend to the reservoirs, *villici* to attend to the pipes, and overseers.

The general supply was to fountains, baths, and other public structures. A private supply could be obtained only by an imperial grant. Not all sections of the city were thus favored at first. Until the reign of Trajan, the inhabitants of the right bank of the Tiber still depended on wells. In general, private supplies were available to leading, prosperous citizens, while others had to employ the services of water carriers or to fetch their own water. Access to a private water supply was granted on payment of a fee or a royalty to the imperial treasury.

According to Pausanias, who wrote in the second century A.D., a public water supply was one of the bare essentials of civic life, and it is clear from the extant remains that many cities throughout the Roman Empire had systems that, on a smaller scale, resembled the water supply of Rome. In general, the water supply was devoted to public buildings, such as baths, and to street fountains. Private supplies were available in varying degree in different cities. At Antioch, many private houses enjoyed this luxury, and Smyrna was reputed to have been as well off as Antioch. Remains of some 200 Roman aqueducts are extant over an area ranging from Spain to Syria and from the Rhine to North Africa.

Many ancient cities, among them Athens and Rome, had sewerage systems. Progressive cities of the Hellenistic and Roman periods had a regular system of drains, running under the streets, which carried off surface water and sewage. Josephus, for example, praises the modern system installed by Herod in Caesarea. Indeed, Strabo remarks with surprise that when New Smyrna was built drains were not provided, so that sewage had to flow in open gutters. The maintenance and cleansing of the drains was the responsibility of the *astynomi* who were mentioned previously. Public slaves performed these tasks and also cleaned the public conveniences provided by Pergamon and other large cities.

During the Republican period, the Roman sewerage system was supervised by the censors. Under Augustus, special officials were appointed, the *curatores alvei et riparum Tiberis,* to whom a *comes cloacarum* was later added. The great sewer of Rome, the *Cloaca maxima,* is said to have been constructed by the Roman king Tarquinius Priscus, but it probably dates from early Republican times. It drained the marshy ground at the foot of the Capitoline hill and emptied into the Tiber, where it was about 10 feet wide and 12 feet high. The *Cloaca maxima* is still part of the drainage system of modern Rome. The system of sewers of which it formed a part is a worthy counterpart of the Roman water supply. Rome also had public latrines, of which there were no less than 150 at the time of Constantine. In the poorer quarters of the city, however, the streets stank of the contents of the chamberpots that were emptied out of the upper stories of the multiple dwelling houses. Despite the achievements of the Romans, the dark sides of public health in the overcrowded Roman slums should not be overlooked. The masses were not always permitted to enjoy the available hygienic facilities.

CLIMATE, SOIL, AND HEALTH. Even before Greek thought became dominant in Rome, the need for locating new towns on salubrious sites had been recognized. According to the Roman architect Vitruvius Pollio, liver inspection by the augurs was employed for this purpose. Several animals that had grazed on the land that was being considered for the settlement were slaughtered and the livers examined. If the liver was greenish-yellow, the area was regarded as unhealthy for man. This awareness of the close relationship between environment and health was later reinforced by Greek ideas, which found a theoretical underpinning in the Hippocratic work on *Airs, Waters and Places*. Vitruvius, in his book *De Architectura* (*On Architecture*), stresses the importance of determining the salubrity of a site and gives exact indications for the selection of places suitable for the founding of cities and the construction of buildings. He also gives considerable attention to the position, orientation, and drainage of dwellings.

Especially worthy of note in this connection are the empirical observations made by the Romans on the relation between swamps and disease, specifically malaria. In the first century B.C., Marcus Terrentius Varro (116–27 B.C.) had warned against locating farms near marshy places, "because there are bred certain minute creatures which cannot be seen by the eyes, which float in the air and enter the body through the mouth and nose and there cause serious diseases." This view was followed by his contemporary Vitruvius, and by the agriculturist Columella in the first century A.D. In addition, Vitruvius also noted that towns located near marshes may remain healthy if seawater has a chance to mix with marsh water. This acute observation can be explained today in the light of our knowledge that certain mosquito vectors cannot breed in saltwater.

DISEASE: ENDEMIC AND EPIDEMIC. Despite the important observations made by Vitruvius, Varro, and others and the remarkable achievements of the Romans in public health engineering, the problems of endemic and epidemic disease with which they had to cope were similar to those encountered by other peoples of the Mediterranean basin. Rome experienced epidemic outbreaks of disease at various times in its history from 707 B.C. to the time of Justinian. Unfortunately the available information is so inadequate that it is impossible to offer even a tentative diagnosis for the disease or diseases responsible for the majority of these epidemics. In a few instances, one can hazard an informed guess, and in at least one epidemic we can recognize the disease. This was the epidemic of bubonic plague, which ravaged the Eastern Empire during the reign of Justinian and which appears to have been rivalled in severity only by the Black Death. However, with Justinian we are already at the beginning of the period known to history as the Middle Ages.

Let us therefore glance briefly at the earlier epidemics to see what diseases may have prevailed. Immediately following the eruption of Vesuvius in 79 A.D., a severe epidemic spread through the Roman Campagna. Northern Africa was ravaged by a pestilence that broke out in 125 A.D. The nature of these two epidemics cannot be determined, nor do we know very much more about the series of epidemics, which came later in the second century A.D. during the reign of Marcus Aurelius. Known as the Long or Antonine pestilence, these epidemics began in 164 and prevailed to 180 A.D., ravaging the entire Empire from Syria to the West. Identification of the pestilence is still doubtful, but based on contemporary accounts, three possible diagnoses have been suggested, namely, exanthematic typhus, bubonic plague, or perhaps smallpox. The last named seems more probably to have been the cause of the plague of Cyprian, which lasted from 251 to 266 A.D. In 312 A.D., there was another severe epidemic of smallpox.

Other diseases that undoubtedly occurred in epidemic form from time to time were diphtheria, malaria, tyhoid fever, dysentery, and perhaps influenza. Tuberculosis was present in the ancient world, and Vitruvius mentions "cold in the windpipe, cough, pleurisy, phthisis, spitting of blood" as "diseases which are cured with difficulty" in regions where the winds blow from the north and northwest. Various sore throats were described by classical writers, and it seems plausible to assume that some of them may have been caused by streptococcal infection. The overcrowded *insulae*, the multiple dwelling houses, in which the Roman *proletariat* lived were admirably suited for the spread of many transmissible diseases. Nevertheless, the care that imperial Rome bestowed on water supply and sewage disposal may have helped to prevent outbreaks of typhoid and dysentery, while typhus may have been prevented by the Roman fondness for bathing and the discouragement experienced by *Pediculus corporis* as a result.

THE WORKERS' HEALTH. The Romans were aware that disease could result from occupational hazards. Pliny mentions that some diseases prevailed primarily among slaves. Incidental references to the dangers of certain occupations occur in various poets. Martial mentions the diseases peculiar to sulfur workers; Juvenal speaks of the varicose veins of the augurs and of the diseases of blacksmiths; and Lucretius refers to the hard lot of gold miners.

Indeed, there are more references to miners than to any other occupational group. Various authors comment on the pallor of the miner's complexion. Lucan speaks of the pale seeker for Asturian gold. Silius Italicus, who served as proconsul during the reign of Vespasian, refers to the avaricious Asturian who is as pale as the gold that he tears out of the earth. Statius, who lived at the time of Domitian, echoes this thought when he speaks of the pallor of the miner, returning from his labor, being almost as great as that of the gold, which he collects. The pallor, which these citations indicate was characteristic of Spanish miners, was probably due to the poor ventilation of the mines. It is also likely that hookworm disease was involved. Even today it is endemic in Spain and may have been as prevalent in ancient times.

Galen had personal experience of the occupational hazards of miners. During one of his journeys, he visited the island of Cyprus and spent some time inspecting the mines where copper sulfate was obtained. The miners worked in a suffocating atmosphere, and Galen mentions that he himself was almost overpowered by the stench. The workers who transported the vitriolic fluid out of the mine did so as rapidly as possible to avoid suffocation. Galen goes on to relate that the miners were naked while at work because the vitriolic fumes destroyed their clothing.

Nothing was done to protect these workers but apparently they helped themselves. Primitive respirators were employed to avoid the inhalation of dust. Pliny mentions that minium refiners used membranes and bladder skin as masks before their faces. Julius Pollux (124–192 A.D.) says that the miners of his time covered themselves with bags and sacks, or employed bladders to cover their mouths as a protection against inhalation of dust.

THE PROVISION OF MEDICAL CARE. While the Romans achieved but little in medical theory and practice, their contribution to the organization of medical service was far more important. During the early days of the Roman Republic, medicine was chiefly in the hands of priests. It was then practiced by slaves and later by freed men. Greek physicians began to migrate to Rome in the third century B.C. and were soon much sought after. After 91 B.C., physicians were always to be found there. Under the Republic and the early Empire, however, all medical knowledge and technique benefited only the well-to-do. The poor relied on folk medicine and the gods.

By the second century A.D., however, a public medical service was constituted. Public physicians known as *archiatri* were appointed to various towns and institutions. This practice spread from Italy to Gaul and to other provinces. About 160 A.D., Antoninus Pius regulated the appointment of these medical officials. He decreed that large cities should have no more than 10 municipal physicians, while the middle-sized cities and small towns were to have but seven and five, respectively. The principal duty of these doctors was to give medical attention to poor citizens. Their salaries were fixed by the *decuriones*, or municipal councillors. They were apparently allowed to accept fees from those who could afford to pay, but they were expected to provide free care for those who could not. In addition, they were encouraged to undertake the training of medical students.

Apart from the municipal physicians, medical care in imperial Rome was provided also in several other ways. Many doctors were in private practice. There were also a number of other groups of salaried doctors. Some were attached to the imperial court, others to the gladiatorial schools or to baths. Alexander Severus organized the medical service of the imperial house when he was emperor (222–235 A.D.). In some cases, we find an arrangement whereby physicians were attached to a few families who paid them an annual sum for all attendance throughout the year.

Another important contribution of Rome to organized medical care is the hospital. *Iatreia*, or surgeries, were common among the Greeks; these were the shops or offices of individual physicians. Temples, such as that of Aesculapius at Epidauros, had accommodations for those who sought help from the gods. Under the Republic, the Romans were no better off. In the first century A.D., however, Columella mentions *valetudinaria*, or infirmaries, for slaves; and Seneca tells us that such establishments were used even by free Romans. Excavations at Pompeii seem to indicate that private physicians may have had institutions somewhat like a modern convalescent or nursing home. Galen seems to imply in some passages that in the provinces private establishments developed into hospitals supported by public funds.

This development of public hospitals for civilians was paralleled by the creation of military hospitals at strategic points. In such camps or in nearby provincial towns similar institutions were also created for the imperial officials and their families. Eventually, under the influence of Christianity, motives of benevolence entered into the creation of public hospitals in many localities. The first charitable institution of this kind was established at Rome in the fourth century by a Christian lady named Fabiola. The foundation of hospitals for the sick and the indigent during the medieval period derives from the Roman *valetudinaria*.

BATHS AS WELL AS BREAD AND CIRCUSES. The great appreciation that the Romans had for public and private hygiene is shown not only by the remains of water-supply and sewerage systems, but also of the baths. During the period of the Empire, it was customary to visit the public baths regularly. The largest ones are the Baths of Caracalla, which were also a rendezvous for idlers and athletes. Restaurants existed in conjunction with the baths, and there were rooms for cold, lukewarm, and hot baths, as well as for massage.

A census of baths was taken by Agrippa in 33 B.C. At that time there were 170. The number grew steadily and later approached a thousand. The fee generally charged was about half a cent and children entered free. Up to the time of Trajan, mixed bathing was not formally prohibited, although there were *balneae* exclusively for women. Sometime between 117 and 138, Hadrian issued a decree separating the sexes in the baths. Under the later Empire, there were many abuses and unhygienic practices, for example, overeating and drinking, connected with the baths, but on the whole, they were undoubtedly of immense benefit to the Roman people. Personal hygiene was placed on the daily agenda and made available to the humblest Roman.

PUBLIC HEALTH ADMINISTRATION. The administration of the various public services related to health was not developed into a system until the time of Augustus. For example, under the Republic the great aqueducts were not entrusted to any permanent department for maintenance and fell into disrepair. Augustus set up a Water Board to deal with the water supply. The inscription of a silver coin, *M'Acilius triumvir valetudinis*, indicates the existence of a health commission for a special purpose. There were also separate officials for the baths. Agrippa, the minister of Augustus, was *aedile* in 33 B.C. Among his duties were the supervision of the public baths, including the testing of the heating apparatus as well as their cleaning and policing. At the time of Nero, the *aediles* supervised the cleaning of the streets, for which houseowners were responsible. They also straightened the streets and took care of their maintenance. Control of the food supply was also a function of the *aediles*, who supervised the markets and had the right to forbid the sale of spoiled food. These functions were incorporated into the machinery created by Augustus and his successors for the maintenance and administration of public services within the Empire.

This then was one of the glories of Rome, the development of public health services and their organization on the basis of an effective administrative system, a system that continued to function even as the Empire decayed and disintegrated.

-III-
Public Health in the Middle Ages (500–1500 A.D.)

THE DECLINE OF ROME. The disintegration of the Greco-Roman world from within and under the impact of the barbarian invasions led to a decline of urban culture and with it a decay of public health organization and practice. This cannot be attributed alone to the destruction visited upon cities by the invading Germanic tribes, for even where cities remained inhabited, as in Italy or in the former provinces of the Empire, they declined in wealth and importance. This process is clearly evident in Rome itself. After Constantine moved his residence to Byzantium in 330 A.D., the political and economic decline of the city was accelerated. During the fifth and sixth centuries, Rome was several times plundered and severely devastated. In 410, Alaric took and sacked the city that had ruled the world. While under siege by the Goths in 537, the 11 principal aqueducts of the city were broken. Thereafter, the waterworks were not repaired and decayed because the impoverished city did not have the financial means to carry out the necessary repairs. This state persisted until 776, when Pope Adrian I began a partial restoration. The fate of hygienic establishments in the provincial cities was no different than in Rome. They were destroyed or decayed gradually because little or nothing was done to preserve them.

However, these changes did not occur with equal impact in all parts of the Empire. While in western Europe, the machinery of government broke down and economic decline was accelerated under the stress of anarchy and invasion, the eastern half of the Empire remained relatively unaffected. The prosperous cities of Asia Minor, Syria, and Egypt were still, in the fifth century, almost undisturbed by invaders, and their products and wealth continued to flow to Byzantium. As barbarian kingdoms were established, Roman administrative organization disappeared from the west of Europe. At Byzantium, however, a centralized government continued to exist, a government capable of dealing with the complex problems of a civilized state. On the other hand, except in Italy, where some elements of Roman organization remained, such matters were beyond the ken of the German invaders. In 476, the last puppet emperor in the West was deposed and by the end of the fifth century the process of separation was completed. With the end of Roman rule in the West and the establishment of new political, economic, and social forms, there opened up a new historical period, the period known as medieval.

THE MIDDLE AGES. The period that historians call the Middle Ages covers a time span of about 1000 years, beginning around 500 and ending about 1500 A.D. The Middle Ages were no more homogeneous, however, than any other historical period, and it is exceedingly important at least to be aware of the impressive diversity in time and space covered by the term "medieval." Within the space of those 1000 years, an eventful panorama unrolled against the extremely colorful and varied geographical, ethnological, political, and cultural background of the European cockpit. The problem that confronted the medieval world was to weld together the culture of the barbarian invaders with the classical heritage of the defunct Empire and with the beliefs and teachings of the Christian religion. This intermingling of the newer pagan elements with the culture of the old Europe lasted for many centuries and passed through several stages. Furthermore, not everything that we at present regard as characteristically medieval was actually typical of the entire period and throughout all of Europe. This situation can be particularly well illustrated by the health conditions and standards prevalent at different times during the medieval period.

The East Roman, or Byzantine Empire, carried on the tradition and culture of Rome, and the outlook of the classical world can be found strangely surviving in its medieval environment. With the transfer of the center of culture to the East, Byzantium (or Constantinople as it was renamed) also became the seat of the medical culture of Europe. Here the Greco-Roman legacy was preserved and from this center it was first transmitted to the Arabs in the East and later to the peoples of the West.

The Arabs were initiated into the realm of Greek science and philosophy through Syriac translations prepared by Nestorian and Monophysite Christians, sectarians who were driven out of the Byzantine Empire because of their heresies and who eventually settled in Persia. By the tenth century, all the essential Greek medical writings had been translated into Syriac, Hebrew, or Arabic, and by that time, the Arabs and those who lived under their rule were making their own contributions to medicine and public health.

In the West during the earlier medieval period, the so-called Dark Ages (500–1000 A.D.), health problems were for the most part considered and dealt with in magical and religious terms. Both pagan and Christian sources provided the basis for the supernaturalism of the western Middle Ages. Old pagan customs and rites survived and were used for individual and community health problems. At the same time, Christianity held that there was a fundamental connection between disease and sin. Disease was punishment for sin. Possession by the devil or witchcraft were also recognized as causes of disease. Consequently, prayer, penitence, and invocation of saints were the means employed to deal with health problems. However, since the body was the vessel of the soul, it was important to strengthen it physically so that it might more easily withstand the attacks of the devil. On that basis, there was room for hygiene and public health in the Middle Ages. In light of this situation, it is not surprising that during this period communal activities in the interest of health were undertaken under the aegis of the Church and particularly the monastic orders. In the general breakdown of Greco-Roman civilization in the West, monasteries were left as the last refuges of learning. Whatever knowledge concerning health and hygiene survived was preserved in cloisters and churches and was applied in the hygienic arrangements and regulations of the monastic communities. Such important hygienic facilities as a piped water supply, suitable latrines, heating arrangements, and proper ventilation of rooms were already in existence during the early Middle Ages, but chiefly where large buildings used for dwelling purposes were erected according to a uniform plan, that is, predominantly in the monasteries. Large monasteries that were located on important highways were also hospices for travellers whose reception was an act of Christian charity. All these circumstances led, as early as the ninth century, to the appearance of monasteries that contained an extraordinarily large number of hygienic contrivances. These undoubtedly provided models for the urban communities that began to develop in Europe about the tenth century. THE GROWTH OF CITIES. The medieval cities varied in their origins. Some developed from old Roman settlements, others arose at river fords and on important commercial routes, while still others sprang up near fortified episcopal sees or the castles of feudal lords, which were able to provide protection against enemies. Every city had to be prepared to defend itself against aggression, and its security rested upon both its citizenry and its encircling fortifications. Many public health problems were simply a result of the circumstance that the city was unable to accommodate its growing population within the fortified walls. The encircling fortifications required for the protection of life and property made expansion very difficult and rendered it necessary to use the land within the walls to the greatest possible extent. The result was the crowding characteristic of medieval cities.

Furthermore, for a long time, most of the inhabitants of the cities maintained rural modes of life. For example, large and small animals were kept within the city and the resulting dungheaps were maintained wherever there was room. Streets remained unpaved for a long period, and every kind of waste and filth collected in them. To deal with these and other problems involving the health of the community, all the institutions needed for a hygienic mode of life had to be created anew by the medieval municipalities. It was within this urban environment that public health, thought, and practice revived and developed further in the medieval world.

SANITARY PROBLEMS OF URBAN LIFE. As in the case of earlier communities, a most urgent task of the medieval town was to provide its inhabitants with an adequate supply of good water. At first cisterns, natural springs, and dug wells probably formed the sole sources of supply. When the supply became inadequate, new sources had to be secured, perhaps from a distance. In the East, where the degree of continuity with Roman civilization was greater than in the West, the use of piped supplies appears earlier. At the end of the ninth century, Sultan Ahmed of Egypt had the new city of Cairo supplied with water from a distance. His engineer, Ibn Katib al Faighani, a Christian, brought the water on an arched viaduct from a deep shaft sunk in the southern desert. In the medieval West, especially during the earlier part of the period, such activities were frequently a result of ecclesiastical or monastic initiative. For example, at Southampton, England, in 1290 a supply of water was brought into the town primarily for the use of a Franciscan friary. Twenty years later, the friars gave the use of their surplus water to the town. Dublin, however, in the middle of thirteenth century boasted of a water supply brought in at the cost of the citizens. Lead pipes may have been used, although they are not definitely mentioned before the fifteenth century. Stone water courses and wooden pipes were also used, the latter at Basel in 1266. A fine example of a purely secular urban water supply is that of Bruges, which was installed by the end of the thirteenth century. The system included a complete network of underground conduits supplying public fountains and other outlets at important street intersections. The water was first collected in a reservoir outside the city and conveyed to the Water House, where it was raised to a high-level cistern by means of a chain of buckets on a wheel, an ancient method already employed in Egypt and Rome. Pipes then carried the water to cisterns in the town.

A constant problem of the municipal authorities in the medieval city was to see that the water required for drinking and cooking was not polluted. When the water was obtained from rivers, the citizens were requested not to throw dead animals or refuse into the stream. Tanners were not permitted to wash their skins there, dyers were forbidden to pour their dye residues into it, and the washing of either linen or clothes at the river was prohibited (Douai, 1271; Augsburg, 1453; Rome, 1468). For the provision of drinking water, fountains and wells were distributed throughout the city. Around these, the multifarious activities of the populace centered. In some parts of Europe, especially in Germany and Italy, such fountains were very beautiful and were adopted by various cities as their distinctive emblems. Yet here as well, the municipal administration had to be constantly alert to the problem of pollution. Regulations implemented by severe penalties appeared in fairly rapid succession to deal with these matters and became the basis of an official sanitary code. In most communities, special officials were appointed or elected to deal with the water supply. At Bruges, the custodian of the Water House took an oath to be diligent and faithful, to guard everything pertaining to the water supply, and never under any circumstances to divulge its secrets.

Another important problem was street cleaning and garbage disposal. The removal of garbage was an important hygienic problem and a difficult technical one during the medieval period. One should not forget that a great deal more refuse collected in a medieval house than in a modern one. The mode of life in the medieval city was still not far removed from rural life, and, at the beginning, urban houses were exactly like those in the villages. Besides the quantities of refuse, another important contributory cause of dirty streets was the circumstance that many inhabitants kept large numbers of animals, such as hogs, geese, and ducks. At Paris, the royal palace as well as numerous private houses had their barns. It was only at the beginning of the fifteenth century that several German cities, among them Breslau and Frankfurt am Main, expressly forbade the construction of hog pens facing the street. A similar prohibition was first promulgated in Berlin in 1641. At times, the dirt in the streets assumed such proportions that priests were unable to attend services, and municipal officials could not appear at their meetings.

The struggle carried on by the municipal authorities against such conditions is reflected in the large number of regulations and edicts issued, as well as in the repeated threats, warnings, and imploring appeals addressed to the citizens. In addition, various positive actions were undertaken. Some cities established municipal slaughterhouses to which the slaughter of larger animals was restricted. The earliest reference to this matter is contained in a document from Augsburg dated 1276. To keep streets clean they were paved. This procedure was first introduced in Paris around 1185. Prague saw its first paved streets in 1331, Nürnberg in 1368, Basel in 1387, and Augsburg in 1416. Another important step was the introduction of canalization, that is, the drainage of wastes into covered pits. In Paris, every large house was required to have a *cabinet d'aisance* draining into the canals. Severe penalties awaited those who failed to comply with the law. Milanese municipal ordinances dating from the fourteenth century devote a great deal of attention to sewers and cesspools. These could be constructed only in places approved by the authorities and had to be sunk to such a depth that not even the slightest odor would be detectable. In London the Thames was used for sewage disposal, but the carrying power of the river was limited.

A series of orders and regulations from 1309 on indicate the continuing need for a better solution of the problem. However, even when arrangements were made for scavengers to take rubbish and filth out of London by carts, the inhabitants continued to throw refuse into the Thames.

PROTECTING THE CONSUMER. Medieval urban life centered in the marketplace. Politics, commerce, religion, and art all met and mingled here. Social gatherings, conspiratorial revolts, solemn ceremonies, and all the other manifestations of public life took place on the stage of the marketplace. A wide assortment of goods was offered for sale. Included were food, clothing, shoes, pottery, and leather goods. Great care was taken to keep the market clean because of the widely held belief that dangerous foci of disease could easily arise wherever food, especially spoiled food, was sold. For this reason, the municipal authorities were particularly concerned with policing the marketplace and with the protection of the citizens against the sale of adulterated or deteriorated foods. In Florence, for example, the marketplaces had to be swept free of bones and other refuse every evening. Every Thursday evening and on the eve of a religious holiday, all the tables, benches, and booths had to be removed so that the marketplace could be thoroughly cleaned. Disposal of refuse within a thousand paces of the marketplace was forbidden, and a severe penalty awaited any who transgressed this regulation.

The vigorous manner in which the inspection of food was carried out by medieval communities is an impressive aspect of public health administration during this period. At the same time, it should be noted that generally only the native consumer was protected. *Caveat emptor* (let the buyer beware) still remained the basic rule for stangers. Here are a few examples of the innumerable regulations dealing with this problem. Augsburg in 1276 ordered that meat considered objectionable for some reason must be designated as such and sold at a special stand. In Basel, at the beginning of the thirteenth century, leftover fish were sold at a special stand where food of inferior quality was offered for sale, but only to strangers. In Zürich (1319), fishmongers were required to get rid of dead fish that had not been sold by evening. The Florentines forbade the sale on Monday of meat that had already been on sale the preceding Saturday. However, in this area as well as in others, the medieval scene has its dark as well as its light sides. For example, certain cities, among them Strassburg (1435), sent the meat of sick animals to hospitals. Nevertheless, these apparent inconsistencies should not occasion inordinate astonishment, especially if one keeps in mind that the measures previously described were based not on modern scientific knowledge but rather on empirical observation and medical theories derived from the knowledge of classical antiquity.

DISEASE IN THE MIDDLE AGES. All these measures were taken to protect the people against disease, and thus to deal with a problem that hung like the sword of Damocles over the head of medieval man. Two great epidemics may be considered as marking the onset and the waning of the Middle Ages, namely, the plague of Justinian (543) and the Black Death (1348). Between these two dates, Europe and the Mediteranean littoral were visited and ravaged by larger or smaller outbreaks of disease. Among the diseases that can be identified are leprosy, bubonic plague, smallpox, diphtheria, measles, influenza, ergotism, tuberculosis, scabies, erysipelas, anthrax, trachoma, the sweating sickness, and the dancing mania. Fear of pestilence was ever present in the medieval mind, but when faced by the problem of epidemic disease, medieval man was far from passive. He did what he could to protect himself, but in a manner colored by the prevailing climate of opinion. Thus, his protective measures were based upon a union of medical and religious ideas. Before considering these measures, however, let us look briefly at some of the diseases that afflicted medieval man.

Of the existence of smallpox in the Middle Ages, there is no doubt. The first unambiguous description of the disease occurs early in the tenth century in a treatise by Rhazes (850–923). He distinguished between smallpox and measles, even though he believed that the two conditions were part of one morbid process. Rhazes referred to the disease as widespread throughout the East, and the same opinion is expressed by Avicenna and other Moslem writers of the tenth and eleventh centuries. It is evident from these accounts that smallpox was a disease well known and established in the Near East before the seventh century. There seems to be general agreement among students of the history of smallpox that the disease became epidemic in Arabia toward the end of the sixth century, and then spread through the Mediteranean area into Europe. Epidemics reported for Italy and France in 570 by Marius, Bishop of Avenches, and by Gregory of Tours (in 581) for that city after 573 were probably outbreaks of smallpox. The term *variola*, which now designates smallpox, occurs for the first time in the report of Marius, where it simply means "spotted." Almost all medical writers of the period refer to the disease, and for the most part the Western authors base their accounts on the writings of Rhaze and other Moslem physicians. Smallpox was known in England during the Middle Ages, but from the few existing references, it is impossible to infer anything concerning the prevalence of the disease.

Measles, in all probability, has been widespread over Europe and Asia since the Middle Ages or earlier. As previously mentioned, it was described by Rhaze who considered measles and smallpox to be two conditions arising from a common morbid process. This doctrine was followed by physicians of the Middle Ages and persisted well into the eighteenth century. The name "measles" is itself a product of semantic and nosographic confusion. During the medieval period, smallpox and measles were coupled together as *variolae* and *morbilli*, the latter term—the diminutive of *morbus*—indicating the status of measles as the little disease in contrast with smallpox. According to Charles Creighton, the English name "measles" was introduced by John of Gaddesden (1280–1361) as the equivalent of the Latin term *morbilli*. The English word was itself derived from the Latin *miselli* and *misellae*—a diminutive of *miser*, and originally referred to the leprous. By some stretch of the imagination, Gaddesden coupled the sores of the legs of "the poor and the wasting," which were called *mesles*, with the *morbilli* of medical writers. Eventually, the term "measles" lost its connection with leprosy and became associated with the disease now known by that name.

From the sixth to the sixteenth centuries, the occurrence of diphtheria is shrouded in darkness only fitfully illuminated by scanty and incomplete reports of epidemics of sore throat. According to the Chronicle of St. Denis in 580, a great flood was followed by a plague called *esquinancie* (*squinancia*). For the year 856, Baronius recorded the occurrence at Rome of an epidemic of sore throat (pestilentia faucium). Cedrenus noted an epidemic sickness known as cynanche, which was prevalent in 1004 in some provinces of the Byzantine Empire and was often fatal. A similar epidemic is also mentioned by Baronius for the year 1039 at Rome. Gilbertus Anglicus wrote in the twelfth to thirteenth century of a *squinantia*, which sometimes caused death by suffocation. In the fourteenth century, John of Ardeme seems to have observed similar cases in England, which he called *squynancy*. A severe epidemic of sore throat occurred in 1337 in Holland. A plague fatal to many children prevailed in 1382 in a number of European countries, among them England, Germany, and France. There is no doubt that some of these were epidemics of diphtheria.

Another serious disease that occurred in severe epidemics was ergotism, known during the medieval period as *ignis sacer*, or St. Anthony's fire. First mentioned around 857 in the chronicles of the convent of Zanten, the disease occurred in at least six epidemics up to 1129. During 1128 and 1129, widespread outbreaks occurred in France, as well as in England, Germany, and the Netherlands. Hirsch lists 37 outbreaks in Europe between 857 and 1486, most of them before the fourteenth century. It appears likely that erysipelas and other exanthematic conditions may have been included under the term *ignis sacer*.

Influenza also occurred in epidemic form in various European countries. Outbreaks are recorded in Italy, Germany, England, France, and the Netherlands between 1173 and 1427.

LEPROSY—THE GREAT BLIGHT. Despite the importance of the diseases just mentioned, however, two others take pride of place in the story of medieval public health. These are leprosy and bubonic plague.

Leprosy was the great blight that threw its shadow over the daily life of medieval humanity. Fear of all other diseases taken together can hardly be com-

pared to the terror created by leprosy. Not even the Black Death in the fourteenth century or the appearance of syphilis toward the end of the fifteenth
century produced a similar state of fright. Leprosy had been known to the Hebrews, Greeks, and Romans in the ancient world but had been relatively uncommon. Early in the Middle Ages, during the sixth to the seventh centuries, it
began to spread more widely in Europe and became a serious social and health
problem. It was endemic particularly among the poor and reached a terrifying
peak in the thirteenth and fourteenth centuries. Leprosy probably assumed epidemic proportions as a result of the large shifts in population that the Crusades
produced. Cases were no doubt brought back by the armies returning from the
East. The disease gradually subsided after the fourteenth century, possibly because many lepers died as a result of the Black Death. Nevertheless, it was not
until the sixteenth century that leprosy lost all practical significance.

The need for action to control leprosy was recognized early, and it is out of
this awareness that there developed a form of public health action that is still
with us, namely, the isolation of persons with communicable diseases. When
people suffering from transmissible diseases may directly menace the health of
those around them, the community acting through its institutions feels justified in subjecting the individual to restraints and even sanctions in order to
protect itself. Thus, people suffering from certain communicable diseases have
had to be reported to the authorities, and in certain cases, the freedom of the
individual may be severely circumscribed. The best known case of this kind is
that of Typhoid Mary.

This aspect of public health work began to develop during the early Middle
Ages with the appearance of leprosy as an important health problem. Leadership was taken by the Church, as the physicians had nothing to offer. The
Church took as its guiding principle the concept of contagion embodied in the
Old Testament. Throughout the ancient world and particularly in the Orient, spiritual uncleanness was considered contagious. This idea and its practical consequences are defined with great clarity in the book of Leviticus, which
deals not only with spiritual uncleanness but also with physiological processes,
such as menstruation, or with pathological conditions, such as urethral discharge, through which an individual becomes unclean. Such persons were to be
isolated from the rest of the community until they had undergone specific purification rites. Much more severe was the isolation prescribed for unfortunates
afflicted by a skin disease named zara'ath. Once the condition had been established the patient was to be segregated and excluded from the community. "All
the days wherein the plague shall be in him, he shall be defiled; he is unclean:
he shall dwell alone; without the camp shall his habitation be."

Following the precepts laid down in Leviticus, the Church undertook the
task of combatting leprosy. The Council of Lyons, in 583, restricted the free

association of lepers with healthy persons, a policy that was continued and developed by later Church councils. In 644, the Lombard King, Rothari, issued an edict providing for the isolation of lepers. Gregory of Tours describes a leper house in Paris in the sixth century, and similar establishments were set up at Metz, Verdun, and Maestricht in the following century. After the tenth century, the number of leprosaria grew enormously. At the beginning of the thirteenth century, there were in France alone about 2000 leper houses, while throughout Europe, they numbered about 19,000. The third Lateran Council in 1179 dealt with the disease in great detail, and the policies laid down prevailed throughout the remainder of the medieval period.

THE LIVING DEAD. A leper was a public menace and therefore was expelled from the community to protect its healthy members. Since the disease was incurable, he was an outcast for life. He was deprived of his civic rights and was considered dead socially long before receiving the merciful boon of physical death. The momentous decision whether an individual suffered from leprosy was not taken lightly. The person under suspicion was examined by a special commission, which, during the early Middle Ages, consisted of a bishop, several other clerics, and a leper, who was considered a "specialist" in such matters. Later, the membership of such a commission comprised several prominent physicians and barbers of the city.

The regulations governing the isolation of lepers were very detailed and precise. The awful finality of exclusion from the human community was symbolized by an enactment of the funeral service involving the participation of the leper. He was clad in a shroud, the solemn mass for the dead was read, earth was thrown upon him, and he was then conducted by the priests, accompanied by relatives, friends, and neighbors, to a hut or leprosarium outside the confines of the community. (A very graphic account of this ceremony is contained in *The Golden Hand* by Edith Simon, a distinguished novel of fourteenth-century England.) Lepers were compelled to wear a characteristic costume and to give warning of their approach by means of a horn, a rattle, or a clapper, and they were forbidden to appear in the marketplace or to enter inns or taverns. No barber was allowed to shave them or to cut their hair. Nevertheless, it is astonishing to find such protective measures abrogated on special occasions. Prohibitions to enter a city were frequently revoked at Christmas and Pentecost, so that the lepers might beg for alms and receive the benefits of public charity. However, these exceptions were few in number and hardly mitigated the isolation to which the leper was condemned.

THE BLACK DEATH. Leprosy has been considered at some length because it accomplished the first great feat in direct prophylaxis, namely, methodical eradication of disease by consistently making the affected individuals harmless as carriers of the causative element. The analogy with the more recent campaigns against tuberculosis and venereal disease is clearly evident. Furthermore, this principle of preventive medicine was amplified and carried further in dealing with that other great scourge of the Middle Ages known as the bubonic plague.

Three great pandemics of plague have been recorded in the course of human history. The plague of Justinian was the first of these, the second was the Black Death, and the third, the widespread epidemics of our century. Human plague is basically a problem of urban communities. Consequently, it is not surprising to find few accounts of widespread outbreaks during the early medieval period after the epidemic waves that followed in the wake of the Justinian plague had subsided. Nonetheless, between the sixth and the fourteenth centuries, there are scanty records of outbreaks of plague in Iraq, Persia, and other parts of the Levant, as well as somewhat questionable accounts of the disease in Europe and the British Isles.

While there can be no certainty on the matter, it seems likely that the plague pandemic of the fourteenth century originated somewhere in the hinterland of Central Asia where a reservoir of infection persists among the wild rodents of the steppes. From its original focus, the disease spread westward until by the spring of 1346 it had reached the shores of the Black Sea, whence it was carried on shipboard to Constantinople, Genoa, Venice, and other European ports. The plague reached Europe in the early part of 1348 and then spread to the interior. It reached Florence and other parts of northern Italy and was probably in Avignon by April and in Valencia and Barcelona by early May. It took about three years for the huge plague wave to sweep over Europe. Successive waves of lesser magnitude followed at varying intervals until about 1388.

QUARANTINE. Frequently, panic was the first reaction to the appearance of the Black Death, and salvation was sought in flight, but not everyone could or would flee. For one thing, the ancient idea that pestilence was a sign of divine wrath prevailed widely, and many felt that their only recourse was prayer and penance. Second, communities refused admission to persons from areas where the plague raged. Consequently, measures had to be taken to protect those who were still well and to help them avoid the dreaded pestilence. The experience gained by isolating lepers certainly influenced the measures taken against the Black Death. Since the disease was generally considered communicable, it was combatted on the same principles as leprosy. The chief defense was avoidance of infection; as a result, the principle of isolation underwent a rapid and general development. Patients had to be reported to the authorities. They were then examined and isolated in their houses for the duration of the illness. Every house containing a plague victim was placed under a ban. All who had come into contact with the patient were compelled to remain in isolation. Food and other necessities were provided by the municipal authorities through special messengers. The dead were passed through the windows and removed from the city in carts. Burial outside the city was likewise intended to prevent extension of the epidemic. When a plague patient died, the rooms were aired and fumigated, and the effects of the deceased were burned.

In addition to these measures taken within the community, it was necessary as well to prevent the entry of the plague. The method employed to achieve this objective, and thus to safeguard the community, was to isolate and to observe all suspected persons and objects for a specified period under stringent conditions until it was definitely established that they were not bearers of the plague. From this endeavor grew a basic contribution to public health practice, namely, the institution of quarantine. The first step was taken at Venice, the chief port of entry for commerce with the Orient. Based on the belief that plague was introduced chiefly through infected goods carried by shipping, the Venetians set up a system for segregating suspected ships, goods, and people. As early as March 20, 1348, a council consisting of three men was established to supervise the health of the community and to take whatever measures seemed necessary to safeguard it. (The Venetians were apparently following an established institutional pattern; as far back as the year 1000, there seem to have been overseers of the public health appointed to serve temporarily during epidemics.) These officials were authorized to isolate infected ships, goods, and persons at an island in the lagoon.

From this beginning, the quarantine system was developed and elaborated by the people of Venice and other communities. In 1374, Bernabo Visconti, Duke of Milan, promulgated a decree to prevent the introduction and spread of the plague. The edict ordered that all plague patients be removed from the city to a field where they would either die or recover. Anyone who had attended a plague patient was to be isolated for 14 days before resuming social relations with others. The same period of observation was applied to travellers or merchants who were infected or simply under suspicion of having the disease. In the same year, Venice, again threatened by plague, denied entry to all suspected or infected travellers, vehicles, and ships. Three years later, on July 27, 1377, the municipal council of Ragusa on the Dalmatian coast ordered a 30-day period of isolation for those coming from plague-stricken areas. Later this period was extended to 40 days—hence the term "quarantine," derived from *quarantenaria*. (According to Clemow, a 40-day period was mentioned for the first time at Venice in 1127.) Then, in 1383, Marseilles erected her first quarantine stations at which, after rigid inspection of incoming vessels, all travellers and cargoes from infected or suspicious ships were detained for 40 days and exposed to air and sunshine.

According to Hecker, the reason for the establishment of a 40-day period was that during the thirteenth and fourteenth centuries the fortieth day was generally considered the day of separation between the acute and chronic forms of disease. The *Bible* was also drawn upon to endow the number 40 with special significance. For example, the Flood lasted 40 days and other biblical episodes also extended over 40 days. The number 40 was likewise considered important in alchemy, for it was believed that 40 days were needed for certain transmutations.

Thus, stirred by the Black Death in the middle of the fourteenth century, public officials in Italy, southern France, and the neighboring area created a system of sanitary control to combat contagious diseases, with observation stations, isolation hospitals, and disinfection procedures. This system was adopted and developed during the Renaissance and later periods and is still a part of public health practice today, although in a more rigorously defined form.

WHAT CAUSES EPIDEMICS? A large body of medical and lay literature explaining the origin of the plague and how to combat it quickly appeared in most European countries. From this literature, it is possible to extract the main theories that were held concerning the causation of this terrific scourge and that provided the basis for the administrative activities described. These views were derived in part from observation of the disease and in part from the Hippocratic tradition, which stressed physical factors of the environment in the causation of disease.

It was generally recognized and accepted that the plague was a communicable disease. This view was based on direct observation, but it did not answer all the questions concerning the origin as well as the nature of the epidemic. Thus, if the plague were contagious, what was the communicable element? And how was it produced? Answers to these questions were obtained from the Hippocratic tradition in the form in which it had been systematized by Galen and transmitted to medieval physicians. There was general agreement that some atmospheric alteration, a corruption of the air, brought on the disease. Corruption of the air was caused by decaying organic matter, stagnant and putrid waters, and the like. In his plague tract, for example, Johannes de Tornamiera says: "In times of epidemic, you must first of all avoid corrupted air which may come from marshy, muddy and fetid places, from stagnant water and ditches, from burial places, from stables of draught animals—avoid completely such places." It was believed that, when inhaled, corrupt air, because of its changed nature, attacked the humors of the body thus producing disease. Mass outbreaks of disease occurred when a malign conjunction of the stars caused the atmospheric corruption to become especially virulent. Many writers also stressed the factor of individual predisposition in endeavoring to explain why some persons were stricken in the course of an epidemic and others were not. Emphasis on the individual went hand in hand with stress on the importance of personal hygiene.

Based on these doctrines, medieval people endeavored collectively and individually to deal with the urgent health problems thrust upon them. However, these views are important not only because they provided a theoretical underpinning for medieval public health practice but also because from them developed the epidemiological theories that were to dominate the modern period up to the latter part of the ninteenth century.

THE ORGANIZATION OF PUBLIC HEALTH. While the medieval community did not have an organized public health system in the present-day sense, it did have an administrative machinery for disease prevention, sanitary supervision, and, in general, protection of community health. The character of this machinery is very intimately related to the administration of the medieval municipality. Despite minor variations, early municipal administrations tended to follow one simple plan. The city was run by a council, whose members may be compared to the selectmen of New England towns. The title given these councillors varied from place to place, but the office was essentially the same. In Italy and southern France, they were known as *consuls*, in northern France and the Netherlands they were called *échevins*, and in England, aldermen.

The council carried on the routine administration of the community. Thus, it had charge of finances, organized the provisioning of the city, and ordered and supervised public works. Among its activities, it also dealt with health and welfare problems. Such matters were generally assigned to one or more members of the council, who then acted as a subcommittee. In fourteenth-century Milan, for example, six officials dealt with street cleaning and environmental sanitation. At Amiens in the fifteenth century, two *échevins* were assigned to supervise the fish market; two, the retail sale of meat; two others, to watch over the baking and sale of bread; still others, to scrutinize the activities of the grocers and apothecaries, and so on. These officials served for one year. At the end of each day, they reported their findings so that when necessary immediate action could be taken. The guilds formed an integral part of medieval city government, and in numerous communities, as in Florence, these functions were carried out by guild officials. Toward the end of the Middle Ages, this administrative pattern grew more complex, but its basic character remained the same.

In general, public health administration was not carried out by physicians but by laymen. Physicians were employed, however, for specific duties, such as the provision of medical care to the indigent and in prisons, the diagnosis of leprosy and similar conditions, and to offer expert council in times of pestilence or in medico-legal matters.

THE PROVISION OF MEDICAL CARE. Like other facets of public health, the provision of medical care in the medieval community was determined by the character of the society in which it occurred. Medieval society was relatively static, with well-demarcated social ranks. Each group was organized and its sphere of action rigidly delineated. During the early Middle Ages, physicians were generally clerics for whom the church provided a living so that they could practice medicine as a charitable service. They were permitted to accept gifts but were not supposed to ask for payment. In fact, throughout the Middle Ages, many physicians because of their clerical status did not have to take account of economic considerations. From the eleventh century on, however, laymen began to enter the medical profession in increasing numbers. As early as 934, for example, the Florentine archives mention one Amalpertus, a deacon of the Church who was also a physician. By the first half of the thirteenth century, however, there were 60 physicians in Florence organized in a powerful guild.

Since the lay physicians were not supported by the Church, they had to earn their livelihood in some other way. This they did by accepting a salaried post, either as body-physician to some lord or as a municipal doctor in a town, or by engaging in private practice. In either case, the duties as well as the remuneration of the physician were specifically stipulated. Municipal physicians were required to treat the sick poor, to investigate the occurrence of unusual or epidemic disease, to provide expert guidance in such situations, and to supervise pharmacies. Most salaried physicians also carried on private practice. When doctors treated private patients, they had to follow rigid codes, and fees were charged according to strict and binding fee schedules set up by the guilds.

During the medieval period, a sharp separation developed between physicians and surgeons. The surgeon working with his hands remained a craftsman who learned his skill by being apprenticed to a master. Each group occupied a different position on the social ladder, the surgeons being relegated to a lower status. During this period, however, both physicians and recognized surgeons neglected almost completely diseases that could not be treated except by dangerous surgical manipulations, with the result that alongside the recognized, settled medical practitioners there developed a class of travelling empirics who performed such difficult and serious operations as couching cataracts, repairing hernias, and cutting for the bladder stone. Although these itinerant oculists, lithotomists, and hernia operators did not rate highly in social standing, their services were needed. As a result, various arrangements were made whereby their skills could be used. Consequently, during the later medieval period, in addition to the itinerant practitioners, there were also some who settled in one community. An oculist is mentioned in 1366 at Speyer, and another in 1372 was at Esslingen in Germany. In cities where there were no resident specialists the authorities endeavored to engage the services of such persons, even if only for a certain time during the year. By and large, these conditions persisted up to and during the seventeenth and eighteenth centuries.

HOSPITALS AND WELFARE INSTITUTIONS. The concept of a need for social assistance in case of sickness or other misfortune was highly developed during the Middle Ages. This is as true of the Moslem East as it is of the Christian

West and is most evident in the creation of hospitals. Religious and social considerations were pre-eminent in the development of these institutions.

In the East, hospitals were created by rulers and public officials in urban centers. In the ninth century, during the reign of the Caliph Harûn-al-Rashîd, a hospital was founded at Baghdad. Another hospital was built in the same city in the next century by the Caliph al-Muktadir. A third hospital was founded at Baghdad in 970; it had a staff of 25 physicians and was used to teach medical students. All in all, there are records of some 34 hospitals in countries under Islamic rule. These hospitals were generally well organized and reflected the high state of development attained by medicine in Moslem lands. At Cairo, for example, the hospital founded in 1283 had separate sections for patients with febrile diseases, for the wounded, and for those with eye diseases, as well as special rooms for women. Medical care was provided by a staff of physicians under a director, and there were male and female nurses.

However, these institutions should not be regarded as the models for the hospitals developed in the West. Hospitals established by the Christian Church were scattered throughout the Near East, and when this area came under the sway of Islam these institutions had been taken over and developed further by the Moslems. In the West, the establishment of hospitals also originated from the Church. The monastic orders of the medieval period made the most significant contribution to this development. The manner in which the monks cared for their own sick became a model for the laity. The monasteries had an *infirmitorium* where the sick were taken for treatment, a pharmacy, and frequently also a garden with medicinal plants. In addition to caring for sick monks, the monasteries also opened their doors to travellers and pilgrims. The beginnings of this practice are unknown, but it is quite likely that they go back to the early Middle Ages.

To be sure, these monastic hospitals had little in common with the modern institutions of the same name. Frequently, they were nothing more than small houses where some sort of nursing care was provided. Owing to their dual nature and function, it is difficult to establish how far the monastic hospitals were actually used for the care of the sick. It is likely that all degrees of variation ranging from infirmaries, devoted almost exclusively to the treatment and nursing of the sick, to simple lodging houses existed in the medieval monasteries. On the whole, however, from about the eighth to the twelfth centuries the monastic hospital was almost the only institution in Europe whose chief task was to care for the sick.

Another important impulse toward the creation of hospitals developed in the middle of the twelfth century with the founding of the Holy Ghost Hospital in 1145 at Montpellier. Sanctioned in 1198 by Pope Innocent III, the Order of the Holy Ghost established and maintained similar hospitals throughout

Europe. Hospitals were also established along the routes taken by the Crusaders, and several knightly orders created during the holy wars assumed the mission of founding and maintaining hospitals. The best known of these orders, the Knights of St. John, or the Hospitallers, for example, founded hospitals in places as far apart as Malta and Germany.

During the late Middle Ages, the cities, particularly through the guilds, took an active part in founding hospitals and other establishments for medical care and social assistance. Proud of their community, wealthy citizens sought to outdo one another in advancing and adorning their beloved city. As early as the twelfth century, merchants were devoting a good share of their profits to benefit their fellow citizens. Hospitals, refuges, and homes were established for all sorts and conditions of men, women, and children. The guilds developed funds for the relief of their sick and disabled members. Wealthy guilds built their own hospitals; others paid regular fees to a cloister hospital, which assumed responsibility for the accommodation and care of their sick members.

Originally in the hands of ecclesiastics, the medieval hospital, from the thirteenth century on, came more and more under secular jurisdiction, especially in the cities. This does not mean that the clergy were entirely eliminated. Monks and nuns continued to provide nursing care as they had done before. Administratively, however, the municipal authorities were responsible. At Amiens in the fifteenth century, for example, the master of the Hôtel-Dieu was elected by the community but installed in his office by the resident bishop. The physician of the hospital was chosen and paid by the municipality. Monks and nuns attended to the needs of the patients.

By the end of the fifteenth century, as a result of the development described, Europe was covered with a network of hospitals. For example, in England alone, from the twelfth to the fifteenth centuries, more than 750 hospitals were established, of which 217 were for lepers. Developments on the continent were similar. At the beginning of the fourteenth century, Paris had about 40 hospitals and just as many lepers houses. According to the chronicler Villani, the city of Florence in 1300, with a population of some 90,000 inhabitants, had 30 hospitals and welfare establishments capable of providing medical aid and shelter to more than 1000 sick and needy people. They were staffed by more than 300 monks or other nursing personnel. During the latter part of the fifteenth century, under Lorenzo the Magnificent, there were at least 40 hospitals of various kinds in operation. Indeed, it is no exaggeration to describe the creation of the hospital as one of the great public health achievements of the Middle Ages.

THE REGIMEN OF HEALTH. Health education and personal hygiene were other areas of public health to which the Middle Ages made important contributions. Medieval man was far more occupied with the care of his body than one might imagine. While there was general acknowledgement of the vanity of earthly existence and a belief in punishment or salvation in the next world, the conviction was also held that by means of a correct regimen one could complete the allotted life span of three score and ten. This need gave rise to a whole literature on the preservation of health. Basically, this literature was derived from classical sources. During the early medieval period, such writings were scanty but still common enough to supply rules of conduct to those who sought them. All the monastic orders had regulations covering personal hygiene. It is likely that the influence of the monastic rules penetrated into the ranks of the laity.

As a rule, the medieval treatise on hygiene was addressed to a person of high rank advising him how to live in order to remain healthy. From the twelfth to the fifteenth centuries, a large number of such books were written in Latin or in various vernacular languages. The best known work of this type is undoubtedly the *Regimen sanitatis Salernitanum* (*The Salernitan Regimen of Health*), which probably originated during the twelfth century and was published in England, Italy, and Germany as late as the middle of the nineteenth century. It was written in verse and could easily be memorized. The introductory verses in the Elizabethan translation of Sir John Harrington are indicative of the sound common sense that permeates this classic of health education:

The Salerne Schoole doth by these lines impart
All health to Englands King, and doth advise
From care his head to keepe, from wrath his heart,
Drinke not much wine, sup light, and soone arise,
When meate is gone, long sitting breedeth smart:
And after-noone still waking keepe your eyes.
When mov'd you find your selfe to Natures Needs,
Forbeare them not, for that much danger breeds,
Use three Physicians still; first Doctor Quiet,
Next Doctor Merry-man, and Doctor Dyet.

This didactic medical poem and its literary successors, the popular health books and almanacs which flooded the European countries soon after the beginning of printing, treated every detail of daily life and indicated how to care for every part of the body. Housing, food, and bodily cleanliness were three of the subjects included under personal hygiene. Domiciliary cleanliness occupied little space in the medieval tracts on hygiene, but interest in the nutritional regimen necessary for the maintenance of health was much greater. The virtue of moderation in diet was extolled. The subject of sleep is likewise treated in great detail. In accordance with medieval views, sound sleep prevents disease and promotes a correct composition of the humors. The idea that the evacuation of the corrupt humors from the body would prevent disease was a widespread, popular belief during the Middle Ages and in accord with contemporary medical opinion. To maintain one's health, it was necessary to submit to three procedures: purging, cupping, and bleeding. They were carried out by barbers and bath attendants. Almanacs, bleeding notices, and bleeding letters informed the public of the best time for bloodletting. It was supposed to be performed only during certain seasons and under special astrological constellations.

Mention must be made finally of another municipal institution that occupied an important place in the medieval town, serving both for purposes of hygiene and pleasure. This was the bathhouse, which was licensed by the municipality and provided both steam and water baths. Bathhouses were already in existence in cities and probably also in the larger villages during the thirteenth century. The presence of food and drink, girls and music tended more and more to turn the bathhouse into a place of amusement. Throughout most of the medieval period, however, it was the hygienic center of the city. At the end of the fifteenth century, when syphilis became a new health problem, this communal type of bathing fell into disfavor. The bathhouse was considered a focus of infection and gradually it vanished from the urban scene.

THE MEDIEVAL ACHIEVEMENT IN PUBLIC HEALTH. On surveying the numerous aspects of medieval public health—the efforts to deal with the sanitary problems of urban life, the creation of administrative measures, such as quarantine, the development of the hospital, and the provision of medical care and social assistance—it is impossible not to recognize the magnitude of these accomplishments. These attempts to create a rational system of public hygiene are all the more impressive when one recalls that they were undertaken in a world in which superstition was rampant and much of the scientific knowledge required for the effective handling of health problems was absent. Most significant of all, however, from a historical point of view, is the fact that in the medieval period were developed the basic patterns of thought and practice within which public health would function for the next two and a half centuries.

-IV-
Mercantilism, Absolutism, and the Health of the People (1500–1750)

BRAVE NEW WORLDS. During the pontificate of Leo X, the famous Italian physician, scientist and poet, Girolamo Fracastoro, wrote a didactic poem on syphilis, which was published in 1530 at Verona. The description of this dread and loathsome disease led him to comment on the evils of the age and to consider the proportion of good and evil in the situation of his time when compared with earlier periods. "Although a cruel tempest rages," he reflected, "and the conjunction of the stars has been wicked, yet we are not completely deprived of divine clemency. If this century has seen a new disease, the ravages of war, the sack of cities, floods and drought, yet it has also been able to navigate oceans denied to the ancients, and has reached beyond the bounds of the previously known world."

In balancing the expansion of the horizon, literally and figuratively, against the ravages of disease and war, Fracastoro echoes the powerful surge of a new age, "the age of the discovery of the world and of man," the age of the Renaissance. To the average reader, the Renaissance has long been a period of historical glamour. Generally, the term calls to mind an age of cultured princes and ruthless condottieri, of painters and sculptors gifted with genius, of classical scholars and paid assassins; in short, an age of versatile supermen for whom life itself was a work of art.

There is much in this picture that is true. However, in the history of public health, the Renaissance is significant not for its brilliance and color, but rather because it is the dawn of a new period of history, the modern period, within which public health as we know it developed. From this point of view, the Renaissance can be seen as a stage in the process that led to the disappearance of medieval civilization and its transformation into the modern world. Furthermore, the same period that saw the rise of modern civilization witnessed as well the beginnings of modern science as one of its integral elements, and one that was to exert a profound influence on public health.

CAUSES AND CONSEQUENCES. The process of change, in which the Renaissance was the first phase, was slow and uneven and extended over a period of more than two centuries. There seems to be general agreement that the roots of this transformation lie in the fourteenth and fifteenth centuries, and that these are related to vital changes experienced by Western Europe, in particular Italy, during this period. In short, changes that had been taking place and maturing slowly within the medieval order finally found decisive expression, and in one place after another inaugurated a new political, social, and scientific order.

To understand why this is so, it is necessary to go back into the Middle Ages before the First Crusade. Around this time, as we have seen, and continuing into the twelfth and thirteenth centuries, towns and cities grew up in Europe, but they were most numerous and strongest in northern Italy and Flanders. Engaged in commerce and industry, the inhabitants of these centers developed a new social class, the middle class, or bourgeoisie, whose very name indicates its origin. With this class, a new notion of wealth made its appearance, that of mercantile wealth, consisting no longer in land but in money or commodities of trade measurable in money. Furthermore, as the social standing and political power of the middle class rose and increased, the processes of trade and handicraft slowly began to receive attention as subjects of intellectual inquiry. This attention to problems of commerce and industry played a very important part in creating the environment within which modern science could come into being. In fact, the German sociologist, Simmel, has expressed the opinion that "the money economy first brought into life the ideal of numerical calculability," and that "the quantitatively exact interpretation of nature is the theoretical counterpart of finance." Certainly, it is no accident that detailed statistical information concerning cities is available in Italy during the fourteenth and succeeding centuries.

Moreover, these developments were inextricably linked to the evolution of the national state. The growth and consolidation of central governments was made possible in very large measure by the economic activity of the cities. And it was the intellectual activity of the urban groups, often encouraged and directed by royal patronage, which most profoundly influenced the growth of the secular culture that characterized the Renaissance and of which the new science was one of the most distinctive elements. Desire for wealth as the sinews of war, and an appreciation of the utility of technology in achieving power, led rulers and statesmen to encourage men of inventive ingenuity and technical knowledge.

An exceedingly important part in preparing the way for the opening of the modern period was played by the technological revolution of the Middle Ages. Without the cumulative technological progress of the preceding four centuries, the creators of modern science in the sixteenth century would very likely have been unable to achieve their aims. The development of mines, salt works, foundries, glass works, and other industrial enterprises had a special significance for the shaping of a new intellectual climate favorable for the growth of science. The invention of printing at the end of the fifteenth century made it possible to emancipate such practical knowledge from oral tradition so as to extend and improve it. At the same time, academically trained scholars began to interest themselves in the technical activities of craftsmen. This is clearly evident in the *De re metallica* (1556), a learned treatise on mining by the physician Georg Agricola, in which stress is put on the relation between theory and application, as well as on the social utility of mining. Education began to show the impact of these trends, and practical knowledge was given greater emphasis in the curriculum. Based on these developments and fostered by the favorable conditions already described, natural science made remarkable progress in the sixteenth and seventeenth centuries.

THE OLD PUBLIC HEALTH AND THE NEW SCIENCE. To understand the history of public health during the period of transformation that began with the Renaissance, both its theoretical and practical sides have to be considered. While this period is characterized by the rapid growth and spread of science in various fields, public health as a practical activity received very little, if any, direct benefit from these advances. Nevertheless, during this period, basic knowledge was being acquired on which the foundations of modern public health could eventually be erected.

Scientific advance is never uniform nor simultaneous along an entire front. It occurs rather at different times, in varying ways and in relation to specific areas of knowledge. In some instances, what is required is the discovery and definition of elementary data; in others, where a solid knowledge of elementary factors already exists, fruitful advance can occur through the creation and application of an integrating concept, or by attacking a more complex problem and contributing to its solution. All these aspects may be observed in relation to public health during the period under discussion.

The foundation for an accurate knowledge of the structure of the human body was created through simple, critical observation by Andreas Vesalius, his contemporaries, and his successors. Equally fundamental was William Harvey's discovery of the circulation of the blood which provided a firm basis for consideration of the body as a functional unit. Natural science was characterized during this period not only by the growing use of the experimental method, but also by a disposition to treat natural phenomena mathematically. This trend found expression in several directions; of these the creation of political arithmetic by William Petty was extraordinarily pregnant for the future of public health. Of equal if not greater importance for the further growth of public health were the new developments in epidemiology and clinical observation during the sixteenth and seventeenth centuries. There was an increasing tendency to individualize disease entities on the basis of clinical observation, and a number of diseases were described for the first time, among them whooping cough, typhus fever, and scarlet fever. Finally, the first consistent scientific theory of contagious disease was created by Girolamo Fracastoro.

At the same time, the organization and administration of public health remained practically unchanged. We should remember that there is no absolute contrast between successive periods in history. Each age carries over institutions as well as modes of thought and action from preceding periods. Thus, with minor modifications the public health pattern created by the medieval urban community continued in use from the sixteenth through the eighteenth centuries. With the development of national states, central governments took action sporadically, but, on the whole, public health problems were handled by the local community. As new problems developed and were recognized, they were fitted in some way into the existing pattern.

NEW DISEASES FOR A NEW WORLD. In 1849, the pathologist Rudolf Virchow elaborated a theory of epidemic disease as a manifestation of social and cultural maladjustment. He pointed out that with the dawning of new historical periods "epidemic diseases exhibiting a hitherto unknown character appear and disappear, often without leaving any trace. As cases in point take leprosy and the English sweat." Virchow chose two apposite diseases to illustrate his theory, but he might have picked others, for with the opening of the modern period, the disease picture of Europe changed significantly. Diseases hitherto widely prevalent, such as leprosy, diminished in importance and made way for new or at least previously unnoticed pestilential scourges. Among the epidemic diseases that were observed for the first time, or that were first studied in a more precise way during the sixteenth and seventeenth centuries, were the English sweat, typhus fever, scurvy, some of the acute exanthemata such as scarlet fever and chicken pox, and the disease that was to become a major health problem from the Renaissance to our time—syphilis.

THE ENGLISH SWEAT. Early in August, 1485, Henry Tudor, Earl of Richmond, landed from France at Milford Haven and later that month overthrew Richard III at Bosworth Field. Scarcely had the victor entered London to ascend the throne as Henry VII when a pall of fear and terror fell upon the capital. A communicable disease, apparently hitherto unknown, had broken out among the soldiers of the victorious army and spread rapidly to the surrounding population. The chief characteristics of the disease were high fever with chills, cramps in the extremities and pains in various parts of the body, a feeling of profound anxiety, difficulty in breathing and irregularity of the pulse. Severe cases exhibited delirium, hallucinations, and stupor. The disease lasted from a few to 24 hours. Recovery came after profuse sweats, whence the name, the English sweat.

The sweating sickness spread rapidly to other parts of England, but it did not invade Scotland, Ireland, or the Continent. The disease was exceedingly severe and thousands perished. In London, it killed two successive Lord Mayors and six aldermen in one week. Within a few weeks, however, the force of the epidemic wave was spent, and the disease vanished for some 20 years. The disease reappeared in England in 1508, and again in 1517, 1528, and 1551. The severest outbreak of all was that of 1528, which not only spread rapidly but was also carried to the Continent where it ravaged Germany, Austria, the Low Countries, Denmark, Sweden, Poland, and Russia. There were hundreds of deaths in Strassburg, and in Hamburg, a thousand people are reported to have died within a few days. After 1551, no further epidemics of the English sweat were recorded either in England or in Europe. In 1552, a classic account of the disease was published by John Caius in *A boke, or counseil against the disease commonly called the sweate, or sweatyng sicknesse.* The nature of the sweating sickness has never been satisfactorily clarified. According to some authors, it may have been a form of influenza; according to others, a modified typhus; and still another suggestion is that it may have been due to some virus infection.

JAIL FEVER AND THE BLACK ASSIZES. While the sweating sickness remains a fascinating enigma in the history of disease, other diseases first reported during this period were more important in terms of the havoc wreaked upon the population. One of these was typhus fever, which was first clearly and accurately described in 1546 by Fracastoro in his classic treatise on contagion. Although considered a new disease in the Renaissance, it was probably not new to Europe. Nevertheless, despite indications of epidemic outbreaks during the late Middle Ages, there can be no question that typhus became very prevalent in Europe during and after the sixteenth century. Typhus fever has always been intimately associated with wars, famines, and poverty. It becomes a menace where there is overcrowding and where people cannot keep clean so that they are exposed to the louse that transmits the disease. As a result, it has been frequent in military camps, especially during wars, in jails, on ships, and in hospitals.

Throughout the sixteenth and seventeenth centuries, typhus fever was a constant and dreaded participant in the military campaigns that followed one another in almost uninterrupted succession. During the siege of Granada (1489–1490), the army of Ferdinand and Isabella was ravaged by an epidemic that took 17,000 lives. The modern Spanish name of the disease, *tabardillo*, was already in use at this time. Typhus was also known as spotted or petechial fever and sometimes was named after a country, for example, the Hungarian disease, *morbus Hungaricus.* In 1529, the French army besieging the Imperial forces in Naples was attacked by typhus and almost wiped out. During the Thirty Years' War, typhus contributed greatly to the staggering devastation and useless suffering inflicted upon the helpless mass of people.

The traditional scattering of sweet herbs at the Assizes in England is a relic of epidemiological history, testifying mutely to the fact that typhus, once known as jail fever, was almost an inevitable consequence of going to prison. This connection is strikingly illustrated by a series of outbreaks that have come to be designated in English history as the Black Assizes. The first occurred at Cambridge in 1522 and was followed by others at Oxford in 1577 and at Exeter in 1586. The last of such outbreaks occurred at Taunton in 1730 and at London in 1750. In each instance, a fatal infection, probably typhus, spread from prisoners brought before the court to the judges and other persons present.

THE RED SICKNESS. Characteristic of this period is the increasing individualization of disease based on clinical and epidemiological observation. This trend is evident not only with such diseases as the sweating sickness and typhus but also in the descriptions of scarlet fever and other acute exanthemas. Before the sixteenth century, there is no description of a disease that can be recognized with any probability as scarlet fever. In 1553, however, Giovanni Filippo Ingrassia (1510–1580), who was concerned with problems of public health and legal medicine, described a disease of children, which he differentiated from measles. He stated that is was commonly known as rossania or rossalia, and he described the rash as covering the entire body and consisting of many large and small spots of a fiery red color so that the body appears to be aflame. Although Ingrassia did not mention that the patients suffered from a sore throat, this was evidently scarlet fever.

Nevertheless, the establishment of scarlet fever as a distinct clinical entity was not accomplished until the seventeenth century. In the earlier part of this period, attention seems to have been concentrated on the disease in Germany due to epidemic outbreaks. There are occasional references to a "red sickness" (*Rotsucht*) in popular writings; and in 1624, G. Horst published a book in which he dealt with the "red sickness" as distinct from smallpox, measles, and *röteln* (possibly rubella). Accounts of epidemics at Wittenberg and Breslau in 1627 by Daniel Sennert (1572–1637) and Michael Döring (d. 1644) contain the first clear description of scarlet fever with all its distinctive features. Not only was Sennert the first to note the scaling (desquamation) following the rash, but he was also the first to report serious complications of scarlet fever, particularly the dropsy resulting from inflammation of the kidney.

During the latter part of the seventeenth century, scarlet fever seems to have been prevalent in various parts of Europe and in the British Isles. Indeed, it was in England that the disease finally received the name by which it has been known to the present. In 1676, Thomas Sydenham (1624–1689) introduced into the third edition of his *Observationum medicarum* a short chapter entitled "Febris scarlatina." Apparently his use of this term was simply a translation into Latin of a name in common use at the time. This is evident from the notation of Samuel Pepys in his diary on November 10, 1664: "My little girle Susan is fallen sick of the meazles, we fear, or, at least, of a scarlett fevour." Sydenham described it as a very mild disease, which, as he put it, was hardly more than a name, even though there were occasional fatalities. In general, his description agrees with the character of the disease as we see it today. From Sydenham's day to about the middle of the eighteenth century, scarlet fever seems to have been mild. Despite these descriptions, it continued to be confused with measles until the end of the eighteenth century.

THE RICKETS, OR THE ENGLISH DISEASE. In the early years of the seventeenth century, there appeared an apparently new menace to healthy childhood. "There is a disease of Infants," wrote Dr. Fuller in 1649 "(and an Infant-disease having scarcely as yet gotten a proper name in Latin) called the Rickets. Wherein the Head waxeth too great, whilst the Legs and lower parts wane too Little." Was rickets really a new disease? There is some evidence that it had been known under one name or another long before, indeed in classical antiquity. Valgus and varus deformities of the legs were described by Ambroise Paré in the sixteenth century, so that rickets was probably prevalent in France at the time. Nevertheless, in England, rickets appears for the first time in 1664 in the bills of mortality, and it was not until the middle of the seventeenth century that it was actually brought prominently to public attention as a health problem. The first published description of what we know as rickets today appeared in 1645 as a doctoral dissertation presented by Daniel Whistler for his M.D. at Leyden. "Some twenty-six years ago," he wrote, "the disease was first observed in our country. . . ." This view coincides with the opinion expressed by Drummond and Wilbraham in their study *The Englishman's Food* that, while rickets had certainly been present in earlier periods of scarcity, a marked increase in incidence had occurred during the first two decades of the seventeenth century, owing to the severe economic depression and terrible poverty that prevailed, especially in southern England. Unemployment and rising prices undoubtedly led to decreased consumption of milk and milk products with a consequent reduction in the daily intake of calcium, phosphorus, and vitamin D. Thenceforth, for a period of more than two centuries, the frequency of rickets increased greatly until it became an important public health problem. This increase was very probably connected as well with the growth of town life under conditions where "white meats," especially milk, and sunlight were not easily accessible.

SCURVY—THE BLACK DEATH OF THE SEA. The story of the great geographical discoveries of the fifteenth and sixteenth centuries is a familiar theme. However, the world grown more spacious yielded fresh and unanticipated problems. The sea routes to the Far East and the New World involved longer voyages than had ever been undertaken before, which directed attention to new health problems. Thus, it is no accident that a literature concerned with the occupational health needs of sailors appears in the sixteenth century. The earliest work in English devoted to naval medicine appeared at London in 1598 under the title *The Cures of the Diseased in Forraine Attempts of the English Nation*. Apparently the work of George Whetstone, a soldier and a poet, this booklet deals with scurvy, typhus fever, and possibly yellow fever, heat stroke, prickly heat, and dysentery, all conditions likely to be encountered by sailors in the tropics.

On the long voyages, however, the greatest enemy of the sailor was scurvy, due essentially to a diet deficient in or devoid of vitamin C. Scurvy was not in any sense a new disease. It had been observed during the Middle Ages in besieged towns when the supply of fresh provisions was cut off or in times of scarcity. The disease became an acute problem, however, just as soon as the seafarers of western Europe ventured out into the Atlantic. The Portuguese were among the first to face the ravages of scurvy. On his voyage of 1498, Vasco da Gama lost 55 of his sailors to the dread disease. When Jacques Carrier explored Canada in 1535, his men were attacked by a violent form of scurvy. English experience with this scourge of seamen began about the middle of the sixteenth century on early voyages to Africa. For more than 200 years, scurvy continued to be a widespread disease among seamen. Yet the effect of fresh vegetables and fruit juices in preventing scurvy had been recognized by the Dutch as early as the middle of the sixteenth century. Purchas in 1601, Lancaster in 1605, Woodall in 1617, Cockburn in 1696, and Mead in 1749 all attested to the antiscorbutic value of lemon and orange juice. Up to the middle of the eighteenth century, more than 80 publications on scurvy had appeared, and many of them recommended the use of acid fruits or their juices. Yet it was not until 1795 that the British Admiralty issued their famous order that all men-of-war have a supply of lemon juice.

THE DISEASES OF WORKERS. The interest shown in the diseases of sailors was not an isolated phenomenon. Attention was drawn as well to the health problems of other groups of workers. Indeed, it was during this period that the foundations of occupational medicine were created, thus enabling Ramazzini in 1700 to publish the first comprehensive treatise on the disorders of workers.

As a result of economic and technological developments, miners and metal workers were among the earliest occupational groups to be studied. The increased volume of trade resulting from the growth of commercial enterprise during the fifteenth century created a demand for an expanding currency and for capital. This need could only be filled by a greater supply of gold and silver, and the mines of Central Europe began to do so during the fifteenth and six-teenth centuries. Owing to this demand, the mines were deepened, and the ne-cessity for delving more deeply into the earth affected the miners' health. The deeper the mines became, the greater were the occupational hazards. The ap-pearance at this time of the first books to be concerned with the diseases and accidents of miners is a reflection of these circumstances.

Nevertheless, the very first publication to deal with the hazards of an occu-pational group concerned goldsmiths, not miners. This was a small brochure of eight pages written in 1472 by Ulrich Ellenbog, a physician of Augsburg, and printed in 1523 or 1524. Entitled *On the poisonous, evil vapors and fumes of metals, such as silver, quicksilver, lead and others which the worthy trade of the goldsmith and other workers of metals are compelled to use: How they must conduct themselves and how to dispel the poison (Von den gifftigen besen tempffen und reuchen . . .),* the purpose of the booklet was prophylactic.

The first account of the diseases and accidents of miners appeared in 1556 in the compendious treatise on mining by Georg Agricola (1494–1555). He di-vided the ailments of miners into four groups, those that attack the joints, the lungs, the eyes, and finally those that are fatal, and he discussed the preven-tion as well as the treatment of these conditions. Agricola's account is, how-ever, only incidental to his longer description of mining. In 1567, 11 years after the publication of Agricola's treatise, there appeared at Dillingen, Germany, the first monograph devoted exclusively to the occupational diseases of mine and smelter workers. The author was Theophrastus von Hohenheim, usually known as Paracelsus; the work was entitled *Von der Bergsucht und anderen Berg-krankheiten (On the Miners' Sickness and other Miners' Diseases)*. It consists of three books. The first deals with the diseases, mainly pulmonary, of miners; the second treats of the diseases of smelter workers and metallurgists; while the third concerns itself with diseases caused by mercury. Paracelsus discusses eti-ology, pathogenesis, prevention, diagnosis, and therapy. This monograph ex-erted a definite influence on occupational medicine.

Agricola and Paracelsus placed the study of the occupational health prob-lems of miners on a firm footing. The growing literature on the subject re-flects the significance of their contribution, and while the seventeenth and eighteenth centuries brought forth no important discoveries, the compilation of observations by various authors was in itself valuable. Concurrently, other physicians had written on the hazards of different occupations. There was literature on the health of scholars extending from Marsilio Ficino (c. 1497) through G. Horst (1615) and Grataroli (1652). In the seventeenth century, to mention only a few, J. R. Glauber wrote on the health of seafarers (1657), L. An-tonio Porzio (1685) and Heinrich Screta (1687), of soldiers; G. Lanzoni, of salt workers; and F. Plemp, of lawyers.

This trend, so pregnant with significance for the future, achieved its first, classic statement in the *De morbis artificum diatriba* (*Discourse on the Diseases of Workers*) of Bernardino Ramazzini of Modena, a physician of great skill, learning, and personal charm. His attractive personality is reflected in the introductory poem to his book. In it he describes the work as itching and burning to be published and warns of the dire fate awaiting it. Published in 1700, this work is to the development of occupational hygiene what Vesalius' book is to anatomy and Morgagni's to pathology. Realizing that occupational health was a matter of great social importance, Ramazzini undertook not only to study the morbid conditions caused by occupations but also to call attention to the practical application of this knowledge. In the first edition of his book, he discussed 42 groups of workers, among them miners, gilders, apothecaries, midwives, bakers and millers, painters, potters, singers, and soldiers. The second edition of 1713 was enlarged to include 12 more groups, among them printers, weavers, grinders, and well-diggers. Ramazzini's work has a dual significance. It is a synthesis of all knowledge on occupational disease from earliest times to the eighteenth century, and at the same time, it is also a basis for further investigation. It was thus both retrospective and an intimation of future development. Translated into French, German, and English, Ramazzini's book remained the fundamental text for this branch of preventive medicine until the nineteenth century when new problems were thrust up by the Industrial Revolution.

THE GREAT POX. Among the new or apparently new diseases that characterize the sixteenth and seventeenth centuries, the one that loomed largest was syphilis. Whatever its origin—and this is not the place to discuss this problem—there is no question that the disease appeared in Europe in epidemic form at the close of the fifteenth century, first in Naples whence it spread to the rest of the Continent. Syphilis appeared in Germany, France, and Switzerland in 1495, in Holland and Greece in 1496, in England and Scotland in 1497, and in Hungary and Russia in 1499. Because physicians considered it a new disease, various names were used to describe it. The French called it the Neapolitan disease, while the Italians referred to it as the French disease, *morbus Gallicus,* which became the most common name throughout Europe. In different countries, there were vernacular names as well: the great or French pox in English, *la grosse vérole* in French, and *die Blattern* in German. In 1530, however, Fracastoro published his poem *Syphilis sive morbus Gallicus,* which soon became popular and went through many editions. It recounts the legend of the handsome young shepherd Syphilus, who, for an insult to the god Apollo, was punished by a terrible malady, the French disease. Composed on the model of Vergil's *Georgics,* Fracastoro presented the symptoms, course, and treatment of the disease in polished Latin verse. The popularity of the poem eventually led to the general adoption of the name *syphilis.*

At that time, syphilis presented much more acute symptoms than it does today and was treated like other epidemic diseases. Tolerance in sex matters was generally characteristic of the period from the Renaissance to the eighteenth century, so that there was no stigma attached to the disease and strenuous efforts were made to combat it. No one thought of concealing a syphilitic infection, and the German knight Ulrich von Hutten, even published an account of his case so that others might benefit from his experience. As a result, knowledge about syphilis—its clinical manifestations, its communicable character, and how to treat it—was disseminated rapidly and widely. By 1530, the sexual character of the infection was generally recognized, and vigorous action was taken to control sources of infection.

Some of the first control measures were directed against prostitutes. Brothels were accepted institutions, and prostitution was widely practiced. Rome at the end of the fifteenth century had more than 6800 public prostitutes. The Venetian census of 1509 listed no fewer than 11,654 *femene da partido* in a population of 300,000. As early as 1496, prostitutes were expelled from Bologna, Ferrara, and other cities. In 1507, a statute of Faenza ordered that women desiring to be prostitutes had to be examined first and that those found to have the French disease could not serve. In general, the measures taken to control syphilis were derived from those that had been developed to deal with other epidemic diseases, especially leprosy and plague. Nonresidents who were sick or suspected of having the disease were expelled from the community or prevented from entering it. Sick citizens had to go to special hospitals for treatment. In 1496, Besançon expelled prostitutes and other strangers suffering with the Neapolitan disease. Similar action was taken by Zürich at this time and in 1497 by Nürnberg. In the latter year, Bamberg forbade syphilitics to enter inns and churches or to have any contacts with healthy persons. In 1496, the barbers at Rome were forbidden to serve syphilitics. Special hospitals or other treatment facilities for syphilitics were created early. Arrangements for hospitalization and treatment were made by the municipal authorites at Würzburg in 1496, at Freiburg in 1497, and at Hamburg in 1505. The Confraternity of Ferrara was licensed in 1505 to establish a hospital for syphilitics. A Venetian ordinance of 1552 ordered all those afflicted with the French disease to attend the Hospital of the Incurables for treatment. Many communities also provided free medical treatment for syphilitics, and in most cases, the physicians who treated such patients were required to report them to the authorities.

Possibly as a result of these measures, as well as of the energetic treatment by mercury inunction and the development of some degree of immunity, syphilis in the seventeenth and eighteenth centuries tended to become a more chronic disease. Nevertheless, it remained widespread and a major health problem. As middle-class morality became dominant, the disease began to be considered a social stigma. It went underground, which greatly hindered efforts to control the disease until very recently.

THE SMALL POX. The appearance of new diseases did not mean that previously known diseases vanished. On the contrary, some became increasingly important as community health problems at this time. Thus, there is no doubt of the existence of smallpox in the Middle Ages. With the end of the medieval period, however, smallpox seems to have become more widely prevalent in Europe as well as in Asia, Africa, and the Americas, where it was introduced by European explorers and settlers. On the whole, the disease appears to have been mild and infrequently fatal in Europe. Fracastoro, in his book on contagion, treats smallpox rather lightly as a disease to which almost everyone was subject. There are, however, several reports of epidemics in Italy in the sixteenth century, as for instance, at Mantua in 1567 and at Brescia in 1570, 1577, and 1588. Ambroise Paré refers to smallpox in France, describing cases he had seen in 1586 as well as at other times.

The term "smallpox" appeared in England early in the sixteenth century as the counterpart of the French term *la petite vérole.* The latter was employed in contradistinction to *la grosse vérole,* syphilis. The terms imply recognition of some similarity between the two conditions. The common element is, of course, the eruption that occurs in both diseases.

Toward the end of the Elizabethan period, smallpox began to receive recognition as a common disease in England. In 1629, the first printed bills of mortality for London listed smallpox as a separate disease, and it remained a regular entry from year to year. Throughout the Stuart period, there are frequent references to smallpox, particularly in London, and the increasing severity of the disease is reflected in the rising figures of the bills of mortality. More than 1500 people perished in London alone during the epidemic of 1659. By the end of the seventeenth century, smallpox had come to be regarded almost as an inevitable part of childhood. Infants and young children were reported as having the disease in a milder form, while it was more often fatal to older children and adults. By the beginning of the eighteenth century, smallpox was endemic in the cities and towns of Great Britain and a leading cause of death. Queen Mary died in 1694 during a smallpox epidemic. On the Continent, as in England, smallpox was a continuing threat to the public health throughout the eighteenth century. It smoldered endemically in city and town, flaring up recurrently into epidemic outbreaks.

Smallpox was introduced into the New World soon after its discovery. Thereafter, it appeared in waves from time to time in one or more localities, but its prevalence was never comparable to that in Britain or Europe. Nevertheless, the terror evoked by the disease was vivid. It was the need for informing the public regarding the nature of the disease and the means for dealing with it that led to the publication in 1677–1678 of Thomas Thacher's broadside, *A brief rule to guide the common-people of New-England how to order themselves and theirs in the small-pocks or measles.* This was the earliest medical document to be printed in America north of Mexico.

Everywhere the need for an effective preventive was recognized, and it was in connection with smallpox that one of the great triumphs of preventive medicine, namely, Jennerian vaccination, was achieved in the eighteenth century. The beginnings of this achievement lie in the early eighteenth century and the entire development will be discussed later.

MALARIA AND OTHER DISEASES. Like smallpox, malaria was present in Europe during the Middle Ages, but it is not until the sixteenth century that we are fairly well-informed about its prevalence and distribution. From the sixteenth to the eighteenth centuries, malaria was endemic and frequently epidemic over major portions of Europe. The first European pandemic of the disease is reported for the years 1557 and 1558. During the seventeenth century, England, Spain, Italy, France, the Netherlands, Germany, and Hungary were all heavily infected. According to G. B. Cavallari, in 1602, malaria in Italy killed no less than 40,000 people. England was visited by epidemics of malaria during the second half of the seventeenth century, particularly in 1657 and 1664. Cromwell is reported to have died of malaria. It was during this period, also, that malaria was introduced into the New World. Very probably, the flare-up of malaria during this period was a consequence of the continual wars as well as of the great extension of maritime trade. Europeans had now made permanent contact with some of the worst foci of the disease in Africa, India, and East Asia, and it seems likely that new strains were imported and that parasite carriers spread malaria throughout Europe.

Be that as it may, two significant contributions to the prophylaxis of malaria were made at this time. Sometime between 1630 and 1640, Peruvian bark or cinchona was imported into Europe, thus providing a specific remedy against the disease. Then, in 1717, Giovanni Maria Lancisi (1654–1720), an outstanding clinician, published a volume entitled *De noxiis paludum effluviis (On the noxious emanations of swamps)*. Concerning the epidemiology of malaria, he was interested in the way in which swamps produced the malarial fevers. Lancisi believed that swamps produced two kinds of emanations capable of producing disease: animate and inanimate. The animate were mosquitoes, and these he thought capable of carrying and transmitting pathogenic matter or animalcules. Lancisi thus came close to the vector concept, and in part anticipated the solution of the malaria riddle at the end of the nineteenth century.

Other previously known diseases also appeared in epidemic form during the sixteenth and seventeenth centuries. Indeed, some of the epidemics of this period were among the most severe in history. During the sixteenth century, diphtheria emerged in Europe as a serious epidemic disease, first in the Low Countries, along the Rhine and in France, later in the western Mediterranean area, in the Iberian Peninsula and Italy. Observations made by physicians provided the first adequate clinical descriptions of diphtheria. A series of deadly epidemics that swept Spain and Italy from the end of the sixteenth century led physicians in these countries to accept the communicable character of the disease. Slowly but surely the differentiation of diphtheria as a specific clinical entity was being made. However, toward the end of the seventeenth century, the violence of the disease appears to have abated, and the interest of physicians in it declined. As the eighteenth century advanced, diphtheria again became increasingly prevalent in Europe and broke out as well in Great Britain and America, although nowhere with such virulence as in the Spanish and Italian epidemics of the preceding century.

Bubonic plague continued to smolder throughout Europe during the sixteenth century. As the century advanced, however, the plague seems to have become more widespread; towns that had previously remained untouched were stricken, and the outbreaks became more deadly. It was not until the seventeenth century that the disease recurred with the greatest violence since the Black Death. Under the Tudors and Stuarts, the plague visited England at frequent intervals, reaching its climax in the great epidemic of 1665. The Continent was also severely ravaged. Almost half the population of Lyon was swept away in the terrible epidemic of 1628 and 1629. Moving northward along the valley of the Saône, the country around Dijon was invaded and in 1636 suffered a frightful outbreak, which almost depopulated the region. Italy's experience was similar during the period 1629 to 1631. According to Corradi, between 1630 and 1631, there were one million deaths from plague alone in northern Italy. Milan, in 1630, lost 86,000 persons and no less than 500,000 are reported to have died in the Venetian Republic. Toward the end of the Thirty Years' War, plague spread through Germany and the Netherlands. From 1654 to 1656 the peoples of eastern Europe suffered the brunt of the attack. Toward the end of the seventeenth century, the outbreaks declined in intensity, and, even though bubonic plague still afflicted Europe in the eighteenth century, it was no longer the overwhelming problem of previous centuries.

CONTAGION OR EPIDEMIC CONSTITUTION? Clearly, physicians had sufficient opportunity to study and observe pestilential diseases. Much knowledge was accumulated and gave rise to considerable speculation on the genesis of epidemics and of various acute febrile diseases. Endeavors to explain these phenomena led to the development of conflicting concepts that were to influence public health thought and practice up to our time. The one concept was that of the epidemic constitution, the other that of contagion. Neither concept was entirely new, each deriving in part at least from earlier views.

The idea that epidemics are caused by a constellation of weather conditions and local circumstances was an element in medieval epidemiology and can be traced back to the Hippocratic writings. Hippocrates stressed the meteorological variations and the character of the seasons as the elements determining the rise and fall of epidemic diseases and the variations in their seasonal and annual incidence. This concept of an epidemic constitution, that is, a state of the atmosphere which produces certain diseases capable of spreading as long as the particular constitution lasts, was developed during the sixteenth and seventeenth centuries. The first prominent advocate of this idea was Guillaume de Baillou (1538–1616), a French physician who gave the first clinical description of whooping cough and introduced the notion of rheumatism. In his book, *Epidemiorum et ephemeridum* (*On epidemic and ephemeral diseases*), published posthumously at Paris in 1640, Baillou took Hippocrates as his model and discussed the atmospheric states or constitutions prevailing seasonally and during various years between 1570 and 1579. Thus, he noted that there was a wet spring in 1571 and that many people had colds, pleurisy, and sore throats.

This approach was carried further by the great English clinician Thomas Sydenham (1624–1689). He held the view that acute febrile diseases fell into two major groups: the epidemic distempers produced by atmospheric changes, and the intercurrent diseases dependent on the susceptibility of the body. Plague, smallpox, and dysentery were among the diseases in the former group; scarlet fever, quinsy, pleurisy, and rheumatism among those in the latter. While the acute intercurrent diseases might appear independently of the prevailing atmospheric state, they too could be influenced by the epidemic distempers. Sydenham held that a prominent feature of an epidemic distemper was a so-called stationary fever, which might graft itself upon intercurrent diseases. A characteristic mark was thus set upon all illnesses prevalent during the period of a particular atmospheric constitution. The state of the atmosphere and the hypothetical changes in it which produced disease, Sydenham termed "the epidemic constitution." The epidemic distempers increased in severity and violence as the epidemic constitution waxed and developed its force to the fullest, and then declined as the atmospheric elements yielded to a new constitution, which would prevail for a certain period and be associated with other epidemic diseases. Sydenham was not clear on the postulated atmospheric change, but he believed that it was due to a miasma arising from the earth and was even willing to consider an astrological origin of epidemics.

The influence of the atmospheric-miasmatic view was to last long, and the concept was destined to play an important part in the advancement of public health in the nineteenth century. Edwin Chadwick, as we shall see, adhered to the theory that epidemic fevers were due to miasmas arising from organic matter, and while this idea was erroneous, it provided a basis for action in the interest of the public health. In historical development, things are often neither all white nor all black, and erroneous ideas may be used creatively.

Concurrently, however, there were other physicians and laymen who saw in contagion the principal factor responsible for the rise and spread of epidemic disease. This view was presented in a systematic form in 1546 by Girolamo Fracastoro (1478–1533) in his treatise *De contagione, contagiosis morbis et eorum curatione* (*On Contagion, Contagious Diseases and their treatment*). This book is one of the great landmarks in the evolution of a scientific theory of communicable disease. Fracastoro has been mentioned several times in connection with specific diseases, and it is evident that his work on contagion was based on wide and practical study of plague, typhus fever, syphilis, and other epidemic diseases. His treatise comprises three books: the first presents his theory of contagion, the second discusses various contagious diseases, and the third deals with their cures.

Fracastoro was the first to present clearly a theory of infection as we now understand the term, and he grasped the fact that infection was a cause and epidemics a consequence. Based on objective observation and shrewd reasoning, he concluded that epidemic diseases are caused by minute infective agents that are transmissible and self-propagating. These seeds, or *seminaria*, of disease are specific for individual diseases; like seeds produce like diseases. Disease occurred when the seeds acted on the humors and vital spirits of the body. It is difficult to say just how Fracastoro conceived the *seminaria*, but it is clear that they cannot be equated with living microbes in the modern sense. We are probably closer to his thought if the seeds of disease are regarded as chemical substances or ferments. Furthermore, the seeds of a disease may vary in their ability to invade the body or to persist in the environment, and these changes as they occur help to explain the cyclical behavior of certain diseases. Finally, Fracastoro recognized three modes of contagion: by direct contact from person to person; through intermediate agents such as fomites; and at a distance, for example, through the air. He postulated that under unusual conditions the general atmosphere becomes infected, producing pandemics, and that such conditions might occur in association with abnormal atmospheric and astrological conditions. Fracastoro, like many of his predecessors and contemporaries, believed in astrology.

Some of these ideas were neither new nor original with Fracastoro. The doctrines of animate contagion and of specific seeds of disease had been advanced by others, among them Varro, Columella, and Paracelsus. Furthermore, he did not discover bacteria or predict their existence. What he did, however, was equally if not more significant. By reasoning logically from observed facts, and by using analogies shrewdly when observations were lacking, he crystallized the diffuse ideas of his predecessors and contemporaries. Fracastoro concluded that the contagious element must be particulate, and he worked out a clear and essentially accurate account of the way in which such seeds of disease act. In this manner, he created a contagionist theory of epidemic disease, which was to compete with the atmospheric-miasmatic theory to the end of the nineteenth century.

LEEUWENHOEK AND HIS "LITTLE ANIMALS." Though Fracastoro was able to elucidate the mechanism of contagion, the seeds of disease remained shrouded in mystery. The idea that contagion might be caused by minute living organisms was not seriously entertained, however, until the seventeenth century. The truth began to be discovered, and then very slowly, when the microscope began to reveal its wonders. With the development of the simple magnifying lens, and the beginning of the compound microscope in the sixteenth century, it became possible for the first time to investigate the nature of the minute *seminaria* postulated by Fracastoro.

Even when it was found that minute forms of life too small to be seen with the naked eye swarmed throughout nature, in air, in water, and in soil, these tiny creatures were not at first connected with the causation of disease. The first to observe bacteria and other microscopic organisms was Antony van Leeuwenhoek (1632–1723), the remarkable linen draper of Delft, who communicated his discovery to the Royal Society of London in his famous letter of October 9, 1676. He described the forms known today as cocci, bacilli, and spirilla, but a possible connection between his "little animals" and disease apparently did not occur to him. This is not surprising, for they were found by Leeuwenhoek in harmless vehicles, such as rain water, soil, and healthy human excretions.

While it was a fascinating experience to watch these little creatures wriggle and dart about, it was infinitely more exciting to ask where they came from and how they lived. Many believed that they were spontaneously generated, while others, among them Leeuwenhoek, held that they came from pre-existing germs. Considerable controversy developed around this question, as well as the related problem of fermentation and putrefaction. Minute organisms were found in easily decomposable substances, in sour milk, in rotting meat, or in spoiled bouillon, in short, wherever decay or fermentation occurred. Furthermore, when easily spoiled organic matter was put in a warm place for a short time, swarms of organisms appeared where there were none before. It seemed plausible therefore to conclude that microorganisms were actually being generated from lifeless matter. In line with this trend of thought, it appeared equally reasonable to look upon microscopic organisms as products rather than causes of disease, generated in putrid fevers. Thus, the belief in spontaneous generation was an obstacle to the acceptance of a germ theory of disease. Attempts to solve the problem of spontaneous generation and the nature of fermentation led ultimately to an understanding of the problem of communicable disease, but this did not occur until the nineteenth century.

During this period, however, there slowly multiplied the number of observers who claimed that these microscopic creatures were probably the cause of contagious diseases. As we know, the theory that living organisms might be the agents of communicable disease was not new at this time. Girolamo Cardano in 1557 suggested that the seeds of disease were minute animals, capable of reproducing their kind, and other scientists expressed similar views. It was not until 1658, however, that Athanasius Kircher, a Jesuit, made the first explicit claim to observation of a minute living organism as the cause of plague. Despite its crude and contradictory character, his work attracted attention throughout Europe, and enthusiastic microscopists began a hunt for disease germs. Enthusiasm, however, was not enough to offset the technical and theoretical handicaps under which these investigators labored, with the result that their confusing and contradictory reports soon led to a reaction against the germ theory of disease. The theory did not lack supporters during the eighteenth century; among them may be mentioned the Englishman Benjamin Marten (fl. 1720) and the Austrian M. A. von Plenciz (1705–1786). No acceptable evidence, however, was produced in support of their views, and it was not until the 1830s and 1840s that the germ theory was again revived on the basis of new evidence.

FOUNDATIONS OF PUBLIC HEALTH ADMINISTRATION. The history of public health must concern itself with two components. One is the development of medical science and technology. Understanding the nature and cause of disease provides a basis for preventive action and control. However, the effective application of such knowledge depends on a variety of nonscientific elements, basically on political, economic, and social factors. This is the other major strand in the fabric of public health, and to this component we now turn.

Public health activity from the sixteenth to the eighteenth centuries was shaped by two basic tendencies. On the one hand, administration continued to center in some local unit, chiefly the town, thus retaining the limited parochial quality acquired during the medieval period. A countervailing trend, on the other hand, is the emergence at this time of the great Leviathan, the modern state, whose outlines slowly appear out of the storm sea of politics like a whale coming to the surface. As time went on, the state developed more and more into a centralized national government with a set of political and economic doctrines that in varying degrees influenced the administration of public health. For any adequate appreciation of the relevance of these doctrines to practical affairs, they must be seen as part of a scheme of policy and administration whose supreme aim was to place social and economic life in the service of the state. This was the system that came to be known as mercantilism, or as cameralism in its specifically German form.

From a political standpoint, mercantilism has often and properly been described as the policy of power. The idea of mercantilism is not exhausted, however, in such a description of its content. Mercantilism was much more than this; it was also a conception of society. The welfare of society was regarded as identical with the welfare of the state. Since power was considered the first interest of the state, most elements of mercantilist policy were advanced and justified as strengthening the power of the realm. *Raison d'état* was the fulcrum of social policy. For policy makers in all countries, whether in kingdoms or city-states, the important question was: What course must the government pursue to increase the national power and wealth? As the rulers and their advisers saw it, what was required was first of all a large population; second, that the population be provided for in a material sense; and thirdly, that it should be under the control of government so that it could be turned to whatever use public policy required. While mercantilist doctrine in its application received varying emphasis at different times and in various places, it was recognized everywhere in some degree that effective use of population within a country required attention to problems of health.

For example, with the growth of industry in seventeenth-century England, production came to be regarded as a matter of central importance in economic activity, and labor, one of the most important factors of production, as an essential element in the generation of national wealth. Obviously, any loss of labor productivity due to illness and death was a significant economic problem. Moreover, since population was a factor of production, it was essential to know the number and the "value of people," especially of those occupational groups esteemed most productive. It was the recognition of this need in England in the seventeenth century that led to the first significant attempts to apply statistical methods to the public health. The application of the numerical method to the analysis of health problems was destined to prove extraordinarily fruitful for the study and development of public health.

POLITICAL ARITHMETIC: THE BOOKKEEPING OF THE STATE. Initially, those who undertook to use the statistical approach concerned themselves chiefly with what might be called the bookkeeping of the state. Efforts were made to ascertain the basic quantitative data of national life in the belief that such knowledge could be used to increase the power and prestige of the state. Characteristically, this new field of endeavor was given the name "political arithmetic." This development was not without antecedents. The importance of statistical knowledge with regard to cities had been clearly recognized in the Italian Renaissance, notably at Florence and Venice but had not been developed into a method for the analysis of health problems.

The father of political arithmetic was William Petty (1623–1687), physician, economist, and scientist, who invented the term and was keenly alive to the importance of a healthy population as a factor in national opulence and power. Repeatedly, Petty urged the collection of numerical data on population, education, diseases, revenue, and many other related topics. Full of the idea that analysis of such data could throw light on matters of national interest and policy, he employed mathematical calculations wherever possible. While Petty recognized the importance of a quantitative study of health problems and suggested many topics for investigation, the first solid contribution was made by his friend John Graunt (1620–1674), whose classic book *Natural and Political Observations . . . upon the Bills of Mortality* appeared in 1662. Taking the figures showing the number of deaths in London during the preceding third of a century, Graunt interpreted them by inductive reasoning, demonstrating the regularity of certain social and vital phenomena and bringing to light a number of important facts. Thus, he noted that deaths due to various physical and emotional disorders, and even to certain accidents, "bear a constant proportion unto the whole number of burials." Graunt also pointed out the excess of male over female births as well as the eventual approximate numerical equality of the sexes; the ratio of births to deaths in city and country, and the excess of the urban over the rural death rate; and the variations of the death rate by seasons. Finally, Graunt made the first attempt to construct a life table.

Graunt's work is even more significant, however, because it contains the beginnings of statistical methods of analysis. He recognized that the accuracy of mathematical deductions from data must inevitably be limited in one way or another by the adequacy and precision of the observations themselves. Evident defects in the scanty and imperfect materials available to him led Graunt to test the reliability of his data. As a result, he was able to show that even imperfect data, if carefully, logically, and honestly interpreted, could be made to yield useful information.

Based upon the promising beginning made by Graunt and Petty, the cultivation of political arithmetic, "the art of reasoning by figures upon things relating to government," was continued during the seventeenth and early eighteenth centuries, notably by Gregory King, Charles Davenant, Edmund Halley, John Arbuthnot, Sebastien de Vauban, and Johann Peter Süssmilch. Population continued to be a central object of political arithmetic, and ingenious endeavors were made to calculate the size and to determine the state of various populations. Interest was turned to various elements, including disease, that might cause the number of people to increase or decline. These endeavors, however, yielded little substantial progress. Nevertheless, this period produced a few practical and theoretical contributions pregnant with future significance.

On the practical side this is true of the life, or mortality, table. Graunt's crude effort found a favorable response in other countries, and within a generation of his death businessmen were endeavoring by its use to put life insurance on a sound basis. In 1669, seven years after the publication of Graunt's work, Christian Huygens had already taken up the problem of determining mathematically the probable expectation of human life at any given age. More valuable, however, was the life table published in 1693 by Edmund Halley. This table was directly applicable to the calculation of life annuities, and it is worth noting that the first life insurance companies established in London in the eighteenth century made use of Halley's table. The sound operation of any life insurance plan presupposes knowledge of the rates of mortality and life expectancy, and as the eighteenth century progressed, some improvements were made in the construction of such tables with the result that insurance operations were placed on sounder actuarial lines. This development was likewise fostered by those interested in helping the poor provide for themselves through voluntary sickness insurance schemes, so-called friendly societies. Finally, after the middle of the eighteenth century, the life table found some application in attempts to test the efficacy of inoculation against smallpox.

On the theoretical side, there was the first intimation that the calculus of probability might be applied to the study of political arithmetic. In 1713, following the pioneer work of Pascal, Fermat, and Huygens, there appeared the *Ars Conjectandi*, the important posthumous work of Jakob Bernoulli, in which he developed the mathematical theory of probability and set himself the problem of applying it to "civil, moral and economic conditions." For the most part, however, writers on the calculus of probability paid scarcely any attention to the frequencies presented by the actual statistical material. Nevertheless, the inherent potentialities of the mathematical theory of probability in relation to vital phenomena had been recognized by the early eighteenth century and would eventually be developed in the nineteenth century.

TOWARD A NATIONAL HEALTH POLICY. Political arithmetic was but a means to an end, namely, national prosperity and power. Population was a central interest of political arithmeticians because its basic political and economic importance was an axiom of statecraft, and any impairment of this resource was a matter of high concern. Problems of health and disease were considered chiefly in connection with the aim of maintaining and augmenting a healthy population, and thus in terms of their significance for the political and economic strength of the state. Rulers, statesmen, administrators, physicians, in short, men of affairs, grasped that it was not enough simply to recognize natural fertility and population as major conditions of national prosperity. The acceptance of this premise went hand in hand with the responsibility for removing impediments to the full development of these resources. A major aspect of this responsibility was the creation of conditions and facilities that would promote health, prevent disease, and render medical care easily accessible to those in need of it. Logically, this approach implied the concept of a national health policy, and the implication was accepted and developed in various directions both in England and on the Continent.

While the idea of a national health policy was not systematically developed along theoretical lines in England, bold and penetrating analyses of health problems were made and proposals calling for national action were put forth. A most striking contribution was made by William Petty, the versatile father of political arithmetic, who saw that control of communicable disease and the saving of infant life would contribute most to prevent impairment of population. Furthermore, the achievement of this aim required that medical knowledge be advanced to the greatest degree possible, and in 1676, in a lecture given at Dublin, Petty stressed the duty of the state to foster medical progress. Almost 30 years earlier, he had recognized the crucial importance of the hospital in the training of physicians and in the furtherance of medical research, and to this point he returned again and again. In addition to general recommendations, Petty made specific proposals. Thus, in 1687, he proposed a Health Council for London to deal with public health matters. Another proposal in the same year suggests a hospital of 1000 beds for London. Petty recommended the establishment of isolation hospitals to which plague patients would be removed and where they would receive medical care. To buttress this recommendation, and in general the usefulness of any measures undertaken to combat the ravages of the plague, he undertook to calculate the economic loss due to the disease. Similarly, he advocated the creation of maternity hospitals, having in mind particularly unmarried pregnant women. He also believed that certain occupational groups in the population were of direct concern to the state. In keeping with this point of view are his suggestions that studies be made of occupational morbidity and mortality. Finally, Petty realized that to achieve these aims an adequate supply of medical personnel would be required. Consequently, he proposed that an analysis be made of health needs, using the methods that Graunt had employed, and then on this basis to calculate the numbers of physicians, surgeons, and others necessary to meet these needs.

Petty was not alone in attempting to deal with public health problems on a national scale, or in endeavoring to analyze them quantitatively. Among his contemporaries and successors, these interests were expressed in varying degree. Of these, three deserve mention: the learned diplomant and promoter Samuel Hartlib, the physician Nehemiah Grew (1641–1712), and the Quaker cloth merchant and philanthropist John Bellers (1654–1725). Most remarkable, indeed, is the plan for a national health service set forth by Bellers in 1714 in his *Essay towards the Improvement of Physick*. The substance of his argument and proposals may be summed up as follows: Illness and untimely death are a waste of human resources. The health of the people is extremely important to the community, so that it cannot be left to the uncertainty of individual initiative, which the high incidence of curable disease shows to be inadequate to the task of dealing with this problem. On these grounds, it is necessary to establish hospitals and laboratories to be used as teaching and research centers, to erect a national health institute, and to provide medical care to the sick poor.

Despite their great potentialities, the ideas of these thinkers had no immediately tangible results. Their proposals did not lead to concrete action because they ran contrary to major political and administrative trends. Effective implementation would have required the existence of a well-developed local administrative mechanism operating under centralized control. But it was precisely this network of administration which disappeared after the English Revolution of the seventeenth century. Local officials were in theory representatives of the central government, and a centralized administrative apparatus had been developed under the first Stuarts. However, the Civil War broke the bond between the local authorities and the Crown, and neither the Commonwealth nor the restored monarchy was able to re-establish the old system. Indeed, the outstanding feature of internal English administration from the middle of the seventeenth century to the Poor Law Amendment Act of 1834 is its intensely parochial character. This trend had important consequences for the development of public health, since there was no machinery to deal with the needs of the local community and at the same time to take into account the welfare of the country as a whole. Throughout the eighteenth century, public health problems in Britain continued to be handled on a local basis, and it was not until the nineteenth century with the advent of the new industrial and urban civilization that the problem of organizing the larger community to protect its health became a matter of national concern.

The mercantilist position in relation to health was also developed on the Continent, particularly in the German States, at about the same time. There, however, it emerged as an integral element in the theory of absolute monarchy. The relation between the ruler and his subjects was conceived to be like that of a father to his children. In line with this paternalistic theory, it was recognized that one of the duties of the absolutist state was to protect the people's health. But the people were not much more than the object of governmental care. In matters of health, as in all other spheres of activity, the ruler knew what was best for his people, and by means of laws and administrative measures ordered what they should or should not do. Within this framework, the idea of "police" is a key concept in relation to problems of health and disease. Derived from the Greek *politeia,* the constitution or administration of a state, the term "police" (*Policey*) was already employed by German writers in the sixteenth century. Characteristically, the theory and practice of public administration came to be known as *Polizeiwissenschaft*, the science of police, and the branch of the field dealing with public health administration received the designation *Medizinalpolizei*, or medical police.

An early but pregnant formulation of the German mercantilist approach to public health was offered in 1655 by Veit Ludwig von Seckendorff (1626–1692), a contemporary of William Petty, who served in various administrative posts at the ducal courts of Gotha and Sachsen-Zeitz. According to Seckendorff, the appropriate aim of government is to establish such ordinances as will ensure the welfare of the land and of the people. Since prosperity and welfare manifest themselves in growth of population, means must be taken to guard the health of the people so that their number may increase. A governmental health program must concern itself with the maintenance and supervision of midwives, care of orphans, appointment of physicians and surgeons, protection against plague and other contagious diseases, excessive use of tobacco and spirituous beverages, inspection of food and water, measures for cleaning and draining towns, maintenance of hospitals, and provision of poor relief.

Attention to the obligations of the state in matters of health expanded further during the seventeenth and eighteenth centuries. As in England, various adminstrators, physicians, and philosophers offered proposals dealing with aspects of public health administration. Thus, in his many-sided practical activities, Gottfried Wilhelm von Leibniz (1646–1716), the great philosopher, scientist, and politician, on numerous occasions referred to health problems and to modes of governmental action in such matters. He was one of the first to lay stress on statistical investigation, and during the 1680s published several essays in which he indicated the need for adequate population and mortality statistics. About this time, Leibniz also suggested a Health Council to deal with matters of public health. Governmental supervision of public health was also advocated at the end of the seventeenth century by Conrad Berthold Behrens (1660–1736), a physician of Hildesheim. Based on the premise that governmental authorities are obligated by the law of nature to care for the health of their subjects, Behrens argued that such provision must rest on two major forms of action, prevention of disease, and its treatment when it occurs. Prevention must concern itself with the constitution of the air and with nutrition. Behrens also dealt with infectious diseases and other matters of public health interest. These efforts as well as the contributions of numerous others culminated during the late eighteenth century in the monumental work on medical police of Johann Peter Frank, which will be discussed in the next chapter.

Despite these developments on a theoretical plane, neither England nor any of the Continental countries actually created a national health policy during this period. Indeed, few practical public health measures were enacted that were intended to be applied on a national basis. Among these may be mentioned the various plague orders issued by the English government during the sixteenth and seventeenth centuries. Another kind of action was taken in Prussia in 1685 when a *Collegium sanitatis*, a board of health, was established, possibly as a result of Leibniz' proposal for a medical authority to supervise the public health. It is also worth noting that, in 1688, the Great Elector undertook to determine the number of marriages, births, and deaths in Prussian cities and villages. In France, the practice of collecting statistical data was established by Colbert. It was not, however, until the end of the seventeenth century that a general survey of the population of France was undertaken. In general, governments of this period, however well-intentioned they may have been, lacked the knowledge and administrative machinery to carry out effectively any national health policy and program. As a result, public health problems continued to be handled overwhelmingly on a local community basis, a state of affairs that persisted well into the nineteenth century.

THE TOWN AND THE PUBLIC HEALTH. When examining the efforts of local authorities to solve the problems that confronted them, it is well to remember that they had to operate within narrow limits, most generally, within the framework of town government. Whether they dealt with pestilence or poverty, the authorities were concerned only with the interests and problems of their particular community. This parochial attitude becomes understandable if one realizes that local officials had no control over external causes affecting the health or welfare of the community. If plague was introduced into London by ships or goods from the East, other towns could not stop the ships from entering the port, nor could they secure the disinfection of the goods. All they could do was to try and prevent infected persons or contaminated goods from entering their town. In essence, the towns of the sixteenth and seventeenth centuries faced problems, on a smaller scale, analogous to those that confronted the national states of the nineteenth and twentieth centuries, and that eventually led to the creation of an international health organization.

Within these limits, the town authorities dealt with problems of health and welfare and took such action as seemed suitable. In these areas, local development preceded national policy. The Elizabethan Poor Law, for example, did not create anything new but simply endeavored to organize town practices on a national basis. To understand the problem of public health administration at this time, it is necessary to recall some of the great differences between towns of the sixteenth and seventeenth centuries and those of today. Fundamentally, the town of that date was much closer to the medieval community than to the modern city. The city or town today is almost entirely an industrial or commercial center. Modern urban populations live in miles of continuous streets in standardized housing far removed from a rural setting. Then, the town was a market for surrounding districts, a center for handicraft production and agriculture. Cattle were kept on the town pastures, and gardens occupied a large part of the available space within the city walls.

Public health administration in the Renaissance or seventeenth-century town was handled in much the same way as in the medieval town. Most towns were governed by an organized authority, the Town Council, which was a permanent body, often elected for life. While the constitution of these units varied from town to town, for practical purposes the town authority often exercised some of the powers of a sovereign state. Because the Town Council was generally a permanent body, it was able to some extent to provide a responsible administrative staff to handle such matters as street cleaning, drainage, water supply, and other aspects of public health.

STREET CLEANING AND DRAINAGE. The primary responsibility for keeping the streets clean fell on the inhabitants. In England, most towns insisted on weekly sweeping. At Coventry and Ipswich in the sixteenth century and at Gloucester in the seventeenth century, each householder had to clean and sweep the streets in front of his door every Saturday. At Cambridge, all paved streets had to be swept on Wednesday and Saturday. At Gloucester, four inspectors made rounds on Monday to make sure the job had been done the previous Saturday, and at Coventry the inspection was carried out on Sunday.

The major problem, however, was not the regular sweeping of the streets, but rather how to dispose of sewage and other refuse from both streets and houses. In the interest of cleanliness and public health, the towns endeavored to enforce a number of restrictions. Butchers and fishmongers were forbidden to throw offal into the gutters or into any streams or water courses from which the town might draw water. Punishment was supposed to be visited on anyone who polluted the streets with human or animal excretions. By the middle of the seventeenth century, the town of Gloucester tried to solve this problem by establishing municipal privies. Animals, particularly swine, were not allowed to roam the streets under penalty of a fine for the owners.

Nevertheless, the problem of sewage disposal was not solved during this period. Several methods were employed. In small towns, gardens attached to houses might be used for this purpose. In larger towns, other arrangements had to be made. A common practice in the sixteenth century was to select several places outside the town to which the people were supposed to carry all the waste and refuse. Such a method has obvious disadvantages. Depending as it does on the cooperation of many individuals, it is inefficient. As a result, a number of municipal authorities in the sixteenth century turned to another method, namely, to have scavengers, using carts, collect sewage and other wastes. By the seventeenth century, this method had been adopted by most towns. In London in Shakespeare's time, the scavengers were the officials who supervised the work, while the actual cleaning was done by men called rakers. Two scavengers were appointed to each parish and held office for a year. That the office was not menial may be seen from Dr. Johnson's definition of a scavenger as "a petty magistrate, whose province is to keep the streets clean." Seventeenth-century Dublin had a regular system of scavenging, but its weakness lay in the fact that this work was farmed out to a private contractor, who seldom did more than he was absolutely obliged to in carrying out his contract. It should be noted that this method of dealing with community problems, that is, by contracting with a private person or group, became more and more common and was one of the major administrative problems with which the modern public health movement had to deal.

Street drainage was carried into streams or ditches. As the latter offered an easy way for disposing of wastes, a major problem was to keep them from being polluted and creating a noisome stench. At first, this was an individual responsibility in a number of English towns, but in the course of the sixteenth century, the town authorities assumed this responsibility. That this task was not always effectively carried out may be seen from John Stow's comment in his *Survey of London* (1598) that the town ditch is "now of late neglected and forced either to a very narrow, and the same a filthy channel, or altogether stopped up. . . ."

It is clear that while the town authorities had good intentions, and endeavored to enforce the various ordinances for disposal of sewage and waste, the administrative system was inadequate. This situation was to prevail until well into the nineteenth century.

THE WATER SUPPLY—TOWARD PRIVATE ENTERPRISE. The situation with regard to the town water supply was similar to that just described for drainage and street cleaning. As in the medieval community, a great deal of the water needed by the townsfolk was provided by wells and springs within the town. With the further development and growth of urban communities during this period, these sources in numerous instances proved inadequate and arrangements were made to supply water from a source outside the town. In some towns, where a supply of fresh water had already been delivered into the community during the medieval period, it was often necessary to enlarge it to meet the growing need. Despite additional supplies, there was sometimes a real shortage of water, as at Northampton during the exceptionally dry summer of 1608, when the water was turned off at the public taps from 10 a.m. until 2 p.m. and from 7 p.m. until 6 a.m. Similarly, in seventeenth century Dublin, it was usual for one or more of the regular sources to fail. Once, a district of the city was without water for a whole year because the ancient conduit had decayed and the municipal authorities did not have enough money to have the necessary repairs made.

All through London's history until recent times, the question of water supply continued to be a problem. Here, too, the first sources were wells and natural springs. Later, three rivers—the Thames, the Fleet, and Walbrook—were drawn upon for water supply. Toward the end of Elizabeth's reign, however, the existing sources were inadequate, and the City Corporation was given the power to bring in water from springs in Middlesex and Hertfordshire. Nevertheless, no action was taken until 1609, when Sir Hugh Myddleton, a goldsmith and citizen of London, offered to finance such an enterprise, at which point the Corporation transferred to him the powers they had obtained. As a result, Myddleton organized the New River Company and, with the backing of James I, proceeded to bring water to London. The first water from this source was admitted to the Islington reservoir in 1613. The New River Company was the first of a number of private enterprises that were organized to carry out public functions and represents a new and important departure in the organization of community services. However, this trend did not become truly prominent until the late eighteenth century.

The development of these companies is related as well to technical innovations, particularly the use of pumps. In central Europe, pumps had been used for drainage in mines prior to the sixteenth century. About the beginning of the sixteenth century, however, such pumps began to be used for water supply purposes. The idea seems to have originated in Germany and spread through Europe. Various attempts along this line were undertaken in England during the late sixteenth century, but it was not until the following century that the use of machinery in connection with water supply became common. Altogether, the late seventeenth century and the early eighteenth century saw a marked increase in the installation of waterworks, and companies were formed for this purpose. The public health consequences of this development did not become clearly apparent until the nineteenth century, which will be considered later.

The usual method of distribution was to bring the water direct to a central cistern, and where necessary local cisterns were supplied from this center. The inhabitants drew their water directly from these cisterns. The main cistern was generally housed in a very ornate and elaborate structure, which in England was always called the "conduit." Before the seventeenth century, water was rarely laid on to private homes. People in most of the larger Tudor and Stuart towns obtained their water from the public conduits. During the seventeenth century, however, with increased and improved supplies, more private homes were supplied with water. At Leeds, for instance, at the end of the seventeenth century, a water company was organized to pump water to a reservoir whence it was distributed in small pipes to householders.

Conditions were more or less similar on the Continent and in the New World, particularly in Spanish America. At the end of the seventeenth century, Paris had two main sources of supply, namely, the Seine and the aqueduct of Arcueil, which brought water from a source 15 miles away. The Spanish *conquistadores* and colonizers brought with them the European practices with which they were acquainted. Ancient aqueducts and waterworks dating from the Spanish colonial period can be seen in Mexico today. For example, as one enters the city of Morelia, the capital of Michoacan, from the east, the highway follows a great masonry aqueduct of more than 250 arches built in the sixteenth century to carry water into the city from mountain springs several miles away. Similarly, the most conspicuous architectural and engineering feature on approaching Querétaro is the great aqueduct, built during the colonial period, which supplies the city with water from the neighboring hills.

Most water supplies were more or less polluted by the time the consumer was reached. Toward the end of the seventeenth century, the water of the Seine was reported to be very pernicious to strangers and to affect adversely even the French themselves. Dysentery was the chief complaint. Pollution was prevalent in England as well. In 1765, Manchester forbade the practice of drowning cats and dogs and of washing dirty linen in its Shute Hill reservoir. At York, householders had two or more large water pots. The water, taken from the river, was unfiltered and was left for a day or two to permit the sediment to settle out. While water that had cleared was being used, other pots were settling or being refilled.

The practice of filtration to purify water occurs in the seventeenth century. The idea of using sand for this purpose was proposed by L. A. Porzio in his book on the conservation of the health of soldiers. The application of this idea on a city-wide basis did not occur until the beginning of the nineteenth century. During the seventeenth and eighteenth centuries, however, filters for household use were developed and employed in France.

THE LAME, THE HALT, AND THE BLIND. Like other aspects of public health, the provision of medical care reflects the transitional character of the period. For the most part, it remained a local responsibility. The town or the parish looked after the sick poor and others unable to care for themselves. Care was provided through hospitals and physicians engaged by the community for this purpose. However, while the form was not greatly different than it had been during the medieval period, the management of these services changed greatly in some countries as a result of the Reformation and the rise of the absolutist state.

This was particularly true in England of the hospitals. With the dissolution of the monasteries under Henry VIII, the English hospital system as it had been, disappeared. A number of establishments were taken over by local municipalities, while others were turned to other purposes. Between 1536 and 1539 and the rise of the voluntary hospital in the eighteenth century, few new establishments were built. The hospital remained a combination of an almshouse, an old age home, and a true hospital for the care of the sick. These institutions were administered by the town or the parish as part of the policy of dealing with the poor. Various measures designed to deal with poverty were passed during the sixteenth century, and these measures were finally consolidated in the Elizabethan Law of 1601 (43 Elizabeth, Chapter 2), which remained the basis of English Poor Law administration for more than two centuries. While the law makes no specific mention of health matters, it was intended to relieve the "lame, impotent, old, blind, and such other among them being poor and not able to work." As time went on, however, this simple statement was expanded in practice to include the provision of medical and nursing care. The full development of local action did not come, however, until the end of the seventeenth century and the eighteenth century when internal English administration was almost completely a local matter.

On the continent there were similar tendencies in some countries. In France and Germany, hospitals tended to pass into the control of national or municipal government. As early as the reign of Henri IV, plans had been made to establish institutions for the care of the poor, but little was accomplished. Until well into the seventeenth century, medical relief was provided by local authorities along uncentralized lines. Thus, in 1649, among the activities of the commissioners in charge of poor relief at Paris was the examination and treatment of those suffering from venereal diseases and scurvy. Under Cardinal Mazarin, a determined effort was made to cope with the problem of the poor by establishing *hôpitaux généraux* (general hospitals), a combination of hospital and almshouse. The creation of these institutions reflects the increasing role of the absolute state in dealing with economic and social problems. This trend was carried further under Colbert in various undertakings intended to provide care for the sick and, in general, to improve the health of the nation. In Germany, the maintenance of hospitals after the Reformation became the responsibility of municipal corporations. Later, in the eighteenth century, royal governments exerted an influence by founding new institutions.

Another important trend that developed in the seventeenth century was the view that hospitals should be places for the treatment of the sick and, at the same time, centers for the study and teaching of medicine. This was to have extraordinarily fruitful consequences in succeeding centuries. In this development, Holland led the way. Bedside teaching was established at Leyden in 1626. Later in the century under the leadership of Hermann Boerhaave (1668–1738), this trend was consolidated and developed so that it was able to influence other medical centers, notably Edinburgh in Scotland. As we have seen, this idea was advanced in England by Francis Bacon, Samuel Hartlib, William Petty, and John Bellers, and in the eighteenth century with the establishment of hospitals and dispensaries it was put into practice. This development will be traced in the next chapter.

AN AGE OF TRANSITION. Clearly, the period from the beginning of the sixteenth century to the middle of the eighteenth century is a time of transition. The great scientific outburst of the sixteenth and seventeenth centuries laid the foundation of medical science in anatomy and physiology. Observation and classification made possible the more precise recognition of diseases. At the same time, the possibility and importance of applying scientific knowledge to the health needs of the community was given ideological form. A quantitative approach to health problems developed in relation to the political and economic needs of the modern state. The idea that microscopic organisms might cause communicable diseases began to assume concrete form.

And yet none of these areas of growth that were pushing forward into the future actually had any effect on the handling of community health problems. The community of the sixteenth, seventeenth, and even the eighteenth centuries treated problems of epidemic disease, medical care, environmental sanitation, and water supply in much the same way as the medieval community had done. The administrative pattern that had been set up in the medieval period persisted and would actually not be altered until the nineteenth century. It was during this seminal period, however, that the basis for change was being created.

-V-
Health in a Period of Enlightenment
and Revolution (1750–1830)

A SEED TIME OF HISTORY. The 80 years from 1750 to 1830 form a pivotal period in the evolution of public health. The peculiar interest of these decades
derives from the creation during this period of the foundation for the sanitary
movement of the nineteenth century, a development fraught with momentous
consequences for modern public health.

These 80 years left a legacy that continues to attract our attention because
it continues to affect us. They were a period of upheaval and crucial change,
of revolution and restoration, an intensely confused period marked by a melo-
dramatic and kaleidoscopic variety of incident. It is easy enough to be diverted
by the surface glitter and pageantry of history from the less dramatic but more
far-reaching realities of change as they affect the lives of ordinary men. Beneath the surface, however, general trends revealed the basic unities of the period. During these decades of decision, Europe endeavored to repudiate its past
and to build the future on a new foundation. The great political revolutions in
France and America, the rise and fall of the Napoleonic Imperium, the endeavors to restore the *ancien régime* are the more dramatic expressions of this basic
process of change.

Despite its diversity, despite its complex antecedents and contradictory
goals, the European world during these 80 years had at least one tenuous kind
of unity, one relatively constant factor in its climate of opinion: change was
accepted as inevitable. More and more, men, having experienced sudden social change, found it difficult to conceive society as static. They might dispute
about the desirability of a particular change, or how to go about making a
change, but all accepted change as something that happened to men in society.
This intellectual and emotional atmosphere, as well as the attitudes associated

with it, are ultimately referable to the cultural and economic movements of the eighteenth century known as the Enlightenment and the Industrial Revolution. The situations created by these developments provided the seed-beds in which germinated the new ideas and tendencies that revolutionized public health in the nineteenth century.

ENLIGHTENMENT AND REASON. At its height, the Enlightenment was an international movement, but there is no doubt that its intellectual leadership was French. Although it had originated in the political, social, and economic ferment that characterized the England of the late seventeenth century, intellectual supremacy had passed indisputably to France by the middle of the eighteenth century. Here the heritage of Locke and Newton provided the stimulus that released the genius of some of the ablest intellects and most brilliant writers of the century.

Basic to the thought and action of the Enlightenment was an acceptance of the supreme social value of intelligence and, as a corollary, a belief in the great utility of reason in social progress. The theoretical underpinning for this eighteenth-century confidence in the capacity of human reason came from John Locke's epoch-making *Essay concerning Human Understanding,* and its denial of innate ideas. Since the mind owed everything to environment, to sensations from the outer world, the shaping of the mind and the practical expression of this process in education became matters of profound significance. It was realized that social intelligence could be made effective only if there was an informed public opinion. Characteristic of the period therefore was an eager didactic impulse to make the results of science and medicine available to the public, and in line with this trend, efforts were made to enlighten the people in matters of health and hygiene.

The leaders of the Enlightenment believed that their activities would redound to the greater benefit of humanity, that their ideas coincided with the truest interests of mankind. Inspired by their belief in the perfectibility of man through education and free institutions, the French philosophers Diderot, d'Alembert, Voltaire, and Rousseau directed attention to the reform of social institutions and conditions. The critical thought and humanitarian idealism of these thinkers found its consummate expression in the monumental *Encyclopédie des Arts, Sciences et Metiers* published in 28 volumes from 1751 to 1772. Diderot declared that the aim of the *Encyclopédie* was to collect scattered knowledge, explain it to the contemporary reader, and "hand it down to those who follow us, so that the labor of centuries past may not become lost labor for the centuries which follow." It was a crucible where thinking men tried to fuse theory and practice, so that knowledge might become more readily available for the betterment of man's condition.

Concrete expression of this approach to questions of public health is presented in various articles of the *Encyclopédie* on such subjects as duration of life, the hospital, foundlings, political arithmetic, man, and population. Thus, Diderot, in his article on *Man*, emphasized the importance of infant mortality for growth or decline of population, and he pointed out that a sovereign who was seriously interested in increasing the number of his subjects must take measures to reduce the number of infant deaths. Furthermore, in his article on the *Hospital*, Diderot outlined a public assistance scheme, including old-age insurance and medical care, the latter to be provided through the various hospitals of Paris. In this connection, he stressed the need for reforming and improving the hospitals, especially the Hôtel-Dieu where mortality was exceedingly high.

With the outbreak of the French Revolution, it was expected that the fine hopes and plans of the Enlightenment, the promises implied in Liberty, Equality, and Fraternity, would be realized. For a while, however, the apparent failure of the Revolution and the disappointment of these hopes cast doubt on the doctrines of the Encyclopedists who were regarded as having fathered them. Nevertheless, these ideas were not destroyed, and, because they had their roots in needs and ideals that had not been satisfied, they were destined not to remain in abeyance. In France, the Directory and the Consulate saw the flourishing school of the *Ideologues,* Cabanis, Daunou, Destutt de Tracy, who carried on the work of the Encyclopedists. By far the most significant thinker, however, in the transmission of the thought of the eighteenth century and its transformation into that of the nineteenth century was the Englishman Jeremy Bentham. Combining the intellectual optimism and daring of the Enlightenment with a practical outlook derived from the tradition of Lockean empiricism, Bentham exerted a wide influence on social thought and legislative practice both in England and on the Continent. At the hands of his disciples, the Philosophical Radicals, his ideas were to provide a theoretical underpinning for British social and health policy throughout most of the nineteenth century, thus helping to create the modern public health movement.

OF HUMAN WELFARE. While rulers and men of affairs endeavored to guide their policies by the great mandate of enlightenment, a note of humanitarian protest also made itself heard, and as the eighteenth century approached its close this mode of thought and action became increasingly important for matters of human welfare. On all sides, a new interest was taken in the rights and conditions of men, an interest that expressed itself in an increasing concern with the health problems of specific groups. Appreciation of the social effects and aspects of disease led merchants, physicians, clergymen, and other public-spirited citizens to undertake ameliorative efforts. By the end of the eighteenth century, it had been thrust upon public attention that problems of health and disease were social phenomena of importance to the individual and to the community. The effects of disease upon the body politic had been recognized and efforts had been directed to their solution.

Through practice and theory of the eighteenth century and the early nineteenth century in matters affecting the public health ran the two strains of individual action and social regulation. Consciousness of the need for governmental action in matters of the public health was greatest on the Continent, especially in the German-speaking states; and it was there that the science of "medical police," which embodied this awareness, was systematically developed, culminating in the monumental *System einer vollständigen medicinischen Polizey* of Johann Peter Frank, of which the first volume appeared in 1779; the sixth and last was published in 1817. The idea of medical police as developed by Frank was rooted in a particular political, economic, and social system, namely, enlightened absolutism. At the end of the eighteenth century, this system differed substantially from conditions obtaining in Great Britain, France, and the United States.

Characteristic of Great Britain is the development of private initiative coupled with cooperative action. To a very considerable degree, this phenomenon is related to the limited character of local governmental activity. In many ways, this very aspect of the governmental system gave increasingly greater scope to private initiative, making it necessary and possible to deal on an empirical basis with new problems as they presented themselves. This trend must also be referred to the dynamics of social and economic change. The tempo and character of economic life had been changing in England before the middle of the eighteenth century, but by comparison the industrial and agricultural changes during the latter half of the century were both rapid and revolutionary. Not without reason have these developments been designated as the Industrial and Agricultural Revolutions. These profound alterations in the economic life of the country necessarily disturbed its social structure and gave rise to a new attitude of mind toward problems of community life. Representing essentially the views of the middle class, this distinctive ethos was characterized by two dominant facets: insistence on order, efficiency, and social discipline, and a concern with the conditions of men. It is significant that the hospital and dispensary movement, the infant welfare movement, and other similar activities originated in urban centers, first in London and then in other cities and towns. Wealth, commerce, and industry were largely centered in cities, and at the same time, it was much easier for the middle class to make itself felt.

Out of such activities, there gradually emerged a theory of social action in relation to health. This "New Philosophy," as it was called by Sir Thomas Bernard, may be considered the British counterpart of the concept of medical police. While not so systematically developed, it was an accurate ideological reflection of the activities carried on by laymen and physicians. It reflected a marked interest in the health and welfare problems of the poor, not merely as a matter of charitable sentiment, but rather in order to be able to deal rationally and intelligently with them. It provided a theoretical rationale for the growing social conscience, but it was a humanitarianism with numerous blind spots, a humanitarianism of the successful, tempering sympathy with a firm belief in the sober and practical virtues of efficiency, simplicity, and cheapness. Nevertheless, it produced various reforms, small in scope when compared with what came in the nineteenth century, but highly important as evidence of a new approach and new methods.

AN INCREASE OF POPULATION. "The Eternal Female groaned! it was heard over all the Earth": William Blake wrote these words in 1792 with Revolutionary France in mind. Yet he could hardly have characterized more felicitously the pregnant period in which he lived, a period that, as he wrote, was in travail with the "Giant-brood" of the future. A man born in the early years of the reign of George III, and who survived to be an old man, lived through a period of profound and dramatic change. He lived through a period in which handicraft was replaced by the factory, and handpower, by water and steam. He lived through a period in which England was undergoing a radical transformation from an essentially agricultural country to an industrial one.

A most significant and fundamental element in this change was the remarkable and rapid increase of the population, which began about 1750. The population, which till then had been practically stationary, began to grow rapidly. It is noteworthy that this phenomenon was not limited to England. From 1748 to 1800, for instance, the population of Prussia almost doubled, while that of Berlin increased about fivefold from 1700 to 1797. This growth was generally due to a high birth rate and a falling death rate.

The statistics are very defective, but there can be no doubt about the main trends. Deaths exceeded births in the towns, and yet the towns continued to grow. It is clear that they depended for growth chiefly on increase of the rural population. The large cities, such as London, were regarded as devouring Molochs. A rapidly expanding population means a world of children, and the crux of the matter was infant mortality, which was appallingly high, particularly among the children of the poor. It was apparent that here was a serious and dreadful waste of life, and steps were taken in England and other countries to stem the enormous wastage. An effective movement for reform came into being in England and directed itself against the factors and conditions responsible for infant deaths.

THE CAMPAIGN AGAINST GIN. The English reformers directed their efforts first of all against the traffic in gin. The significance of the campaign against gin resides not alone in its effectiveness, but even more in the circumstance that it was one of the first efforts to secure social reform through organized pressure on Parliament. It is thus a prototype of public health agitation, which was to assume crucial significance in the nineteenth century. Backed by newspaper propaganda, magistrates, and doctors, petitions were presented to the government. Hogarth's *Gin Lane,* only too true as a historical document, was published at this time. Finally, goaded into action, Parliament passed a series of Gin Acts culminating in an Act of 1751, which gave the control of licensing to the magistrates and checked the amount of spirits consumed. The decline in the consumption of spirits had an appreciable effect on the death rate, especially on infant mortality.

A SLAUGHTER OF INNOCENTS. The enormous child mortality was also attacked from several other directions. It was recognized that illegitimacy was common and great numbers of unwanted babies died of neglect or were murdered. Many were abandoned to the parish authorities. Children of the poor faced many hazards even when raised by their parents. In some London parishes around 1750, the mortality of children ranged from 80 to 90 per cent, while that of those younger than 1 year of age was even higher.

Awareness of the problem is reflected in the establishment in 1741 of the Foundling Hospital of London as a result of the efforts of Thomas Coram. In 1748 appeared *An Essay upon Nursing and the Management of Children* by William Cadogen, written for the governors of the Foundling Hospital, in which he upheld the rights of infants to life and liberty and proceeded to lay down sane empirical rules on nursing, feeding, clothing, and exercise. The remarkable Jonas Hanway—merchant, traveler, opponent of tea drinking, advocate of the umbrella, and philanthropist—waged an important campaign against infant mortality, exerting his greatest influence in the cause of the infant parish poor. In 1769, he secured an Act making it compulsory for London parishes to send infants into the country to be nursed. On April 24 of the same year, George Armstrong opened the first Dispensary for the Infant Poor in England. No less than 35,000 children were treated there during the next 12 years.

A similar awakening of public conscience to the problems of childhood took place on the Continent. Infants were looked upon as victims of improper care, and demands were raised for more rational hygienic measures. In France, Nicholas Andry coined the term "orthopedics," in his book *L'Orthopédie ou l'art de prévenir et de corriger dans les enfants les difformités du corps,* published in 1741. He pointed out that many deformities and ailments in children were a consequence of wrong handling. The demand for the correct physical upbringing of infants was supported in 1760 by Jean Charles des Essartz in his book *Traité de l'éducation corporelle en bas-age, ou réflexions pratiques pour les moyens de procurer une meilleure constitution aux citoyens.* More effective than all medical arguments was *Émile,* the educational novel by Jean Jacques Rousseau published

TABLE I
Average Mortality Rates for the British Lying-In Hospital

Year	1749–1758	1779–1788	1789–1798
Maternal mortality rate per 1000 live births	24	17	3.5
Infant mortality rate per 1000 live births	66	23	13

in 1762. Its influence extended far beyond the borders of France. The decree passed by the French National Convention, June 28 to July 8, 1793, providing for the welfare and health of children and expectant mothers, represents the culmination of this development.

A tendency to promote the welfare of children is evident also in Germany where it is best expressed in the writings and proposals of Johann Peter Frank and his contemporaries. Here the trend was to achieve reform by administrative action. At the same time, health education was not neglected. Illustrative is B. C. Faust's *Gesundheitskatechismus*, which was published in 1794, enjoyed numerous printings and was also translated into various languages.

Paralleling the infant welfare work of this period were the efforts to improve obstetrics and reduce maternal mortality. William Smellie helped to improve the professional standing of obstetricians. Prior to 1739, when Sir Richard Manning-ham established a ward for lying-in women, there had been no provision in London hospitals for obstetrical patients. This example was soon followed by others. In 1747, for instance, Middlesex Hospital set aside a ward directed by an obstetrician. Then, in rapid succession, the British Lying-In Hospital was founded in 1749, the London Lying-In Hospital in 1750, Queen Charlotte's in 1752, and several others were rapidly added to these. An outstanding contribution to the improvement of obstetrical practice was made by Charles White of Manchester, whose demand for cleanliness in obstetrics anticipated the later contributions of Holmes and Semmelweis in the prevention of puerperal fever.

Some idea of the effect of these developments in obstetrics may be obtained by comparing mortality rates for different periods. In Table 1 the average figures for the British Lying-In Hospital indicate the trend.

Around 1810 or 1820, the death rate began to rise again, continuing into the "Hungry Forties" of the nineteenth century.

ALL MANNER OF CONDITIONS AND MEN. Concern with the health of specific groups is evident as well in the attention devoted to the working conditions and diseases associated with certain occupations. Bernardino Ramazzini had published his classic treatise on the diseases of workers in 1700, but it was not until after the middle of the eighteenth century that further significant contributions to occupational welfare were made. During the latter half of the century, naval and military medicine occupied the attention of various British, French, and German physicians. Notable for improving the health of seamen, especially the eradication of scurvy from the Royal Navy, are the contributions of James Lind (1716–1794), Gilbert Blane (1749–1834), and Thomas Trotter (1760–1834). Lind recommended the use of lemon juice to combat scurvy, and made other suggestions to improve the living conditions and personal hygiene of seamen, thus helping to reduce the incidence of typhus fever. In France, the work of Lind was adopted by Poissonier-Desperrières, the French authority on naval medicine. The diseases of soldiers and their prevention occupied the attention of John Pringle (1707–1782) in England, and of E. G. Baldinger (1738–1804) and J. P. Brinkmann (1746–1785) in Germany.

In the German-speaking lands considerable attention was paid to the diseases of miners and metal workers. The health conditions of workers in general were considered by Z. G. Huszty in 1786, E. F. Hebenstreit in 1791, and George Adelmann in 1803. In England, Robert Willan (1757–1812) described various skin diseases in workers—dermatoses of shoemakers and metal workers, grocer's itch, eczema of washerwomen, and baker's itch.

During the first decades of the nineteenth century, France took the lead in this field of public health. In 1817, for example, Kerandren (1769–1857), a naval surgeon, published a volume on naval hygiene, based on numerous detailed studies. A. L. Gosse (b. 1791), anthropologist and participant in the Greek war of liberation, published two treatises on dangerous trades in 1816 and 1817. Another expression of this interest was the publication in 1822 of Patissier's translation of Ramazzini's treatise, enriched by his own observations. In 1825, F. E. Fodéré (1764–1835), an original and forceful public health thinker, published his *Essai historique et moral sur la pauvreté des nations* (*Historical and moral essay on the poverty of nations*) in which he discussed the health hazards created by the big factories of St. Etienne and Marseilles. Then in 1829 there appeared a journal devoted to public health, which immediately acquired an international reputation and still appears today. This publication, the *Annales d'hygiène publique et médecine légale* (*Annals of public hygiene and legal medicine*), devoted considerable space to occupational health.

This endeavor to project hygiene from a personal to a public plane is strikingly illustrated by the investigations of John Howard (1726–1790) in the course of which he laid bare the appalling condition of English prisons. As High Sheriff of Bedfordshire, he had become familiar with prison conditions and had undertaken the task of investigating the state of the jails. In 1777, he published his famous account of the *State of the Prisons,* in which he gave a full report of his inquiries and proposed remedies for the evils he had revealed. Howard's investigations in many respects anticipate and are prototypical of the work of the sanitary reformers of the nineteenth century. They illustrate the effectiveness of approaching social evils in terms of their consequences for the health of the community, and they bear striking testimony to the value of inquiry in dealing with such problems. Through his revelations of the relation between jails and jail fever, Howard aroused public opinion and made possible improved conditions. He thus showed that people are galvanized into action when the facts about social disease are forced upon them and that an aroused public opinion could be employed as a lever to compel reform. Howard devoted his life to prison reform, journeying throughout Europe in this cause, and ironically enough, he died of jail fever at Kherson in the Ukraine. In England, Howard's work was continued after the Napoleonic Wars by Elizabeth Fry, Thomas Fowell-Buxton, and other Quaker philanthropists.

LUNACY AND CONSCIENCE. "Man is born free, and everywhere he is in chains!" Rousseau's angry cry was not uttered with the mentally ill in mind, and yet to no other group of his time could it be applied with greater accuracy. In the eighteenth century, madmen were locked up in jails, workhouses, and madhouses, and insanity was attributed to sin and the activities of the devil as well as to a variety of other causes, among them retention of bodily excretions, emotional disturbances, bad diet, and lack of sleep. Ignorance, superstition, and moral condemnation dominated the treatment of the insane.

Here and there voices had been raised in earlier centuries in an effort to penetrate the dense pall of ignorance and fear that shrouded in mystery the nature of mental illness. Among these were Paracelsus, Johann Weyer, Reginald Scot, and Felix Plater in the sixteenth century, and a number of other physicians and philosophers in the seventeenth century. For the most part, however, these were voices crying in the wilderness and it was not until the latter part of the eighteenth century that evidence of change began to appear. By the end of the century, forces had been set in motion, which were to alter radically the care and treatment of the insane.

Lunacy reform was not an isolated movement. It was part of the larger concern with the rights and conditions of men and is thus connected with the other reforms of this period: reform of the penal system, concern for the care of children, improvement of working conditions, and improvement of the public health. Motivated by the ideas of the Enlightenment and the new spirit of humanity in community life, it is not surprising to find proposals and action for reform appearing almost simultaneously in various European countries, particularly in France and England.

In 1774, after having investigated conditions in the madhouse at Pforzheim, G. F. Jaegerschmid (d. 1775) proposed that less disturbed patients be given more freedom, and that restraint be employed only in the case of violent patients. Furthermore, he insisted that properly trained nursing personnel be employed to care for the patients and that this staff should report regularly to a supervising physician. These proposals were not realized, but in 1788, Vincenzo Chiarugi (1759–1820) brought about reforms of this type in the hospital of St. Bonifacio at Florence. Chiarugi's reforms, when considered chronologically, antedate those initiated by Philippe Pinel in France and William Tuke in England. However, since he first described his work in his treatise on insanity published in 1793–1794, and since it was written in a rather difficult Italian, it was relatively inaccessible to others and did not produce the effect it might have had on the practice of his day.

More profound and far-reaching was the influence of the Retreat founded at York in 1792 by the Society of Friends. The project for the Retreat was the brain-child of William Tuke (1732–1822), a tea and coffee merchant and a Quaker, who was roused to action by the evil conditions at the York Asylum, an institution for the insane founded in 1777. Built to accommodate 30 patients, the Retreat was opened in 1796. Here Tuke introduced a regimen based on common sense and Christianity. Every effort was made to provide a family environment for the patients. Good food, fresh air, exercise, and occupation replaced brutality, chains, and semistarvation. Tuke proved that kindness was a more effective therapy than rigorous confinement. His work was directly influential in the United States, where the example set by the Retreat was followed in the creation of the Friend's Asylum, opened at Frankford, Pennsylvania, in 1817, and of the Bloomingdale Asylum, opened in 1821 in New York.

The year after William Tuke conceived his project a similar step was taken by a French physician under more dramatic circumstances, in the midst of revolutionary turmoil and the alarms of war. The physician was Philippe Pinel (1745–1826) who in 1793 had been appointed physician to the Bicêtre in Paris, where men were confined. Convinced that a regimen based on kindness, sympathy, and a minimum of mechanical restraint was more effective in the treatment of the insane than the brutal methods prevalent in his day, Pinel in 1793 removed the chains from 53 lunatics. The results were encouraging. Three years later, he became physician to the Salpêtrière, the second largest asylum in Paris, where incurable women were kept. Here he introduced a similar regimen and demonstrated conclusively the value of humane treatment for the mentally ill. Pinel presented his system of moral treatment and its results in his classic *Traité médico-philosophique sur l'aliénation mentale* (*Medico-philosophic treatise on insanity*) published in 1801. His work exerted a weighty influence, not alone in France but throughout the European Continent as well as in Britain and America.

One of the more significant results of the reform of the treatment of the insane was that it led to the establishment of asylums. In England, the pioneer work of Tuke and others first took form during the early nineteenth century in the County Asylum Act of 1808, and the amending acts of 1815 and 1819. The first county asylum to be built was at Nottingham, which was opened in 1811. By 1815, three county asylums were in operation, and by 1842, there were a total of 16. In general, these institutions exhibited definite progress in the use of humane methods and the development of professional standards for the care of the mentally ill. This movement for the creation of special institutions for the insane during the first three decades of the nineteenth century may be observed in the United States as well. These hospitals eventually made possible the scientific study of mental illness.

HOSPITALS AND DISPENSARIES. The development of asylums paralleled the rise of general hospitals and dispensaries. At the beginning of the eighteenth century, hospitals scarcely existed in England, except in London, and even there accommodations were inadequate. Provision for the sick poor was needed, however, especially in the metropolis. London was growing, wages were high, and workers were attracted to the city. Many of them, unable to establish the needed residence requirement, were ineligible for parochial relief when sick. There were two older hospitals, St. Bartholomew and St. Thomas, but these were overcrowded and unable to care for all those in need. Recognizing the problem, a group of London laymen and physicians in 1719 organized the Charitable Society in Westminster to provide for such sick persons as were unable to obtain proper care. This was the beginning of the Westminster Hospital, which was soon followed by the establishment of other institutions. Guy's (1724), St. George's (1733), London (1740), and the Middlesex (1745) were established. Thus, by 1760, most of the great London general hospitals had been established. By 1797, the seven general hospitals had 1970 beds.

About the middle of the century, special hospitals were created. The London Hospital had been founded "for the relief of all sick or diseased persons, and in particular manufacturers, seamen in the merchant service, and their wives and children." Still more specific was the object of the Middlesex Hospital, which was founded in 1746 for smallpox patients and to encourage inoculation. The same year also saw the establishment of the Lock Hospital for patients with venereal disease. Mention has already been made of provision for obstetrical patients and foundlings. St. Luke's, for the reception of mentally ill persons, was established in 1751.

From 1760 to 1800, the growth of hospitals in London slowed down, but thereafter, the process of development was resumed. During the first four decades of the nineteenth century, 14 hospitals were founded in London. While some were general hospitals, it is noteworthy that most of them were special hospitals. Thus, the London Fever Hospital was founded in 1802; the Royal London Ophthalmic Hospital, in 1804; the Royal Chest Hospital, in 1814; the Royal Ear Hospital, in 1816; and the Royal National Orthopaedic Hospital, in 1838.

The influence of these trends was soon felt and paralleled outside London. The first provincial hospital was the one founded at Winchester in 1736. The movement thus started to spread rapidly to Bristol (1737), York (1740), Exeter (1741), and Liverpool (1745). By 1760, there were 16 provincial hospitals, of which 14 were general in character. By 1800, there were 38, and by 1840 there were 114. Similar forces were at work in Ireland and Scotland, and, by the end of the eighteenth century, hospitals were to be found in most of the cities and larger towns.

Even while hospitals were being founded, it was realized that these institutions would have to be supplemented by some other kind of establishment. To fill this need, the dispensary was developed. The dispensary idea may be traced to the seventeenth century, but it was not until 1769 that the dispensary came into being. This was the Dispensary for the Infant Poor, opened by Dr. George Armstrong at a house in Red Lion Square, Holborn, London. There was no provision for home visiting, although it was suggested that this might be done later. The opening of Armstrong's dispensary was followed in 1770 by the founding of the General Dispensary by the Quaker physician John Coakley Lettsom and a group of associates. The distinctive feature of the General Dispensary was that provision was also made for medical care in the home. In a sense, the provision of domiciliary care was not really new. At least in the field of obstetrics, arrangements of this kind had been made more than a decade earlier. William Smellie, the founder of scientific midwifery in Britain, had initiated a scheme by which he and his students attended poor women gratis in their homes. At the General Dispensary, this approach was applied to all medical patients who could not come to the dispensary. Following the example set by Lettsom, dispensaries sprang up in London and the provinces. From 1770 through 1792, 15 were founded in London, and, from 1715 through 1798, 13 were established in the provinces. By 1840, there were 23 dispensaries in London, and 80 dispensaries had been opened in the provinces.

The beginnings of hospitals in the Americas may be traced to the sixteenth century, when the Spanish *conquistadores* founded institutions like those prevailing in Europe at the time, and others were established in succeeding centuries. These were created under the auspices of the church or the temporal authorities, municipal or national. The English colonies in America followed the pattern set by the mother country. The first successful effort to establish a general hospital occurred in Philadelphia toward the middle of the eighteenth century, with the opening of the Pennsylvania Hospital in 1751. The second oldest hospital in the United States, the New York Hospital, was opened in 1791. Despite these beginnings, the development of hospitals in the United States was slow. The chief reason for this lag was that there were few cities and large towns. By 1825, New York City had two more hospitals, one general and the other an eye and ear infirmary. General hospitals had also been established in Boston, Baltimore, Cincinnati, and Savannah.

The hospitals and dispensaries founded in Great Britain during the eighteenth century and the early nineteenth century were significant factors in promoting health and saving lives. While it is not easy to define this influence statistically, it seems clear that these institutions helped to spread medical information and to impress on people the rudiments of hygiene. Furthermore, they were not governmental undertakings; they were the outcome of voluntary efforts by private citizens and were financed by subscription and bequest. Clearly, neither the voluntary hospital nor the dispensary was an outgrowth of experience with the social and economic changes brought about by the Industrial Revolution. Nevertheless, the establishment of these institutions helped to create a pattern of behavior that was to become familiar in the endeavors of the nineteenth-century public health movement to cope with the health problems brought by industrialization. This pattern is characterized by several stages: First, a social evil is recognized by an individual or a small influential group. Secondly, studies, local experiments, or improvements are undertaken through individual initiative. Thirdly, these endeavors then act to enlighten and mold public opinion and to attract the attention of government to the problem. Finally, such agitation leads to governmental action and if successful to legislation.

The growth of hospitals was not restricted to England or America during this period. Municipal growth in France during the eighteenth and the early nineteenth centuries necessitated a considerable extension of hospital facilities. By 1830, Paris had no less than 30 hospitals housing some 20,000 patients. The Hôtel-Dieu alone had 1000 beds. Similar developments occurred in the German-speaking countries, although not to the same extent. It should be noted, however, that on the Continent these institutions were founded and administered under government auspices.

Valuable as these hospitals were, they left much to be desired. Nursing was primitive, hygienic conditions in many instances were poor, and owing to false concepts of economy wards were overcrowded. Toward the end of the eighteenth century, steps were taken to change matters. John Howard, the prison reformer, also studied the state of hospitals and offered proposals for improvement. Under the influence of James Lind, the pioneer of naval hygiene, ventilation was improved, better sanitary accommodations were installed, and a much higher standard of cleanliness was introduced. In Ireland, the reform of hospitals was first undertaken seriously at the beginning of the nineteenth century. Conditions in French hospitals were much poorer than in the English establishments. Indeed, on the eve of the Great Revolution, it was proposed that the Hôtel-Dieu in Paris be abandoned, and its patients moved to new hospitals to be established. The need for improvement was recognized by the revolutionary governments, and in 1793, the Convention passed a decree that every hospital patient should have his own bed and that beds should be separated from each other by a distance of three feet. By the early nineteenth century, conditions were considerably better. Conditions in German and Austrian hospitals were similar to those in France, but here, too, changes for the better did not occur until the first decades of the nineteenth century.

IMPROVEMENT OF TOWN LIFE. By modern standards, most cities and larger towns of the eighteenth century were extremely unsanitary, dirty, and pervaded by nauseating smells. Jonathan Swift's London lodging, for example, had "a thousand stinks" in it. Urban sanitation was poor, indeed worse in some respects than it had been in the seventeenth century. Streets and alleys were frequently foul and ill-cleansed. Sewage and household refuse were commonly flung out of doors and windows; and slaughtering was carried out in public places. This is vividly portrayed in Swift's verses:

Now from all parts the swelling kennels flow,
And bear their trophies with them as they go;
Filth of all hues and odors seems to tell
What street they sailed from by the sight and smell;
Sweepings from the butchers' stalls, dung, guts and blood,
Drowned puppies, stinking sprats, all drenched in muck,
Dead cats and turnip-top come tumbling down the flood.

Nonetheless, the second half of the eighteenth century began to see considerable improvements in British cities and towns. These changes were most marked between 1750 and 1815, that is, during the first impact of industrialism and during a prolonged period of war, which brought with it violent economic fluctuations and other social evils. From the 1760s onward, first London and then other communities developed and put into effect schemes for civic improvement. Deteriorated and obstructive buildings were pulled down, and streets were drained, paved, and lighted. Narrow, tortuous thoroughfares were widened and straightened. Brick buildings replaced timbered houses, with the result that some horrible slums disappeared. As the newer quarters with wide streets and open squares appeared, the wealthier class gravitated to them leaving the older unsanitary sections to the poor. During the 1780s, the pavements, the street lights, the water supply, and the sewers of London were noted with admiration by visitors. Of course, such observations should not be judged by modern standards, but rather compared with contemporary conditions in other cities. (By our standards, London was then still dark, dingy, and dirty.)

The example set by London spread to the provinces, and other towns undertook improvements. The Westminster Paving Act of 1762 may be taken as a point of departure in this development. Manchester obtained a similar act in 1776, and soon its streets were able to bear comparison with those of London. Liverpool not only improved its streets but also even began a campaign against cellar dwellings. The extent of this movement may be gauged from the fact that between 1785 and 1800 no less than 211 other communities embarked on schemes of civic improvement.

Some improvement was made in urban water supplies and sewerage. Steam pumps and iron pipes were gradually introduced. However, up to the first decade of the nineteenth century, the mains continued to be made chiefly of wood. During the first 30 or 40 years of the century, a need for increased and better urban water supplies was widely felt, and as the growth of the iron industry now made possible a more extensive use of that material, iron pipes and mains began to be introduced. After 1827, the use of iron was made compulsory. The West Middlesex Water Company—one of the London suppliers— substituted iron for wood in 1808. Dublin after vacillating between wood and iron finally went "cast iron" in 1809, with replacement of the wooden mains being carried out over the following five years. In 1805, the lead pipes of Lichfield were replaced by cast iron. The New River Company in London was also replacing its wooden pipes with cast iron at about the same time. It is of interest to note that in 1826 the estimated cost for laying cast iron pipes at Gloucester varied from about 5 s. per yard for 2 inch diameter to 10 s. a yard for 5 inch diameter. In London, about the same time the cost for a 2 foot 6 inch diameter cast iron pipe in 9 foot lengths was £8 per yard.

Despite these advances, however, various inadequacies still remained. Because of inefficient methods of jointing and the resultant leakage, an intermittent supply remained common until well into the nineteenth century. This was particularly true in the poorer sections. Generally, a standpipe was the source of supply for a number of houses. At Bath, at one time during this period, there were only three standpipes for the use of the poor, and these provided water only during certain hours in the morning. At York, during the earlier nineteenth century, one half of the city was supplied for two hours on Mondays, Wednesdays, and Fridays, and the other half, on the alternate days. No water was supplied on Sundays. Efforts were also made to improve the quality of the water supplied, but with little success. For the most part, water came from polluted rivers and surface sources. At London, in 1827, it was shown that the intake of the Grand Junction Water Co. was only three yards away from the outlet of a large sewer. Similar conditions existed in other communities. Slow sand filtration of water supplies was introduced in London in 1829 by James Simpson, engineer of the Chelsea and Lambeth Water Companies. He made use of a small reservoir with layers of large and small stones, gravel, and sand in that order from the top down. Although the filter depends on the gradual formation of a film of algae, diatoms and other microscopic living forms, its biological nature and action were not understood until much later. The primary purpose of the sand filter at this time was to remove gross pollution and to clarify the water.

The development of community water supplies in the United States paralleled closely the British pattern. When the Manhattan Company was organized in 1799 to provide New York City "with pure and wholesome water," bored logs were used to transport the water, and lead pipes carried it into the houses. In 1797, the Watering Committee of Philadelphia undertook to use steam pumping, and in 1817, the same group imported cast iron pipes to replace bored logs. At Lynchburg, Virginia, in 1829, cast iron pipes were used for what is said to be the first high-pressure water main in the world.

W. G. Smillie has noted as a general rule that in the United States the establishment of a community water supply has preceded the development of a sewerage system by a period of years, ranging from 5 to 50. This generalization applies as well to the British scene in a broad sense. Many years were to elapse before community water supplies would be employed to dispose of household wastes. The idea of using running water to carry off excreta had appeared at an early period, and in the sixteenth century, Sir John Harington, courtier and poet, had invented a water closet, which he persuaded Queen Elizabeth to install in her palace at Richmond. However, it remained an amusing freak. In the eighteenth century, water closets while no longer a novelty were still a rarity. Occasionally, such contrivances would be installed in the private homes of the well-to-do. Thus, two were put in the Bloomsbury house of the Duke of Bedford in 1771 when new bathrooms were made. It was not till the closing decades of the eighteenth century that the water carriage system of drainage began to become common. Twenty years later, in 1791, John Howard, on visiting Guy's Hospital, noted with surprise and satisfaction that the new wards each had a closet, the water being turned on by an ingenious arrangement when the door opened. The provinces lagged behind London. As late as 1808, the inhabitants of Exeter emptied their sewage into the gutters, and in the entire town, there was only one water closet. However, the introduction of this amenity soon created more problems than it solved, since the cesspits were cleaned out very infrequently and the contents seeped out into the soil saturating the ground over large areas and polluting springs and wells used for water supply. Furthermore, it was deceptively easy to dispose of sewage by allowing it to discharge into the sewers that existed under many cities by this time. The only thing the matter with this solution was that the sewers were designed to carry off rainwater; in consequence, as the practice became more general, rivers and lakes in or near all the larger towns were turned into nothing less than open sewers. This was to be one of the major problems facing the sanitary reformers of the nineteenth century.

Clearly, at the end of the eighteenth century and the beginning of the nineteenth, the conditions of urban life began to improve. Nonetheless, this movement was quite uneven, and much still remained to be done. Accumulation of sewage, pollution of water supplies, overcrowded and inadequate housing: in short, all the things that agitated the reformers of the Victorian period. However, the situation could be tolerated as long as towns were not growing too rapidly, and the movement for civic betterment and improvement of health kept pace with existing conditions. However, as towns began to grow at an increasingly rapid rate under the impact of industrialism, and this growth was not properly controlled or regulated, the existing evils got out of hand to an extent that more than counteracted the earlier gains. Statistically, the situation is reflected in the movement of mortality. After about 1815, the death rate, which had declined during the later eighteenth century and the early nineteenth, again began to rise. Britain provides the earliest and most striking instance of this development, although similar accounts could be given for the United States and various Continental countries somewhat later.

Complicating the situation was the circumstance that the community recognized little corporate responsibility for the well-being of its members. The old order that had come down from the Middle Ages was in the last stages of disintegration, and the new order was just making its appearance. One consequence of this process was that urban government in Britain throughout the eighteenth century was in a bad way. Newer towns like Birmingham and Manchester were not incorporated and lacked fully developed municipal institutions, but towns with municipal corporations were not much better off. Many of them dated from Tudor days, and some were even older. Although they had dealt reasonably well with urban hygiene during the earlier period, by the later eighteenth century, they were demonstrably inadequate to the purposes of local government. Indeed, the typical municipal corporation of the eighteenth century hardly regarded itself as an organ of local government. (As the Webbs have pointed out, the very term "local government" did not appear until after the middle of the nineteenth century.) The typical corporation accepted no responsibility for the proper development of sanitary and health services, or other civic amenities. As a result, when increasing population and urgent community problems began to force the question of municipal organization and action upon public attention, new organs were developed to achieve the desired end. The most common way of getting new services developed was not by means of the existing municipal corporations, but to set up, alongside of them, new and independent authorities. The long succession of local Improvement Acts in the eighteenth and early nineteenth centuries makes clear that, under various names, town after town set up such special bodies of Improvement Commissioners, created by Parliament with power to levy taxes. (The situation is, indeed, analogous in some respects to that in the United States at present where independent authorities are created to build utilities, such as highways and bridges, or to deal with problems that exceed the boundaries of older governmental jurisdictions, e.g., the Port of New York Authority or the Tennessee Valley Authority.) It was these Commissions, which in the latter part of the eighteenth century introduced the municipal services and improvements, that have already been described. While mainly concerned with lighting, cleaning, and paving streets, removing sanitary nuisances, and regulating traffic, attention was also focused on health problems.

Action by official agencies of this type complemented and was intimately related to the voluntary activities connected with maternal and child welfare, hospitals, dispensaries, and prisons. Both trends illustrate the combination of private initiative and cooperative action so characteristic of Britain at this time. Peculiarly illustrative is the story of the Manchester Board of Health. Manchester, the first industrial city, was created at this time by the impact of industrialization on the cotton industry. An epidemic of typhus fever in 1784 attracted attention to the factories and the health problems connected with them. In consequence, a group of Manchester physicians headed by Thomas Percival was asked to look into the problem. Their report to the County Justices on the health of Manchester contained recommendations for remedial action. Little was done, however; other epidemics occurred, and the situation grew worse. Finally, in the winter of 1795–1796, the spread of typhus terrified the inhabitants to such an extent that Dr. Percival and his associates again met and formed the Manchester Board of Health. The members of this body were fully aware that the repeated epidemics were connected with the cotton mills, many of whose workers were children, and they recommended legislation to regulate the hours and conditions of work in factories as well as needed measures to prevent or reduce the spread of disease.

This approach to community problems fitted in well enough with the opinion generally held in England about the scope of government. Except in external relations, foreign policy, and commerce, private enterprise was to an ever-increasing degree the principle that replaced public activity. This is nowhere more evident than in the provision of water supplies. Toward the end of the eighteenth century, private water companies became more and more common in Britain, reaching a high between 1800 and 1835, when the Municipal Corporations Act began to reverse this trend. By about 1830, there were eight companies supplying London. In 1819, Edinburgh handed over its water supply to a private company for a sum of £30,000. In Bath, the municipality supplied water, but in 1845, there were in addition seven water companies supplying parts of the city. This tendency to leave the provision of water to private enterprise was not limited to Britain. The United States followed the British practice. Municipal ownership and operation of such public utilities was not common in American communities in the first part of the nineteenth century. From 1800 to 1817, there were only 17 community water supplies in the United States, and all but one were privately owned. To find public functions turned over to private companies organized for profit is not surprising in a business-minded community. Indeed, this type of thinking is still very much with us in demands that systems for the generation of electric power developed through governmental activity be turned over to private operation and distribution.

To supplement one authority or agency by another was often the most effective means of achieving some immediate improvement in the condition of a town or part of a town. In the long run, however, this approach could not deal effectively with the larger problem, which was being broached at this very time: How to organize life in a complex industrial and urban society? A major aspect of this problem was the organization of the community to protect its health, and the lesson had yet to be learned that this could not be accomplished on a piecemeal, hit-or-miss basis. The need for centralized organization and administration had not yet been recognized, and, for the time being, authorities multiplied and proliferated. During the 1830s, for example, the government of London was divided between the City Corporation and the city companies, seven boards of commissioners for sewers, nearly 100 paving, lighting, and cleansing boards, about 172 vestries of one sort or another, boards of guardians appointed under the Poor Law Act of 1834, as well as a bewildering collection of other authorities. The parish of St. Pancras alone had 21 paving and lighting boards on which sat 900 commissioners. Many of the boards in this parish, as well as in others, were frequently irresponsible and extravagant and often corrupt. To top it all, there was no agency to deal with health. Various aspects of the public health were the responsibility of diverse authorities. This was the situation that existed when the reform of local government was undertaken after 1830, and it provided the context within which the movement for sanitary reform took its origin.

HEALTH IN NATIONAL POLICY. In the more advanced countries of the world today, the health of the people has become a major concern of government, and the provision of services for the promotion and maintenance of health is a fundamental part of an impressive edifice of social services. This concern finds expression in the concept of national or community health and is the product of a long period of evolution.

Taking as a point of departure the mercantilist position in relation to health, a few far-seeing men had been led in the seventeenth century to adumbrate the idea of health as a significant element of national policy. On a theoretical plane, this idea had been developed in varying degree in different countries. However, owing to lack of knowledge and administrative machinery, it had nowhere been possible to develop and to implement a health policy on a national basis. While this goal was not actually achieved until the late nineteenth century, significant advances in this direction were made during the period under scrutiny. The most characteristic developments are to be found in the German-speaking lands, in revolutionary France, and in Great Britain.

A HEALTH CODE FOR ENLIGHTENED DESPOTS. On the Continent, particularly in the German States, interest in health as a question of public policy entered upon a new stage of development during the second half of the eighteenth century through the creation of a concept of medical police. Influenced by the doctrines of political philosophers and the theoreticians of police science, physicians adopted the police concept and began to apply it to health problems. As far as is known, the term "medical police" was first employed in 1764 by Wolfgang Thomas Rau (1721–1772). The idea of medical police, that is, the creation of a medical policy by government and its implementation through administrative regulation, rapidly achieved popularity. Efforts were made to apply this concept to the major health problems of the period, which reached a high point in the work of Johann Peter Frank (1748–1821) and Franz Anton Mai (1742–1814).

Frank is best known at present as a pioneer in public health and social medicine, although among his contemporaries his reputation was based to an equal if not greater degree on his activities as a clinician, medical educator, and hospital administrator, and this reputation was, indeed, well deserved. In 1766, he had already conceived a plan to write a book on all the measures to be taken by government for the protection of the public health, that is, on medical police. The first volume of this work appeared in 1779; the sixth and last was published in 1817.

Carrying out the idea that the health of the people is the responsibility of the state, Frank presented a system of public and private hygiene, worked out in minute detail and based on enormous erudition and rich practical experience. A spirit of enlightenment and humanitarianism is clearly perceptible throughout the entire work, but as might be expected from a public medical official who spent his life in the service of various absolute rulers, great and small, the exposition serves not so much for the instruction of the people, or even of physicians, as for the guidance of the officials who are supposed to regulate and supervise for the benefit of society all the spheres of human activity, even those most personal. Frank is a representative of enlightened despotism. The modern reader may, in many instances, be repelled by his excessive reliance on legal regulation, and by the minuteness of detail with which Frank worked out his proposals, especially in questions of individual, personal hygiene. Nonetheless, he clearly realized that regulation and police intervention have their limits.

To summarize Frank's *System* is no simple task. Nevertheless, by making use of the womb to tomb arrangement, which he employed, as well as some of the categories of modern public health practice, it is possible to give some impression of the entire work. Population policy was a matter of high concern in the eighteenth century, and the *System* appropriately opens with a consideration of population. This introduction on the general problems of population is followed by a detailed consideration of procreation, marriage, and pregnancy. According to Frank, it was the duty of public officials to promote marriage. As part of such a program, he proposed a bachelor tax, a suggestion that has been realized in our time. As far as possible, Cupid should have the assistance of the law. Frank was imbued also with the importance of training and education for marriage. From marriage, he logically turns his attention to pregnancy. Insisting that all labors be attended by a trained person, he urged that the midwife be consulted prior to the expected date of confinement. Among other measures, he proposed legislation to enforce a reasonable period of bed rest during the puerperium, and to free the mother for several weeks from any work in or outside the house, which might prevent her from giving the necessary attention to her child. When necessary, the state should support the mother for the first six weeks after the delivery.

Problems of infant and child health are considered next. It is not possible here to deal with the multifarious details of the child welfare program outlined by Frank. However, mention must be made of the discussion of the care of school children and the necessary police supervision of educational institutions. With his customary thoroughness, Frank covers the welfare of school children, ranging from accident prevention to mental hygiene, and from the lighting, heating, and ventilation of school rooms to athletics.

In the third volume of his *System*, Frank turns to the hygiene of food, clothing, recreation, and housing, including sanitation. Food is considered in even greater detail than maternal and child health. Each item of the diet is followed from its point of origin till it reaches the consumer's table. En route, various relevant topics, such as the animal diseases that contraindicate the use of flesh for food, as well as others, not quite so relevant, are discussed and debated. Problems of sanitation are considered in relation to housing, sewage and garbage disposal, and water supply. In considering the hygiene of communities, Frank insisted that municipal authorities had no more vital task than that of keeping cities and towns clean. For the disposal of garbage and refuse, he urged the establishment of dumping grounds at a considerable distance from the town. He also pointed to the need for public comfort stations and for building and locating toilets that would not contaminate any sources from which drinking water was obtained.

In the fourth and fifth volumes, Frank turned to several problems that today, for the most part, are treated separately from public health. Of considerable interest, however, is his discussion of accidents and his position that many accidents are preventable. From this premise, he concludes that the health authorities should initiate a program to deal with the factors responsible for such occurrences. In fact, in this area, contemporary public health is just realizing the importance of the problem of accident prevention.

In addition to the six volumes mentioned, three supplementary volumes appeared in 1822, 1825, and 1827, respectively. Among other topics, these volumes deal with vital statistics, military medicine, venereal disease, hospitals, and epidemic and communicable diseases. Difficult as it is to summarize a work as vast as Frank's *System*, it is clear that he achieved his objective of formulating and presenting systematically a coherent, comprehensive health policy.

The publication of Frank's *Medicinische Polizey* exerted an unusually strong influence, and the work helped to spread the idea of medical police beyond the borders of the German States. It was among German officials and physicians that the greatest interest was aroused. This impact is most significantly revealed in the draft of a health code submitted to the government of the Palatinate in 1800 by Franz Anton Mai, physician and humanitarian, who throughout his career was active in proposing measures to improve the health of his countrymen. The scope of Mai's code is as broad as that of Frank's treatise. Composed in 1800, it was approved by the Elector, the medical faculty of the University of Heidelberg, and the medical officials of Mannheim. Nevertheless, Mai's proposal was not realized, due in considerable measure to political conditions, the alarms and excursions of war, and the ineffectual character of government in the German States in the early nineteenth century. Nonetheless, its value resides in the effort to put into practice what Frank preached—the creation of an integral code of law governing all aspects of health and intended not only to maintain but positively to promote health.

The topics covered by the code indicate its comprehensive character. These include hygiene of housing and of the atmosphere, hygiene of food and drink, medical aspects of recreation, hygiene of clothing, the health of various occupational groups, health and welfare of mothers and children, accident prevention, first aid, prevention and control of communicable disease, both human and animal, organization of medical personnel and provision of medical care, and health education. Mai placed great emphasis on education, not only of the people but also of physicians and other medical attendants. He felt that doctors, midwives, and others who dealt with questions of health and disease were the logical health educators. In fact, the first section of the code, dealing with the duties of a health officer, proposed that this official instruct either the children in the schools or their teachers in the maintenance and promotion of health. Furthermore, the health officer would enlighten adolescents on the danger of sexual excesses. As one reads this section, it appears that Mai intended the health officer to be a kind of community health educator who would provide instruction in health matters for young couples about to marry, for wandering students and journeymen, and such other groups or individuals as might require it.

The achievements of Frank and Mai represent the high point in the development, exploration, and attempted application of the idea of medical police. Seen in retrospect, however, the imposing concept of medical police was already hollow when peace and more settled conditions returned after Napoleon's downfall. Theory notwithstanding, the social purposes and ends of medical police were already outmoded and reactionary. During the early decades of the nineteenth century, this concept was an ideological superstructure set upon the crumbling foundations of absolutism and mercantilism. In short, to undertake to apply this concept to the health problems of the new industrial society was to offer a solution in terms of a remedy even then ready to be discarded.

This does not mean, however, the denial of any important achievements and permanent effects to the idea of medical police. For one, the development and exploration of the concept of medical police was a pioneer endeavor in the systematic analysis of the health problems of community life. Secondly, a definite body of knowledge was collected and these efforts stimulated further study of such problems. To France and England, however, fell the task of developing, under the new conditions of the early and middle nineteenth century, the fundamental problems of health organization defined by Johann Peter Frank and the other workers who created the concept of medical police. It was in these countries that health policies were first developed and applied on a national scale.

HEALTH AND THE RIGHTS OF MAN. There were good reasons for the enthusiasm with which the French people welcomed the States-General in 1789. Here was an opportunity to air grievances that had accumulated during two centuries of arbitrary rule and to deal with problems clamoring for solution. By the last decade of the eighteenth century, it was obvious to many Frenchmen that profound changes were needed to deal effectively with problems of health and welfare.

The Constituent Assembly, the first of the revolutionary governments, faced a twofold task, to liquidate the old regime and, at the same time, to construct the new France. The Declaration of the Rights of Man promulgated by the

Assembly abolished the privileges of the *ancien régime*, and it proclaimed the freedom and equality of the individual and the sovereignty of the nation and the law. How could these general principles be turned into specific acts? In this spirit, the physician members of the Assembly wished to reconstruct the health system just as the other deputies were intent on rebuilding the political structure of the state. On September 12, 1790, on a motion by Joseph Ignace Guillotin (1738–1814), the physician after whom the guillotine is named, the Constituent Assembly created a Health Committee (*Comité de salubrité*). In his motion, Guillotin demanded that medical practice, teaching, forensic medicine, health police and sanitary services in city and country, epidemic diseases, and even animal diseases should all be controlled by a Health Commission. The Committee, which was set up, was charged to look into all matters "relating to the art of healing, and its teaching, to health establishments in city and country, such as schools and the like, and in general to all subjects likely to be of interest for the public health." As part of the work of the Health Committee, Jean Gabriel Gallot (1743–1794), its secretary, in 1790 laid before the Constituent Assembly a plan for the complete reorganization of the medical system, as well as a plan for the erection of hospitals in the country. However, the Assembly adjourned without having taken any action and left to its successor the task of fulfilling this duty.

The Legislative Assembly, which had been set up under the constitution of 1791, merged the Health Committee with the Committee on Mendicity to form a Committee of Public Assistance. Although one section of the new committee was concerned with public health, it paid more attention to the provision of assistance, inclusive of medical care, to the needy. Under the Convention, the need to overcome foreign foes, internal anarchy, and civil war absorbed the energies and attention of the revolutionary government. Nonetheless, the Convention recognized the obligation of the state to protect the health of its citizens.

In 1791, Rochefoucauld-Liancourt, chairman of the Committee on Mendicity, had presented to the Constituent Assembly a plan for a national system of social assistance. Liancourt recognized full well the important role of sickness as a cause of indigency, and his plan specified that each rural district would have a physician or surgeon appointed by the department, who would care for the indigent, supervise the health of children receiving assistance, and perform some of the duties of a local health officer. At stipulated times, they would inoculate the children and adults on their panels against smallpox. In the event of serious or epidemic disease, they would report to the welfare bureau of the district or department and request consultation from physicians attached to these bodies. Each year these district physicians would be required to report to the district office their observations and reflections on the climate and the soil, on the epidemics that had occurred, and on the treatment of these diseases, and they also had to make a comparison of births, marriages, and deaths.

In 1793 and 1794, the Convention passed a series of laws that established a national system of social assistance, including medical care. As part of this system each district was to have three medical practitioners who would perform some of the functions envisaged by Liancourt. Application of these laws was incomplete, however, for the available resources were limited, and those available were more urgently needed to provide the sinews of war. Following the downfall of the Robespierrists in Thermidor, the Convention and then the Directory retreated from this policy.

Further steps to create a nationwide system of public health began early in the nineteenth century. Up to the eighteenth century, French cities and towns had boards of health (*bureaux de santé*) that dealt with epidemic outbreaks. In 1802, however, Dubois, the Paris prefect of police who was responsible for public health administration, at the suggestion of Cadet-Gassicourt, a well-known hygienist, organized a health council (*conseil de salubrité*) to serve in an advisory capacity. Originally composed of four members, the number was increased to seven in 1807, and additional members were added in later years. The function of the council was to study public health problems referred to it by the administrative authorities and to make recommendations as to actions that should be taken. The Paris council covered a wide range of problems: sanitation of markets, dissection halls, public baths, sewers and cesspits, prison conditions, first aid for victims of drowning or asphyxiation, medical statistics, industrial health, epidemics, and adulteration of food. From 1829 to 1839, the Council dealt with 443 problems.

The Parisian example did not evoke any immediate response in other towns. Slowly, however, as the impact of industrialism came to be felt in urban life, a few cities began to set up similar councils: Lyon in 1822, Marseille in 1825, Lille and Nantes in 1828, Troyes in 1830, and Rouen and Bordeaux in 1831. In some departments, local district councils were set up. This spontaneous movement did not, however, lead to the formation of a national system at this time. In 1822, the French government created a superior health council of 12 members to advise the minister of commerce on health matters. This body never amounted to much, and it was not until the revolution of 1848 that a national system of public health administration was established in France. In 1793, the triumph of the machine and the concentration of capital were still in the future, but it was in terms of the situation created by these developments that the men of 1848 endeavored to apply the ideas of their predecessors to the organization of community health.

A PAROCHIAL HEALTH POLICY. During the latter part of the eighteenth and early nineteenth centuries, community health problems in Great Britain continued to be handled by local authorities. Local government was carried on by the counties and by the parishes into which the counties were divided. These administrative units provided the frame of reference for thought and action in matters of community health. Indeed, the outstanding feature of internal British administration during this period was its intensely parochial character. This had important consequences for the development of public health, since there was no machinery to subordinate the interests of the parish to the welfare of the larger community.

The state was not entirely oblivious or indifferent to matters of health in the eighteenth century. Experts were consulted when epidemics threatened the country, as in the instance of Richard Mead (1673–1754), who in his *Short Discourse concerning Pestilential Contagion and the Methods used to prevent* it, published in 1720, advised the English government on methods of dealing with plague should it spread from France, where there was then an epidemic. Although only trivial financial contributions were made to medical institutions, it helped them with some of their legal problems. In nineteenth century Ireland, for example, laissez-faire notwithstanding, Parliament authorized the grand juries to make presentments for hospitals and dispensaries and made contributions to them from the national treasury.

There was no central administrative agency to deal with health problems on a national scale, nor was there any accepted policy upon which an organized health program might be based. This does not mean that such ideas were absent. Adam Smith, in the *Wealth of Nations* (1776), makes a cursory comment indicating that he would have favored health legislation had he known of effective techniques for dealing with health problems. Even more significant is the proposal made by Jeremy Bentham in 1820 in his *Constitutional Code,* the great project for a practical Utopia on which he spent the final years of his life. He proposed a cabinet of 14 members, among whom there would be a Minister for Health, who would deal with environmental sanitation, communicable diseases, and also the administration of medical care. While Bentham's idea did not come to fruition at this time, it foreshadowed the future. Bentham was a massive influence on the leaders of sanitary reform in England, on Edwin Chadwick, Southwood Smith, and others who would create public health in the sense that we know it today. Bentham was favorably impressed with the French system of administration that had arisen following the Revolution, a system that carried on the policy of centralization developed under the Old Regime but in a more efficient way. This administration contrasted favorably with the illogical patchwork of jurisdictions that made up English local government and with the inefficient and sometimes chaotic efforts of local officials who in complete independence of the central government dealt with public health and other vital social services. Bentham died in 1832, and his disciples lost no time in implementing his ideas.

THE BOOKKEEPING OF LIFE AND DEATH. When Bentham set up his hypothetical government in 1820, he took care to provide a Central Statistical Office. At this time, the significance of statistical information was generally recognized as a result of developments that had occurred over the preceding 70 or 80 years.

The need for accurate numerical data concerning the people of a country was increasingly recognized in the eighteenth century, and efforts were made by several European states to determine the numbers of their populations and their characteristics. It was Sweden that first gave political arithmetic a solid basis through the collection of official population statistics. Based upon a study by Per Elvius, mathematician and secretary to the Swedish Academy of Science, legislation was approved in 1748 requiring the parish clergy to prepare tabular records of the population. These tables were eventually sent to the central government where they were condensed into a general summary for the entire country. This summary was prepared by a committee which, in 1756, was made a permanent agency called the Tabular Commission. Its most active member was Per Wargentin, who, in 1766 published mortality tables for the nine years 1756 to 1763. Based on observation of the living population as well as on deaths, these were the first mortality tables for an entire country.

It should also be noted that the Constitution of the United States provided for a decennial census, and that the first census was carried out in 1790 by direct enumeration. Censuses had been taken even earlier in specific colonies, for example, in Connecticut in 1756 and in Massachusetts in 1764.

Britain and the German States lagged behind Sweden and France in the official collection of official statistics. In England, various private individuals continued to make observations on vital statistics and to calculate estimates of population. On the basis of such data, mortality tables were constructed. Among the best known of these are the Northampton Table of Richard Price and the Carlisle Mortality Table drawn up by Joshua Milne upon John Heysham's study of vital statistics at Carlisle. Private efforts to collect and compare vital statistics also characterize the situation in the German States. While official censuses were undertaken quite regularly, as in Prussia under Frederick II, and the clergy were required to maintain registers of births, deaths, and marriages, these materials were not subjected to analysis by any public agency. In 1741, Johann Peter Süssmilch (1707–1767), a Prussian pastor published a large collection of German and foreign data, a work that is actually a rather complete compendium of the statistical literature available at the times.

Knowledge in this field was still vague and not precise. This situation was due not only to the inadequacy of the available data, but also to a lack of proper methods for dealing with them. A modern work on statistics is concerned in large measure with methods of evaluating errors of sampling, that is, with techniques that will enable the investigator to test the data thoroughly for bias so that this factor may be taken into account in any inferences to be drawn from the material. In the eighteenth century, however, such methods were not applied; in fact, they were just beginning to be developed. An important step in this direction was taken by Laplace, the famous mathematician. In 1786, he proposed to estimate the French population from the birthrates in a selected group of ressperative districts. Furthermore, Laplace outlined a method for assessing the accuracy of the result by determining the probable limits of the deviation from the true numbers.

This important contribution by Laplace was not, however, the first attempt to apply more precise mathematical methods to vital phenomena. The merits of variolation against smallpox provided the subject matter for heated controversy during the greater part of the eighteenth century, and it was in relation to this practice that the first attempts were made to determine by statistical means the value of a prophylactic measure. The most significant approach was made in 1760 by the mathematician Daniel Bernoulli. In an essay communicated to the Royal Academy of Science in Paris, he undertook to analyze the mortality caused by smallpox and to show the advantages of inoculation as a preventive measure. Bernoulli endeavored to determine how many years would be added to the average life span if smallpox were eliminated as a cause of death; in short, he was concerned with the mathematical problem of obtaining a measure of the influence of a specific disease on the duration of life.

The last years of the eighteenth century and the early decades of the nineteenth century have all the earmarks of a period of transition. The era opened up by Graunt and Petty was nearing its close, but the curtain of time had not yet risen sufficiently to reveal in detail the period of Quetelet and Farr, which was to follow. Indeed, the very name "political arithmetic" was being replaced at this time by a new term, "statistics," which had first been employed in 1749 by Gottfried Achenwall to designate the descriptive analysis of the political, economic, and social organization of states. The purposes and ends upon which the concept of political arithmetic had originally been premised were now in large measure outmoded, but fundamental political, economic, and social upheavals, notably the French Revolution and the Industrial Revolution, were thrusting forward new needs, problems, and goals to be handled by statistical means.

As yet, there was no close contact between the calculus of probability and the statistical investigation of health questions. However, the importance of bridging the gap between these areas was recognized by Condorcet, the Encyclopedist and revolutionary, who spent the last months of his life in projecting a history of the progress of the human mind. In this paean to the unlimited perfectibility of man, he prophesied that preventive medicine would eventually lead to the disappearance not only of communicable diseases but also of those due to nutrition, occupation, and climate. Condorcet conjectured that the calculus of probability would be a powerful instrument. Condorcet's work appeared posthumously in 1795. Twelve years later, in 1807, his friend Phillippe Pinel presented a report to the Institut National in which he undertook to prove statistically the value of his "moral treatment" of patients at the Salpêtrière.

Despite the best intentions, however, the use of probability theory in the study of health problems made little headway at this time. Nevertheless, there was a continuing interest in a numerical approach to questions of health and disease. Fed by various sources, this interest provided a fruitful basis for the development of a new period in the late 1820s. Medical and socioeconomic trends and influences were involved in this process. Problems of epidemic disease and public health provided an important stimulus to a continuing interest in the numerical method. As the industrial system developed and spread, its effect on the mass of the people aroused increasing concern. This interest in the social problem created by industrialization was an important motivating element in fostering the statistical analysis of health questions. It had been recognized much earlier that health conditions were in many ways causally related to the socioeconomic environment. The problem now became that of explicitly connecting poor health with deleterious social conditions on the basis of numerical data.

In addition, other conditions were favorable to this development, particularly in England and France. Between 1801 and 1831, four general censuses were carried out in England, and, perhaps even more important, civil registration of vital statistics was established in 1831. Even prior to the passage of the Registration Act, its significance for the statistical study of health problems had been apparent to men like Edwin Chadwick and William Farr. Under the latter's direction, the quality of the enumerated data was improved and a solid basis for statistical analysis was created.

THE GEOGRAPHY OF HEALTH AND DISEASE. The survey method of studying community health problems is an important tool in the modern public health armamentarium. Nevertheless, it is no recent innovation, but rather the product of a development extending over a period of more than 200 years. Interest in the relation of geographic factors to health and disease goes back to Herodotus and Hippocrates. Despite this long tradition, however, it was not until the eighteenth century that this interest was channeled into the development of health surveys.

This development was most marked at first in the German language area of central Europe and then appeared in England, France, Italy, Spain, and other

European countries as well as in the New World. Several factors were involved in the process. One was political. Far back in the Middle Ages, surveys had been made for specific purposes. The Domesday Book, for instance, provided a complete review of the resources of the kingdom conquered by the Normans in 1066. Later, other rulers made surveys of the resources and revenues of their domains. Typical is the survey carried out by a German prince, Wilhelm IV, Landgrave of Hessen-Cassel, who ruled from 1567 to 1592. This trend was reinforced by the mercantilist point of view. Thus, a memorandum of September 1678, prepared by Gottfried Wilhelm von Leibniz (1646–1716) for Duke Johann Friedrich of Hannover and headed "Thoughts on State Administration," proposed the creation of a "political topography or a description of the present condition of the country."

This should include the number of cities, towns, and villages, as well as the total population of the country and its acreage. There should also be an enumeration of the number of soldiers, merchants, artisans, and journeymen, as well as information on the relation of the crafts to each other. Then there should be a listing not only of the number of deaths but also of the causes, as in England. (Leibniz was influenced by Petty and Graunt, and the imprint of political arithmetic on his thought is quite clear.)

Other potent influences derived from the Hippocratic work *Airs, Waters and Places,* which was still a fundamental source of epidemiological theory, as well as from observations on the occurrence of diseases in different parts of the world collected by travellers. As Europe expanded in the Americas, Asia, Africa, and Australia, as scientific travel and colonial undertakings increased, there was a need for information on health conditions in these areas.

As a result, regional surveys or medical topographies began to appear. In Central Europe, such monographs were prepared by medical officers as part of their official duties. The medical officer in the German States was generally obliged to visit the towns and villages of his district, to examine mineral springs and watering places, to supervise the apothecaries, surgeons, midwives, and bathmen, to combat quackery, and to provide medical care for the needy. Various official physicians were instructed to prepare reports on their districts, dealing with such subjects as health conditions, meteorologic and hydrographic data, plants, and the mode of life of the inhabitants. Most noteworthy is a decree to this effect issued in Baden-Durlach on February 7, 1767. As a result, an increasing number of medical topographies dealing with various German cities or districts began to appear during the late eighteenth century. This trend was given even greater impetus by the publication in 1779 of J. P. Frank's first volume, and the appearance between 1792 and 1795 of the first medical geography by L. L. Finke (1747–1828 or 1829). The third volume of the latter work contains a manual for the preparation of medical topographies. This is of some interest as the first of its kind and because the next 50 years were to see an overwhelming production in this field.

Around the end of the eighteenth century, there appeared an increasing number of books and articles devoted to the diseases of particular regions. In 1776, Lionel Chalmers, a physician of Charleston, published *An Account of the Weather and Diseases of South Carolina.* William Currie, in 1792, presented a *Historical Account of the Climate and Diseases of the United States,* and Joseph Gallup in 1815 published *Sketches of Epidemic Diseases in the State of Vermont.* Other examples are Ludwig Formey's *Versuch einer medizinischen Topographie von Berlin* (1796), the *Observaciones sobre el clima de Lima y su influencia en los seres organizados, en especial el hombre* (1806) of Hipolito Unanue, and the *Topographie médicale de Paris* (1822) by C. Lachaise. It is not possible here to mention all the significant contributions, but in general, these monographs dealt with the physical geography and natural history of the region; food, housing, and customs of the inhabitants; and the relation of these factors to the occurrence of endemic, epidemic, and sporadic diseases. In 1830, for instance, a committee of the New York State Medical Society proposed a plan for a "Medical Topographical Survey of the State" and pointed out that since the chief object of medical topography is "to ascertain the influences of climate, soil, different occupations, and normal and physical causes, in the production or modification of diseases," attention must be directed to the age, sex, constitution, occupation, and diet of those most liable to be affected "by endemic or epidemic diseases."

These monographs combine epidemiological studies, sanitary surveys, and social investigations. As such they prepared the way for the more specialized surveys and analyses along those lines that were carried out during the middle and late nineteenth century. In terms of method, the work of Villermé, Chadwick, Shattuck, Snow, Budd, Panum, Virchow, and Pettenkofer derived from the medical topographies of the eighteenth and early nineteenth centuries. We shall see in the next chapter how and under what circumstances this tool was used.

ADVICE TO THE PEOPLE ON THEIR HEALTH. The didactic impulse of the Enlightenment expressed itself in an endeavor to enlighten the people in matters of health and hygiene. This health education movement was international in scope, and while it was adapted to suit local circumstances, its central characteristics were more or less the same in all countries—everywhere the same appeal to reason coupled with a belief in progress and perfectibility.

Illustrative of the many books and pamphlets written to further health education are S. A. Tissot's *Avis au peuple sur sa santé,* which appeared in 1762, went through 10 French editions in six years, and was translated into several languages, and B. C. Faust's *Gesundheitskatechismus,* published in 1794, which has already been mentioned. The latter was so popular that 150,000 copies were sold, and it was even translated into Latvian. In the United States, several periodicals concerned with health education were published during the early nineteenth century. The first of these was the *Medical and Agricultural Register,* established in 1806 and edited by Daniel Adams. It gave advice on personal hygiene as well as on agricultural matters; its life was short. In 1830, a group of physicians issued the *Journal of Health,* which ceased publication after four years. For the most part, it concerned itself with personal hygiene. In addition to such publications, there were numerous home medical guides. One of the most popular was William Buchan's *Domestic Medicine; or The Family Physician,* which first appeared in 1769 and then passed through 19 editions. Buchan was a Scotsman, but his work enjoyed wide popularity as well in the United States and was also translated into German. Southwood Smith, one of the most active of the English sanitary reformers, introduced the general public to a knowledge of the human body and its functions in *The Philosophy of Health* (1835). In this work, he made physiology the basis of a series of health rules.

Despite the earnest conviction, humanitarian devotion, and millennial enthusiasm that these apostles of health brought to this enterprise, it could be successful only to a small degree. For one thing, the spread of health knowledge did not, and could not as yet, concern the working masses in town and country. Scrutiny of the social context of the Enlightenment reveals it as a middle-class movement. The advocates of health education addressed themselves for the most part to the upper and middle classes, not to the peasants and artisans. Furthermore, the humanitarianism of the Enlightenment tended for the most part to neglect underlying economic factors. In Manchester, for instance, Ferriar told the poor "to avoid living in damp cellars," overlooking the fact that most of them could hardly afford anything better. There can be little doubt that the intellectual fabric of the Enlightenment is shot through with Utopian strands. During this period when the philosophy of history was imbued with and dominated by the idea of progress and the history of mankind was considered to be an unbroken ascent from barbarism to civilization, the concept that the rational ideals of the present are the realities of the future was entirely acceptable and logical. If to this sense of the inevitability of progress is added an expectation of human salvation from a revolution in social morality based on a rational way of life, as well as a desire to persuade others of the necessity and reasonableness of such a change, one begins to understand the great emphasis on education in matters of health and hygiene. Simply to demonstrate how to better conditions would in the course of time be sufficient to improve them. Nonetheless, these early efforts at health education are important because they helped to prepare the way for the health campaigns of the middle and late nineteenth century. Indeed, in this area of health education, there is virtually no break in continuity up to the present.

THE PREVALENCE OF DISEASE. Richard Mead, the English physician and hygienist, commented pithily that "as nastiness is a great source of infection so cleanliness is the greatest preventive." This is the point of view that underlies the emphasis on improvement of the environment, on education for personal hygiene, and, eventually, for sanitary reform. But how relevant was this approach to the major disease problems of the period? An answer to this question requires a picture of disease prevalence during the latter part of eighteenth and early nineteenth centuries.

The threat of plague still hung heavy over England in the eighteenth century even though the disease had disappeared after the dreadful visitation of 1665. But while the plague remained only a threat, other epidemic scourges claimed their victims at periodic intervals. In Great Britain, on the Continent, and in the Americas, smallpox was a continuing threat to the public health throughout the eighteenth century and into the nineteenth century. For Americans, the threat of yellow fever was equally serious during the eighteenth and nineteenth centuries. It struck again and again in the main ports, but the worst disasters occurred in the period following the terrible epidemic in Philadelphia in 1793. Charleston, Baltimore, New York, and New Orleans were all invaded, during the closing decade of the eighteenth century, and New York was again attacked in 1805 and 1822. "Fever" was another prominent scourge. Under this term were lumped together a variety of febrile conditions; today, we know that most of these were cases of typhus fever and typhoid fever. Toward the end of the eighteenth century as cities and towns initiated civic improvements, and the living conditions of the better-situated urban dwellers improved, the incidence of fever among them declined. It continued to prevail, however, among the poor, and toward the close of the eighteenth century as the first impact of industrialism began to be felt in England and epidemics appeared among the workers in the new factories, the problem of "fever" again came to the fore. In 1783, the first special fever wards were opened at the Chester Infirmary, and in 1796, a fever hospital was opened at Manchester. From 1800 to 1815, there was some decline in the incidence of "fever," but thereafter, the problem once again became acute.

Opinions concerning the nature and spread of disease continued to be held along much the same lines as in earlier centuries. Direct contagion, defect of bodily constitution, and climatic and terrestrial conditions were all called upon for an explanation. Contagionist and noncontagionist viewpoints alternated in the public favor, and during the early decades of the nineteenth century, the latter position had achieved dominance. The idea that animate organisms might be involved in the causation and propagation of contagious diseases receded into the background and played practically no part in the sanitary movement of the mid-nineteenth century.

VARIOLATION—LIKE CURES LIKE. Although smallpox, yellow fever, and "fever" filled people with terror chiefly because of the dramatic fashion in which they appeared, thousands of individuals, for the most part infants and children, were dying of scurvy, rickets, tuberculosis, whooping cough, scarlet fever, and diphtheria. Nonetheless, it was with the former that physicians and others interested in public health occupied themselves. Furthermore, one of the most significant and pregnant victories of preventive medicine was won in 1798 with smallpox.

By the beginning of the eighteenth century, smallpox was endemic in the cities and towns of Britain and the Continent and was a leading cause of death. It smoldered endemically in city and town, flaring up recurrently into epidemic outbreaks. The impact of the disease is reflected in various statements and estimates dealing with smallpox mortality, and its effects on the population. According to William Douglas, writing in 1760, smallpox was a chief cause of the high infant mortality in Europe. What this meant may be seen from Rosén von Rosenstein's statement in 1765 that "the smallpox carries off yearly the tenth part of Swedish children." In Berlin from 1758 to 1774, there were 6705 deaths from smallpox. Of these, 5876 occurred in children in the first 5 years of life. The London bills of mortality show that 50 per cent of all deaths occurred among children younger than 5 years.

In light of this situation, it was no accident that when a practical possibility of preventing smallpox was suggested it was tried. This possibility was first suggested in England in 1714. It had been known for centuries that an attack of smallpox almost always conferred immunity to subsequent infections. Based on this principle, an effective prophylactic procedure against smallpox had been developed and had long been used in various parts of the world, especially in the East. In this method, smallpox matter from a mild case was inoculated into a healthy individual so that a mild attack would occur; this would then provide protection against any severe attack in the future. The practice was first brought to the attention of English physicians by Emanuel Timoni (d. 1718), a Greek of Constantinople. This was followed by several other accounts. Medical men recognized their importance, but to the public at large, they were "virtuoso amusements."

There the matter stood until 1721 when the operation was furthered by Lady Mary Wortley Montagu (1689–1762). While living in Constantinople, where her husband was the British ambassador, she had had her small son inoculated in March 1718. In the spring of 1721, three years after her return from the Levant, a severe smallpox epidemic broke out in England. Lady Mary decided to have her 5 year old daughter inoculated and had the operation performed in the presence of several physicians, who were tremendously impressed by the result. A number of physicians, among them Sir Hans Sloane, advocated the practice. Popular interest was heightened when the royal family became actively interested, so that in April 1722, the royal children were inoculated.

With royalty setting the fashion, further impetus was given to the practice of inoculation. Despite such influential endorsement, however, the subject was soon embroiled in violent controversy. Two opposing factions developed, sermons were preached for and against the new procedure, and a bitter pamphlet war ensued. While most of the opposition was essentially irrational, the claim that inoculation could spread smallpox was correct. In addition to the danger of spread, there was also the disquieting fact that some inoculated individuals came down with severe attacks, some of them fatal. Despite the controversy, however, inoculation continued to be practiced.

In 1743, inoculation, or variolation, as it is also known, was advertised actively by James Kilpatrick, a physician of Charleston, South Carolina. Partly through his influence, and also because of the increased prevalence and severity of smallpox during the latter part of the eighteenth century, inoculation became a well-established practice. Voltaire was the most ardent exponent of inoculation in France. Despite his agitation, however, inoculation did not become a general practice in France until after 1750. The spread of inoculation to other parts of Europe followed a similar chronological pattern. Inoculation was introduced in Sweden and Denmark around 1754 to 1756, by the king in the former country. Because of its close relations to England, the method was introduced early into Hanover, where the first inoculation was carried out in 1722. However, it was not introduced into the other German States until later in the century. Frederick II of Prussia, for instance, arranged in 1775 to have the practice of inoculation taught to 14 provincial physicians.

As the practice of inoculation gradually came into favor in England and then spread over Continental Europe, a parallel drama was being enacted independently in the American colonies. Smallpox was introduced into the New World soon after its discovery. Thereafter, it appeared in waves from time to time in one or more localities, but its prevalence was never comparable to that in Britain or Europe. Nevertheless, the terror evoked by the disease was equally vivid. It was the need for informing the public regarding the nature of the disease and the means for dealing with it that led to the publication in 1677–1678 of Thomas Thacher's *A brief rule to guide the common-people of New England how to order themselves and theirs in the small-pocks or measles.* As in England, the need for an effective preventive was recognized, so that when the reports of Timoni and others appeared, the seed fell on a receptive soil in America. Two men, the Reverend Cotton Mather (1662–1728) and the physician Zabdiel

Boylston (1680–1766), both of Boston, introduced the practice. Mather had learned about inoculation not only from the English publications but also from slaves brought from Africa. In April 1721, ships from the West Indies brought smallpox to Boston. Mather proposed to the physicians of Boston that they undertake inoculation. Only Boylston responded by inoculating his son, Thomas, aged 6, and two Negro slaves, a man and a boy. The result of the trial was successful and Boylston proceeded to inoculate others. By September, he had inoculated 35 persons with no deaths. These events touched off a bitter controversy in Boston. Nevertheless, despite prolonged opposition, the practice was gradually accepted, and when Boylston died in 1766, he had seen inoculation come into general use, not only in Boston, but elsewhere in the colonies.

As early as 1722, the selectmen of Boston had insisted that Boylston should not inoculate without a license and the consent of the authorities. By 1760, legal safeguards regulating the conditions under which inoculation could be performed had been set up. During the Revolution, inoculation was practiced widely, and General George Washington ordered the entire American army to be inoculated. In this he was no doubt influenced by John Morgan, physician-in-chief of the American armies, who in 1776 wrote a *Recommendation of inoculation according to Baron Dimsdale's method.* Inoculation hospitals were established at various points for this purpose.

There is no question that inoculation had been shown to be of value in preventing smallpox. It was relatively effective in the American colonies where the population was less dense and proper precautions against spread could be taken. This was not the case in Great Britain. Except for the rich who could go to special isolation hospitals, it was agreed that the method could not easily be applied on a mass basis. To be sure, physicians such as John Coakley Lettsom (1744–1815) and John Haygarth (1774–1827) proposed means for making inoculation available to poor people. In 1798, however, Edward Jenner published his revolutionary discovery of vaccination, and the need to solve these problems disappeared.

THE COW POX AND A COUNTRY DOCTOR. Edward Jenner (1749–1823) was a country practitioner who had studied under John Hunter, the celebrated surgeon, and had then returned to his native Berkeley. According to his own statement, Jenner had long been interested in the relation between cowpox and smallpox. As a country doctor, he also practiced inoculation. In the course of his work, he found patients in whom inoculation would not take since they had already had the cowpox. Taking this as a point of departure, Jenner had the idea that it might be possible to inoculate an individual with cowpox matter from another person who had contracted the disease naturally; and then that matter from this individual might be used to inoculate other individuals, and so on. In 1796, an opportunity to try out this idea presented itself. Jenner inoculated a boy, James Phipps, with cowpox matter taken from the hand of a milkmaid, Sarah Nelmes, who had acquired the infection naturally. Then after several weeks he inoculated the boy with smallpox, but it failed to take—James Phipps was immune to smallpox. Jenner first offered his observations to the Royal Society, but the paper was refused. He then published his work in 1798 under the modest title, *An inquiry into the causes and effects of the variolae vaccinae, a disease discovered in some of the western counties of England, particularly Gloucestershire, and known by the name of the Cow pox.*

While the initial reception accorded to the *Inquiry* was not promising, it was not neglected for long. Confirmation soon came from Henry Cline, a London surgeon who was a friend of Jenner, and from George Pearson (1751–1828), a physician to St. Thomas's Hospital, who later opened the first dispensary for public vaccination. The new practice was rapidly adopted, and by 1801, at least one hundred thousand persons had been vaccinated in England alone. The spread of vaccination all over the world was astonishingly rapid, and within a few years, Jenner's *Inquiry* had been translated into the principal European languages. C. F. Stromeyer and G. F. Ballhorn in 1799 began to vaccinate in Hanover and by 1801 had performed 2000 operations. In 1799, too, Benjamin Waterhouse (1754–1846), first professor of the theory and practice of physic at the Harvard Medical School, received a copy of Jenner's *Inquiry*. Impressed with the new method of vaccination, he secured some matter from England and vaccinated his children as well as several domestic servants, seven persons in all. Waterhouse then extended the practice to others and in 1800 published an account of his work under the title *A prospect of exterminating the smallpox.* Thomas Jefferson was an active supporter of Water-house and contributed considerably in establishing vaccination as a public health procedure. In New York, Valentine Seaman was the first advocate of the new practice and in 1802 organized an "Institute for the Inoculation of the Kine Pox." Its purpose was to provide free vaccination for the poor.

Although vaccination was generally accepted, this did not occur without opposition. Some opposition arose from vested interests, such as the established inoculators. Other opponents had valid scientific objections. Some claimed that vaccination transmitted other diseases. Still others objected on religious grounds. Finally, when an attempt was made in England to render vaccination compulsory, the argument was raised that this would be an infringement by the state upon individual liberty. In the face of all this, however, vaccination fought its way to general acceptance.

A WORLD OF COAL AND IRON. Jenner's discovery provided a potent instrument for the control of one important health problem: smallpox. Nevertheless, the full import of vaccination for the conquest of communicable diseases could not yet be appreciated, and this would have to await the work of Pasteur, Koch, and their contemporaries of the latter part of the nineteenth century. However, numerous other questions of community health still remained to be solved, but these would be approached in terms of situations and needs created by the industrial developments of this period.

It is now a commonplace that the transformation in the structure of industry, which has become known as the Industrial Revolution, was not a single event that can be located within two or three decades. The essence of this transformation was the change in industrial production associated with the harnessing of machines to nonhuman and nonanimal power. While this change was drawn out over a long period of time, there is no doubt that in England the crucial stage in this process took place during the period we are considering. The introduction of the steam engine into industry and the development that resulted created a qualitatively new situation. By the 1830s, Great Britain had come under the domination of iron and coal, heavy industry had reached a high pitch of activity, and a new social class, the industrial workers, was beginning to express itself politically and socially. Thus, as the Age of Enlightenment became the Age of Economic Man, a welter of new and unsolved problems thrust themselves upon public attention.

The Industrial Revolution found England without any effective system of local government. Towns were not organized for any of the more significant purposes of administration, and the country districts were no better. Thus, while industry flourished and Coke-towns mushroomed, the health and welfare of the workers deteriorated. It was the discrepancy between this social fact and the prevailing philosophy of economic liberalism that brought into focus the need for grappling with problems of public health.

The sanitary reform movement of the nineteenth century, out of which public health developed, began in England because both the Industrial Revolution and its evil effects on health were felt there first. Nevertheless, wherever industrialism developed, whether in France, Germany, or the United States, the consequences were similar and called for similar remedies. The human cost of industrialization in terms of ill-health and premature death was great, and the sanitary reformers endeavored to reduce it by organizing the community to protect the health of its members. However, their approach to this problem was largely guided and governed by situations, ideas, and methods created between 1750 and 1830.

-VI-
Industrialism and the Sanitary Movement (1830–1875)

THE SATANIC WHEELS. ". . . black the cloth In heavy wreathes folds over every Nation: cruel Works Of many Wheels I view, wheel without wheel, with cogs tyrannic Moving by compulsion each other. . . ."

With bleak and bitter rhetoric, Blake the poet painted the driving machines that in his day were beginning inexorably to change the world he knew. With pitying mind and poetic vision, he foresaw the growth of industry and the attendant evils of a mechanical society. With this vision, he penetrated to the heart of the matter. Historically, the factor that played a predominant part in determining the development of the modern world, and with it of modern public health organization and activity, has been the rise of an industrial economy, the phenomenon to which Jérôme Blanqui in 1837 gave the name "Industrial Revolution."

As significant as industrialization was in the late eighteenth century, it was a mere beginning in contrast to what followed in the nineteenth century. Industrialized countries, such as England, France, and Belgium, introduced technical innovations in old industries and expanded them to new ones. At the same time, less industrialized countries, such as the German States and the United States, entered the field and by the end of the century were contending for positions of leadership with their older rivals.

Expanding transportation and new means of communication kept pace with the growth of industrialization. Road and canal systems were developed in most countries. In England, this development had already started in the late eighteenth century, and by 1830, there were about 20,000 miles of good roads as well as nearly 5000 miles of river-canal routes. France undertook the same task following the downfall of Napoleon. This was also the period of internal improvements, the great era of road and canal building in the United States. While such systems were being constructed, the "iron horse," the railroad locomotive, appeared on the scene to revolutionize transportation. As in so many aspects of industrialization, Britain was first again and by 1850 had more than 6000 miles of track in operation. On the Continent and in the United States, railroad building began in earnest during the 1830s. By the middle of the nineteenth century, the United States had 9000 miles of track, about 3000 more than Great Britain.

Industrialization was also furthered by the need for precision tools. As more complex machines were developed and introduced, engineers required efficient machine tools and increasingly accurate workmanship. Thus, progress in technology, the growth of transportation, and the expansion of the market led to the organization of industry in the factory system with all its advantages as well as its evils. Factories had existed long before the Industrial Revolution, and factory organization may be traced back in European history at least to the sixteenth century. Toward the end of the eighteenth century, however, factories began to increase in number, and in the course of the nineteenth century, the factory became the characteristic institutional form for the organization of production. The factory became the production center for machines, tools, and other articles of consumption. To the factory flowed the elements of production and from it went forth the finished product.

As the new industrial system grew, more and more workers were needed to man the factories. Steam power and the new machines could not be brought to the homes of the workers, as had been done with the means of production under simpler forms of industrial organization. Labor had to be brought to the factory wherever it was located, and it was in relation to this problem of the labor force that the question of community organization for health protection was to be raised and the means provided for dealing with it. Modern public health took its origin in England, because it was the first modern industrial country. To understand how this came about, we must turn to the foremost social problem that agitated England during the early nineteenth century, the problem of poor relief.

THE OLD POOR LAW. The Elizabethan Poor Law had laid upon the parish the duty of providing relief for the indigent. Each parish was responsible for the maintenance of its own poor and consequently attempted to reduce this burden as far as possible. It was believed that this could be accomplished by arranging to employ the poor. This approach was in keeping with the contemporary desire to stimulate national prosperity by using the unemployed poor in manufacture. Between the Restoration and the end of the eighteenth century, scores of books and pamphlets were written on this subject, and many projects were suggested to deal with the problem. The avowed aim of these projects was to create centers of manufacture in the form of workhouses where the poor could learn to support themselves. The first of these establishments was created at Bristol in 1696, and, during the earlier eighteenth century, there was a steady increase in the number of workhouses. While the enthusiastic belief in the efficacy of workhouses to deal with poverty was never realized, many of the plans and programs developed in this connection also turned attention to health problems, particularly the provision of medical care. At the same time, it must be kept in mind that, with the passage in 1662 of the Act of Settlement and Removal, the mobility of the laboring poor was severely limited.

However, despite various activities along the lines described, the problem of the laboring poor as a fundamental social and economic question remained unsolved. By the second decade of the nineteenth century, augmented by agricultural and industrial change, poverty and social distress were more widespread than ever. Nevertheless, the situation remained basically unchanged until 1834, when the drastic and revolutionary Poor Law Amendment Act was passed, ushering in a new period of thought and practice in relation to social welfare and public health.

MOBILIZING THE LABOR FORCE. The revolutionary changes in governmental structure and policy brought about by the Poor Law Amendment Act of 1834 were rooted in specific practical and theoretical considerations. The foremost social problem facing England during the first quarter of the nineteenth century was the organization and financing of poor relief. Assistance to the destitute was administered by 15,000 separate parishes, varying widely in size, population, and financial resources. Furthermore, to all intents and purposes, each parish was autonomous. Within this patchwork system of local authorities, annual expenditures for relief of the poor mounted steadily. From £2,000,000 in 1784, the cost climbed unceasingly to £8,000,000 in 1818, and still amounted to £7,000,000 in 1832, even though the price of bread had decreased by one-third since 1818. At the same time, the new industrialists felt themselves hampered by the "irrational" restrictions of a system handed down from a pre-industrial period. Mobility of the laboring population was an essential requirement for the burgeoning industrial civilization. The labor force had to be available in adequate quantity in the places where it was most needed, and consequently, the industrialists demanded a labor market open to the free play of supply and demand. This condition already existed to a considerable extent in the north of England. In the agricultural south, however, while the enclosure movement was driving the peasantry off the land, various obstacles still prevented the achievement of the desired goal. The rationalization of agriculture uprooted the peasant laborer and undermined whatever traditional social security he had. At the same time, the settlement laws tied him to his parish, so that some form of social assistance was required to relieve the unemployed or underemployed rural worker. The various forms of poor relief employed for this purpose helped to maintain a reserve of rural labor and prevented it from moving into the towns.

Naturally, such stagnant pools of labor and the system that produced them were anathema to the new industrial middle class and to those who voiced its interests and ideals. Since the system of poor relief was alleged to be the chief obstacle to a perfectly elastic supply of labor for industry, the remedy proposed was to do away with assistance to the able-bodied poor, and thus to free labor for economic self-interest. This approach was firmly rooted in specific theoretical positions, namely, the doctrine of philosophical necessity, the political economy of Smith, Malthus, and Ricardo, and the Benthamite philosophy of law and administration.

THE DOCTRINE OF PHILOSOPHICAL NECESSITY. The concept of philosophical necessity was based on faith in a natural order of society. The world of man was believed to be as ordered and regular as the Newtonian universe. Consequently, any effort to tamper with social processes was contrary to nature. The sharpest formulation of this doctrine in relation to the poor was expressed by Joseph Priestley. In his opinion, "individuals when left to themselves are, in general, sufficiently provident and will daily better their circumstances." Poverty and idleness ought to be governed by reason and necessity, and not by any legal provision for the poor, which could act only as an incitement to idleness. If government held aloof and permitted necessity to operate unchecked, material progress would result in decreased poverty and increased education, which in turn would lead to moral improvement. Consequently, any attempt to provide relief through the Poor Law was actually an obstacle to self-help, a sin against philosophical necessity, and an impediment to progress. Instead, the poor should be compelled to fend for themselves and stimulated to help themselves by being provident.

THE VIEW OF POLITICAL ECONOMY. The second strain of doctrine derived from the economic theoreticians of the new order. Political economy developed with the industrial age as the science that established and expounded the laws by which the new economic system operated. According to Adam Smith and the other political economists, the motive for economic activity was the powerful and pervasive force of self-interest. This motive, it was held, was guided by the force of competition and the mechanism of the market. Given free play, the interests of different individuals would thus be harmonized and would lead to a system of spontaneous cooperation. This would mean more productivity, and more productivity meant greater well-being. In short, as a basic principle, it was accepted that unfettered private enterprise was the mainspring of social progress. It was in this context that the Poor Law was regarded as a hampering, antisocial impedient to be removed so as to liberate the immense potential of individual initiative. Maximum self-help by individuals would do more to improve the condition of the poor than any legal assistance.

Nevertheless, this was not an ideal of freedom in a vacuum. It was recognized that desirable economic ends and harmonious relations between individuals were not likely to come into being without a firm framework of law and order. In other words, if things were just left to take their course, chaos and not ordered economic activity would result. Consequently, it was necessary consciously to create the environment within which such factors as competition and the market could properly function. Such a position implies that the hand of the law-giver and the administrator is the invisible hand that guides men in their economic and social action. This concept is at the heart of Jeremy Bentham's legal and administrative philosophy. The problem was to devise means whereby private interests can be brought to coincide with the public interest.

BENTHAM AND THE PHILOSOPHIC RADICALS. These ideas found their most potent and practical expression among the group known as the Philosophic Radicals, whose great teacher and prophet was Bentham. They were a small band of intellectuals who proposed to deal with public problems on a rational scientific basis. Their approach to specific political, economic, or social questions was hard-boiled, but curiously admixed with a considerable degree of naiveté. They contributed greatly to the development of the social sciences in their day, and on the basis of these studies called for a whole series of reforms. The schemes for which this group of highbrows labored so mightily included parliamentary reform, free trade, law reform, birth control, and reform of education. Even though a small group with little emotional appeal (in fact some of the group were heartily disliked by their contemporaries), they managed to put through a large part of their program. Directly or indirectly, the Philosophic Radicals exercised a profound influence on their contemporaries; and many of the far-reaching changes in the English government as well as in economic and social legislation between the 1820s and the 1870s were reforms of the kind for which they argued and fought.

ENTER MR. CHADWICK. Their opportunity came in 1832. Almost the first action of the reformed Parliament was the appointment of a Royal Commission to inquire into the operation and administration of the Poor Laws. Through the appointment of Edwin Chadwick, an ardent Radical and favorite disciple of the master, first as Assistant to the Commission and later as a Commissioner, Benthamite thought was brought to bear directly on the Poor Law inquiry. In Chadwick's mind, Bethamism and classical political economy were fused to produce a dynamic social philosophy ready to be urged to action by propitious circumstances. That Chadwick did not shirk his opportunities is evident even from a superficial examination of the history of nineteenth-century England. As *The Times* put it ironically in 1854:

"Future historians who want to know what a Commission, a Board whether working or Parliamentary, a Report, a Secretary of State or almost any other member of our system was in the nineteenth century, will find the name of Chadwick inextricably mixed up with his inquiries. Should he want to know what a job was in those days he will find a clue to his researches in this ubiquitous name. . . . Ask—Who did this? Who wrote that? Who made this index or that dietary? Who managed that appointment, or ordered that sewer, and the answer is the same—Mr. Edwin Chadwick."

THE NEW POOR LAW. The Report of the Commission appeared early in 1834, having been written by Chadwick and his friend Nassau Senior, the economist. The Poor Law Amendment Act, which became law on August 14, 1834, incorporated the principles of the Report and implemented them. The provisions of the Act may be divided into two parts, those concerning the principles on which relief was to be administered, and those dealing with the new administrative machinery it created. The principles on which relief was to be granted were openly deterrent. No able-bodied persons and their families were to be given assistance except in a well-regulated workhouse. In addition, the lot of the able-bodied pauper was to be made "less eligible" or, in other words, more miserable than that of the worst-situated laborer outside the workhouse. On the administrative side, the outstanding feature was the endeavor to secure centralization, uniformity, and efficiency. In place of the parish offices, the Act provided for three paid Government Commissioners and a paid secretary who would constitute a central Poor Law Commission. The body would issue orders and regulations to guide local poor law officials in the administration of the law. The unit of local administration was to be the union of parishes, and in each union, the law would be carried out by an elective Board of Guardians.

The significance of the New Poor Law as a focal point of social change can hardly be overestimated. The immediate objective of the Act was to reduce the poor rates, but its broader aim was to free the labor market as a precondition for investment. The market economy was asserting itself and clamoring for human labor to be made a commodity. This end was achieved, and it is no exaggeration to say that the social history of the nineteenth century was determined by the logic of the market system as established by the Poor Law reform of 1834. It was no accident that men began to explore the problems of community life with a new anguish of concern in the following decades. For the fact is that the setting of the labor market simultaneously broached the larger question of how to organize life in a complex industrial and urban society.

URBAN GROWTH AND THE PROBLEMS OF TOWN LIFE. A major aspect of this question was the organization of the community to protect its health. The problem of the public health was inherent in the new industrial civilization. The same process that created the market economy, the factory, and the mod-

TABLE 2

The Percentage of the Population of England and Wales Living in Urban Communities

Year	London	Other Urban Centers over 100,000 Population	Towns of 20,000 to 100,000 Population
1801	9.73	0.00	7.21
1831	10.64	5.71	8.70
1861	13.97	11.02	13.22

ern urban environment also brought into being the health problems that made necessary new means of disease prevention and health protection. It is significant that public attention was first attracted to these problems at Manchester, the first industrial city. Here a series of epidemic fevers had brought sharply to the notice of the community the significance of factories and congested dwellings as providing conditions in which such diseases could flourish and spread. During the winter of 1795, the spread of typhus, as we have seen, led to the formation of a voluntary Board of Health. Despite its multifarious activities and recommendations, however, opposition to and neglect of its program rendered the Board ineffectual. At the same time, as the nineteenth century progressed, the growth of unhealthy conditions far outran attempts at improvement.

This situation was generally true throughout the country. More and more English people lived in towns and worked in factories, and as this new way of life spread, health conditions deteriorated, leaving far behind any voluntary, piecemeal efforts to cope with the problem. Thus, between 1801 and 1841, the population of London leaped from 958,000 to 1,948,000; between 1801 and 1831, that of Leeds expanded from 53,000 to 123,000, and that of Huddersfield, from 15,000 to 34,000. What this meant for the entire country is indicated by Table 2, which gives the percentage of the population of England and Wales living in urban communities of various sizes from 1801 to 1861. This rapid growth was soon reflected in mounting death rates. Between 1831 and 1844, the mortality rate per thousand population of Birmingham rose sharply from 14.6 to 27.2; of Bristol, from 16.9 to 31; of Liverpool, from 21 to 34.8; and of Manchester, from 30.2 to 33.8.

The basic factor behind these bald figures was that the rapid growth of the urban population outpaced any increase in available housing. As towns shot up suddenly, the problem became one of packing in as many people as possible, as fast as possible, somewhere, somehow, anyhow. Especially in the older districts of towns and cities every bit of available space was built on, with the result that excessive densities became common features of urban communities. The interaction of several basic elements facilitated, indeed promoted, this characteristic development.

Financial considerations exerted a dominant influence on the mushrooming towns and cities, and this fact makes possible a clearer understanding of why they developed as they did. There was virtually no planning in any sense. Manufacturers erected factories in accordance with their requirements and as workers and their families streamed into the area, speculative builders ran up housing on any land available near the places of prospective employment. Housing for workers was thus built entirely as a commercial undertaking, which had to compete for investment capital with more remunerative alternative possibilities. Builders supplied a demand at a level that was effective and profitable and had no concern with the quality of the houses they created or with the needs of those who lived in them. The Select Committee of 1840, pointed out that despite the heavy financial burden it imposed on the community, inferior housing built back-to-back in congested areas was increasing constantly for the simple reason that it was profitable.

In addition, for large numbers of working people, there was in fact no real choice as far as residence was concerned. Over and over again, during the nineteenth century, evidence was produced to show that they were compelled to live in the congested urban districts because their employment was so often of a casual nature that they had to be on the spot or lose the opportunity of earning the pittance needed for subsistence.

Finally, social changes that accompanied the growth of urban communities tended to accentuate and to prolong overcrowding, congestion, and neglect of the poorer districts. As the new population crowded into any locality, those of higher incomes tended to leave the area to the newcomers. As the opportunity arose, they moved to other districts, frequently suburban and rural. These movements of population were facilitated by the new means of transportation. A Dundee minister, writing in 1841, noted that "the newly-opened railways offer new facilities for uniting the business of the town with family residence in the country, and threaten, ere many years, to convert Dundee into one great workshop, with the families of its workmen wholly detached from the notice or sympathy of the families of any upper class." Today, one of the most prominent trends in the distribution of population in countries like the United States and Great Britain is the settlement of people on the fringes of great cities and the adjacent rural areas, the creation of suburbia and "exurbia." It is clear, however, that this development is only the most recent form of a process extending back about a hundred years, which has been accelerated in our time by the introduction of the internal combustion motor. Beginning in the 1840s and 1850s a much more spreading city appears, and rare colonies of commuters begin to cluster here and there. However, this was only for the few who could afford such luxury. The less fortunate continued to live within the city, the majority of these in wretched slum districts. These districts were intersected by narrow lanes from which in turn sprang a maze of small and ill-ventilated courts. As a result, the workers huddled in a dense maze of tenements so closely packed that there was barely room for access to their doors.

Conditions were still further aggravated, however, by the prevailing assumption that provision for the various physical and social needs of the inhabitants would almost automatically come into existence. It was taken for granted that individuals would either make arrangements to deal with their needs, or that someone would be interested in dealing with them for pecuniary reasons or because of moral principle. The realism of these assumptions may be gauged by the circumstance that shops and saloons, especially the latter, were among the earliest public facilities to be supplied. Saloons filled the vacuum created by the absence of any other provision for recreation and relaxation. In this connection it may be noted that Manchester did not have a single public park until 1845, and the situation of other towns was similar. Indeed, it was not until the last third of the nineteenth century that much was done to purchase and to lay out public parks. For most of the nineteenth century, many towns were characterized by the excessive number of saloons that came into being under these conditions. Birmingham in 1848, for instance, had one public house to every 166 inhabitants.

At the same time, there was little interest in sanitary arrangements, since expenditures for such facilities were not considered remunerative. Furthermore, the infrequency of sewage and garbage removal, as well as the neglected state of the courts and alleys around which the houses were built, gave rise to the practice of using them as places of deposit for all the residents of a given court. As a result, there was scarcely a court that was not occupied by a communal cesspool or dunghill. Houses in the poorer districts had no water closets, and many had no privies. These conditions were not restricted to the homes of the working classes, but they were worst there. In "Little Ireland" in Manchester, there were two privies to 250 people. Nearby Ashton had one district with only two privies for 50 families, and such instances could easily be repeated for other communities. Instead of water closets or privies, there was a "necessary," a kind of tub that had to be emptied every morning. Even with this facility, the situation was grim. In one Manchester district, the needs of some 7000 people were supplied by 33 "necessaries," that is, supplied after a fashion. Since there was in most cases no access to the back yard except through the house, all the dirt and filth had to be carried through rooms, passageways, doorways, and over pavements, which were defiled as a result. This cloacal inferno was even intensified by the rapid migration during the 1840s of thousands of starving Irish who streamed through the port of Liverpool to huddle in the cellars and hovels of factory towns and cities like Birmingham, Bristol, Leeds, Manchester, and others.

The overcrowding in these dwellings can be imagined. Manchester had 1500 cellars where three persons, 738 where four, and 281 where five slept in one bed. In Bristol there were 2800 families, of whom 46 per cent had one room each. Liverpool had 40,000 people who lived in cellars and 60,000 in close courts as described. These figures must be seen against the background information that out of a population of 223,054 in the 1841 census, 160,000 belonged to the working classes. In short, more than 70 per cent were workers and more than 60 per cent of these lived in crowded, dirty, insanitary conditions. London was somewhat better than the newer manufacturing communities, yet it too had large slums where people lived under the most degrading conditions. Nor should one think that such conditions were limited to Great Britain. Equally dismal and brutal conditions were to be found from the 1830s onward in France, Belgium, Prussia, and the United States, in fact, wherever the new industrial system took root and developed. In all these countries, the response was similar—a demand for sanitary reform.

REDUCE TAXES BY PREVENTING DISEASE! As the new urban communities with their congested districts grew, more and more people became aware of their novel, powerful, and alarming qualities. Evidence of the effect of the new towns on health began to appear in England in the 1830s partly in statistical form as the information from the decennial census initiated in 1801 was supplemented by that from the compulsory registration of births, marriages, and deaths introduced in 1837. Attention was drawn to the condition of the towns as a result of several developments. The health of factory workers had become a matter of concern as early as the end of the eighteenth century, owing to a series of epidemics in Manchester. Parliament took up the matter, and in 1802, despite opposition, Robert Peel, himself a mill owner, secured the passage of the Health and Morals of Apprentices Act to improve the condition of the child workers in the cotton mills. While this Act was largely ineffective, it did establish the principle that the State had an interest in the health and welfare of the factory workers. Furthermore, the matter did not rest there. Agitation continued, but it was not until 1830 that the movement for factory reform, initiated by Richard Oastler and Michael Sadler and carried on by Lord Ashley, began to make itself felt. Following a study by a commission of which Edwin Chadwick was a member, the Factory Act of 1833 was passed, marking the real beginning of factory legislation in Great Britain. This movement and its consequences will be examined more closely later, but it is important to note that in the course of this campaign attention was drawn not only to the deleterious aspects of factory labor but also to the deplorable conditions under which the workers lived. In 1831, C. Turner Thackrah, a surgeon of Leeds, in his pioneer work *The Effects of Arts, Trades and Professions and of Civic States and Habits of*

Living on Health and Longevity, revealed that the deplorable working and living conditions prevailing in the city of Leeds were responsible for higher sickness and death rates than those of the surrounding countryside.

This interest in the condition of the towns was further strengthened by the cholera epidemic of 1831 and 1832. It soon became apparent at this time that the disease sought out the poorer districts, the places where sanitation was most neglected, the areas most befouled by excremental filth and other accumulated dirt. Furthermore, it was equally evident that the disease was not limited to the lower classes, and the conclusion to be drawn was quite clear. Without being his brother's keeper, anyone who valued his life felt it eminently desirable not to have virulent diseases and the conditions that fostered them too close at hand. In this light, therefore, the cholera epidemic might be considered a partial blessing in disguise, since it directed attention to the health of towns just when the problem was again becoming acute. The New Poor Law, however, provided the final stimulus, which concentrated attention on the health problems of urban communities. Filth, disease, destitution, and the demand for a reduction in the burden of poor relief are the roots from which the movement for sanitary reform sprang.

Unconsciously, the creation of the Poor Law Commission in 1834 also brought into being the instrument that was to open up fully the question of the health of the population and to provide the means for dealing with this problem. Chadwick was appointed secretary to the Commission, and while his interests and activities were directed at first to the limited goal of reducing the poor rates, he had a much deeper sense of the causes of pauperism. Among the members of the Royal Commission of Enquiry into the Poor Laws, he was the only one to investigate the health of the pauper population. Furthermore, he had a concept of preventive social action applicable to the problems of poverty and disease. Around 1824, Chadwick had become acquainted with Southwood Smith and Neil Arnott, two medical men who were also friends and disciples of Bentham. "From Arnott and Smith," he wrote in 1844, "I derived a strong conviction of the superior importance of the study (as a science) of the means of *preventing* disease, and I was the better enabled to perceive some of the important relations of the facts expressed by vital statistics which were brought before me in my public investigations." Recognizing that pauperism was in numerous instances the consequence of disease for which the individual could not be held responsible, and that disease was an important factor in increasing the burden of the poor rates, Chadwick concluded that it would be good economy to undertake measures for the prevention of disease. He stated his position frankly in a letter to Southwood Smith around 1848.

"The sanitary measures," he wrote, "had strictly and exclusively an official origin . . . they arose as a consequence, though an indirect and perhaps an accidental one of measures directed by Government in 1832, viz. the Enquiry into the administration of the Poor Laws; in the course of some investigations with the view to discriminate the causes of pauperism, excessive sickness, and its preventable causes were suggested by circumstances which appeared in the course of that enquiry and are noticed as one of the topics of examination in my report, laid before Parliament with others . . . afterwards, under the Administrative Commission, in 1838 when a heavy amount of claims appeared as a consequence of the prevalence of an epidemic, I felt it my duty to call the attention of the Commissioners to the preventable nature of the causes of a large proportion of these cases, and recommended a special investigation of them. . . ."

This approach was reinforced by Chadwick's "sanitary idea," his deep-rooted conviction that health was affected for better or worse by the state of the physical and social environment. In fact, before the crucial study of the sanitary condition of the population was undertaken, he circulated a letter of instruction to medical officers pointing out the need "to ascertain the existence and extent of the visible and removable agencies promoting the prevalence of such diseases as are commonly found connected with defects in the situation and the structure or internal economy or the residences of the labouring classes." Furthermore, Chadwick saw clearly that accurate statistical information could be exceedingly important in disease prevention. He tried to set up a Bureau of Medical Statistics in the Poor Law Office, and when the Registration of Births and Deaths Act was passed in 1836, he saw immediately and listed the uses to which it could be put. This list illustrates clearly how problems of pecuniary profit, disease prevention, environmental causation, and governmental action were all intimately intertwined in the thought of a leading sanitary reformer. Thus, Chadwick thought the Act could make possible: "(a) The registration of the causes of disease with a view to devising remedies or means of prevention, (b) The determination of the salubrity of places in different situations with a view to individual settlements and public establishments, (c) The determination of comparative degress of salubrity, as between occupation itself and occupation in places differently circumstanced, in order that persons willing to engage in insalubrious occupations may be the more effectually enabled to obtain adequate provision for their loss of health. (d) The collection of data for calculating the rate of mortality, and giving safety to the immense mass of property insured, so as to enable every one to employ his money to the best advantage for his own behalf, or for the benefit of persons dear to him; and that without the impression of loss to anyone else, (e) The obtainment of a means of ascertaining the progress of population at different periods, and under differing circumstances, (f) The direction of the mind of the people to the extent and effects of calamities and casualties; the prevention of undue interments; concealed murder, and deaths from culpable heedlessness or negligence."

It is within this context that the fundamental document of modern public health, the *Report ... on an inquiry into the Sanitary Condition of the Labouring Population of Great Britain,* appeared in 1842.

THE SANITARY CONDITION OF THE PEOPLE. In 1838, the Poor Law Commission reported to Lord John Russell, the Home Secretary, that three medical inspectors had been employed to look into the prevalence and causation of preventable disease in London, and they offered the opinion that "the expenditures necessary to the adoption and maintenance of measures of prevention would ultimately amount to less than the cost of the disease now constantly engendered."

The three physicians mentioned in the report were James Philips Kay (1804–1877), Neil Arnott (1788–1874), and Thomas Southwood Smith (1788–1861). Their collaboration with Chadwick at this time was no mere coincidence. All three were concerned with health problems in urban communities and were among the first to look into their extent and to reveal their nature to a wider public. At the time of the first cholera epidemic in 1832, Kay had published a brief pioneer work, *The Moral and Physical Condition of the Working Classes of Manchester,* in which he reported the results of a survey carried out among factory workers. In 1835, he had become an Assistant Poor Law Commissioner. Arnott and Smith were fellow Benthamites with Chadwick and had also been active in studying health conditions. Both were interested in fevers, and Smith had been on the attending staff of the London Fever Hospital since 1824. The latter had also been a member of the Factory Commission in 1833 and was to continue to play a very important part in the movement for sanitary reform.

Nor was it a coincidence that these men were interested in "fever," the portmanteau term that included typhoid, typhus, and relapsing fevers. The diseases in this as yet undifferentiated group had apparently subsided toward the end of the eighteenth century, but during the second and third decades of the nineteenth century, there were severe outbreaks first in Ireland and then in Scotland and England. It was observed that not only was the working population more severely attacked than other elements of the community, but that these outbreaks created an economic loss, which adversely affected the whole community. Over a seven-year period, for example, 12,895 people had been patients at the Glasgow Fever Hospital. It was estimated that each of these patients had lost an average of six weeks employment, which at 7s. 6d. per week totalled £29,004. To this had to be added the cost of medical and nursing care, which was about £1 per patient. When the patient died, there was the additional heavy burden of funeral costs. Moreover, widows and orphans were frequently left to swell the ranks of paupers for whom some sort of provision had to be made. It was this recognition of the economic and social costs of preventable disease, which provided the stimulus for action to better public health.

Efforts to deal with this problem were necessary and desirable on grounds of economy as well as humanity. This was after all the Age of the Economic Man. Discussing the impact of disease on the workers, the Select Committee on the Health of Towns declared in 1840: "The property which the country has in their useful labours will be so far lessened, and the unproductive outlay necessary to maintain and restrain them so far augmented." Furthermore, the Committee went on to say, ". . . some such measures are urgently called for, as claims of humanity and justice to great multitudes of our fellow men, and as necessary not less for the welfare of the poor than the safety of property and the security of the rich." In short, disease and destitution might be considered as part of the inscrutable plan of the Almighty, but when they injured or killed the worker and interfered with the sacred industrial machine, it was time for men to take notice and to act.

To investigate these problems and to provide a firm basis of fact for remedial action were the purposes of the famous sanitary surveys, both public and private, of the nineteenth century. The survey as a tool for obtaining information was well known and had been employed during the eighteenth and early nineteenth centuries particularly in the form of the regional health survey, or medical topography. It had also been applied to more specific purposes as in Howard's studies of hospitals and prisons, in Percival's investigation of fever among Manchester factory operatives, and in the examination of the old Poor Law. Furthermore, France as a leader in public health during the early nineteeth century produced several studies of health problems employing the survey method, which were known in England. In 1828, Pigeotte studied the health of textile workers in Troyes, and the same year Villermé's report showed that morbidity and mortality rates in Paris were closely related to the living conditions of the different social classes. Two years earlier, Villermé had published his study of mortality in different sections of Paris, which pointed to a definite relationship between poverty and disease. Chadwick and his collaborators took the survey and employed it to focus attention on the need for sanitary reform and to emphasize the importance of a systematic study of health problems as a basis for administrative action.

Initially, the surveys undertaken by the Poor Law Commission were limited to London. In 1839, however, the Government instructed the Commission to examine the health of the working population throughout England and Wales. Somewhat later the investigation was extended to Scotland. Over the next three years, a vast amount of information was collected throughout Great Britain. Detailed reports were obtained from the various Poor Law districts, and these provided the basis for the report published in 1842 on the sanitary condition of the working population. The final report of the inquiry was presented in three volumes, of which the synoptic volume, summing up the findings and proposing steps for remedial action, was the work of Chadwick. This document is no armchair production. It is filled with vivid details of existing conditions, and contains a serious effort, district by district, to correlate these conditions with variations in mortality rates and economic status. Most significant of all, however, was that the *Report* presented with dogmatic clarity a plausible epidemiological theory that fitted many of the known facts, and from this basis derived the principles on which sanitary reform and community health action in Great Britain and the United States, and to a lesser extent on the Continent, was based for the next 50 to 60 years. To the early public health workers, these principles constituted the law and the gospel of community health action, and for the most part they are as valid today as when they were first enunciated. Indeed, any health program in an underdeveloped country today is to a considerable degree based on the principles set forth by Chadwick more than a hundred years ago.

The report proved beyond any doubt that disease, especially communicable disease, was related to filthy environmental conditions, due to lack of drainage, water supply, and means for removing refuse from houses and streets. Attention was further focused on these problems by Chadwick's adherence to the theory that epidemic fevers were due to miasmas arising from decaying animal and vegetable matter. "The defects which are most important," wrote Chadwick, "and which come most immediately within practical legislative and administrative control, are those chiefly external to the dwellings of the population and principally arise from the neglect of drainage." Thus, the problem of public health was reoriented by definition. It was declared to be an engineering rather than a medical problem. Thenceforth, filth was no longer simply a matter for private disgust; it was raised to the status of an important public enemy of the community health. As Chadwick saw it, what was needed was an administrative organ to undertake a preventive program by applying engineering knowledge and techniques in an efficient and consistent manner. In the *Report*, he stated his position bluntly and without qualification. "The great preventives," he wrote, "drainage, street and house cleansing by means of supplies of water and improved sewerage, and especially the introduction of cheaper and more efficient modes of removing all noxious refuse from the towns, are operations for which aid must be sought from the science of the Civil Engineer, not from the physician, who has done his work when he has pointed out the disease that results from the neglect of proper administrative measures, and has alleviated the sufferings of the victims." It is clear, however, that Chadwick recognized the need for a physician to point out the location, nature, and course of infection in a given area, and in line with this idea suggested in the *Report* the appointment of "a district medical officer independent of private practice, and

with the securities of special qualifications and responsibilities to initiate sanitary measures, and reclaim the execution of the law."

THE HEALTH OF TOWNS COMMISSION. The immediate consequence of
Chadwick's *Report* was the appointment by Sir Robert Peel in 1843 of a Royal
Commission for Inquiry into the State of Large Towns and Populous Districts.
Its report was to public health what the Poor Law Report of 1834 was to public
assistance, and, as in the earlier instance, Chadwick played the leading role in
the work of the Commission. He drafted the major part of the first report issued by the Health of Towns Commission, and the administrative and operational proposals in its second report were his own. The Commission laid bare
for all who would see the appalling conditions that prevailed. Overcrowding
and congestion, poverty, crime, ill-health, and heavy mortality were shown to
be conditions commonly found together.

By this time the facts were not entirely new. In 1840, a Select Committee on
the Health of Towns had conducted the first general investigation of the subject
by a public body and had issued a report that struck with the force of novelty.
It had in fact been a prelude for Chadwick's report, and its recommendations
anticipated those of the Health of Towns Commission. The Select Committee had proposed the appointment of permanent boards of health in all urban
communities over a certain size, the appointment in large towns of an inspector to enforce sanitary regulations, a general sewerage act, and a general act to
regulate all future building. Furthermore, it suggested that within this general
framework special attention be given to the need for an ample water supply,
to the inspection and regulation of common lodging houses, the problem of
crowded burial grounds in populous areas, and the provision of public bathing
facilities for the poor.

After an exhaustive investigation, the Royal Commission presented two reports to Parliament, the first on June 27, 1844, and the second on February 3,
1845. These contained a number of recommendations to be embodied in new
legislation. Most important was a proposal to give the national government
power to look into and to supervise the execution of all general measures for
regulating the sanitary condition of larger urban communities. This proposal
implied, of course, the assumption by the central government of a basic responsibility for the public health, and it involved the creation of a new government department. The Commission further proposed that in each locality the
necessary arrangements for drainage, paving, and cleansing, and for the provision of ample supplies of water be placed under a single administrative body.
It also recommended new legislation to lay down regulations about buildings
and street widths. While the revelations of the Commission proved sufficiently
shocking to the public, there was no precipitate action on the part of the gov-

ernment to improve conditions. Legislation to implement the recommendations of the Commission was delayed in part for immediate political reasons,
and in part because the need to keep property inviolate imposed limits on the
extent to which reform might be undertaken.

Meanwhile, across the nation, the health of cities and towns, and particularly the welfare of the working population, became increasingly a matter of
concern. The reformers turned staunchly to the task nearest at hand. The revelations of the 1830s and 1840s led to activities of various kinds by a number
of different groups. Some of them even received recognition through legislative enactments of limited application. Among these voluntary groups were
the Metropolitan Association for Improving the Dwellings of the Industrious
Classes, and the Society for the Improvement of the Condition of the Labouring Classes, founded in 1841 and 1844, respectively, and both concerned with
providing better dwellings for the poor. Another was the Association for the
Promotion of Cleanliness among the Poor, which set up model bath-houses
in the east end of London. Then there were the organizations dedicated to
sanitary reform, whose objectives were to disseminate knowledge of urban
conditions and to organize public opinion in support of legislative action for
improved public health. Most significant of these was the Health of Towns Association, founded in 1844 by Southwood Smith, with Chadwick hovering in
the background. This group was particularly influential because of its membership, which included the great social reformer Lord Ashley (later the Earl of
Shaftesbury), Robert A. Slaney, who had in large measure been responsible for
the Select Committee of 1840, the Marquis of Normanby, and others.

These groups employed and developed further the approach and methods
initiated by the reformers of the eighteenth century. They created a pattern of
action involving the enlightenment and molding of public opinion, as well as
an endeavor to attract the attention of government to achieve remedial legislation. This approach to health problems was used by public health workers
throughout the nineteenth century and remains today an integral part of community action for better health. Essentially, these efforts represent early types
of community health education and organization, and it is important to note
that these aspects of current public health practice have their origin in the beginnings of the movement for sanitary reform.

A bill to improve the sanitary condition of urban communities had been
introduced in the House of Commons by Lord Lincoln in 1846 but had been
deferred owing to the resignation of the Prime Minister and criticism from
the Health of Towns Associations. A year later, another bill based on the recommendations of the Health of Towns Commission was introduced by Vis-
count Morpeth. Again no action was taken because of opposition from those
whose pecuniary interests were likely to be affected, as well as owing to weak-

nesses in the proposal. Meanwhile, however, the government was being forced to give way by pressure of circumstances, and to enact a number of legislative measures more limited in application. England was stirred by Chartism at this time, and the specter of a proletarian uprising, casting an ominous shadow on the middle-class mind, acted as a persuasive argument toward some degree of reform. Then, in 1846, Liverpool, where sanitary conditions were exceptionally bad, was suddenly confronted by an influx of hordes of starving and diseased Irish, fleeing the famine. Compelled by the emergency to seek greater powers, the municipality succeeded in having Parliament enact the Liverpool Sanitary Act, the first comprehensive sanitary measure passed in England. It gave the town council power to appoint a Medical Officer of Health (a most significant step to which we shall return), a Borough Engineer, and an Inspector of Nuisances. Other legislative measures concerned with urban improvement and enacted at this time were the Nuisances Removal and Diseases Prevention Act of 1846, the Baths and Washhouses Act passed in the same year, and the Towns Improvement Clauses Act of 1847. These legislative measures form a prelude to the Public Health Act of 1848.

At the same time, Southwood Smith and his Health of Towns Association were waging a strenuous educational campaign to arouse an informed public opinion to exert pressure on the government. Imbued with a burning zeal for social reform and a desire to get things done, Smith addressed himself directly to the English people to demand action. His pamphlet, *An Address to the Working Classes of the United Kingdom on their Duty in the Present State of the Sanitary Question* (1847), declared that "for every one of the lives of these 15,000 persons who have thus perished during the last quarter, and who might have been saved . . . those are responsible whose proper office is to interfere and endeavor to stay the calamity—who have the power to save but who will not use it. But their apathy is an additional reason why you should arouse yourselves .... Let a voice come from your streets, lanes, alleys. . . . That will startle the ear of the public and command the attention of the legislature." This appeal was one of the factors that influenced the government to push Lord Morpeth's bill. It was urged on also by an equally, if not more potent, propagandist, the cholera epidemic of 1848. Concern about the public health grew more tense as the year advanced, for by the summer the cholera was creeping closer to Britain. In June, it was raging in Moscow, and by September, it had reached Paris and Hamburg. In the history of public health, epidemics occupy a prominent place among the situations that precipitated action in the interest of the community's health. England in 1848 was no exception, and on the last day of August, the Public Health Act received the Royal Assent.

THE GENERAL BOARD OF HEALTH. Earlier efforts by local authorities to improve sanitary conditions had been hampered by the absence of a central agency to which they could turn for guidance and aid. This difficulty was now overcome by the creation of the General Board of Health. As the Public Health Act was to continue in operation for five years, the Board was limited essentially to a trial duration for this period. In view of Chadwick's Benthamite orientation and his experience with the Poor Law Commission, it is not surprising that when the Board was created in 1848 it followed the model of the Commission. Unfortunately, it was too much like the Poor Law Commission, both in structure and personnel. The latter, having become discredited, had been replaced the year before, with the result that the Board of Health attracted to itself some of the onus of hostility that had grown up around the Poor Law.

The final passage of the Public Health Act had been obtained by the usual methods of political compromise, with the result that it was enacted by Parliament in an emasculated form. For the most part, it was a permissive act, and it did not extend to London. The General Board of Health was empowered to establish local boards of health either when petitioned by not less than one tenth of the taxpayers or compulsorily when the average mortality rate in an area over a period of seven years exceeded 23 per 1000. Authority was given to the local boards to deal with water supply, sewerage, control of offensive trades, provision and regulation of cemeteries, and a number of other matters. To carry out these functions, each board was empowered to appoint an officer of health, who was required to be a legally qualified medical practitioner, as well as an inspector of nuisances, a surveyor, a treasurer, and a clerk. In addition, the central Board had some general powers to institute surveys and investigations of the sanitary conditions of particular districts.

EXIT MR. CHADWICK. The creation of the General Board of Health is a major landmark in the history of public health. Despite its brief existence and the handicaps under which it operated, the Board achieved much. Chadwick, Shaftesbury, and Southwood Smith were named to the Board of Health and proceeded to tackle the difficult problems confronting them with vigor and zeal. The report of its activities from 1848 to 1854 testifies sufficiently to the energy, determination, and intelligence with which the commissioners and their staff carried on their work. Several achievements of the Board may be mentioned. In 1851, sponsored by Shaftesbury, the first housing acts, the Laboring Classes Lodging House Act, and the Common Lodging Houses Act were passed by Parliament. Sewerage systems and proper water supplies were established in numerous communities as a result of the missionary work of the Board. Most significant of all, perhaps, was the establishment of the Medical Officer of Health. The example set by Liverpool with the appointment of W. H. Duncan (1805–1863) was followed by the City of London in 1848 when it appointed John Simon (1816–1904) to a similar post. During the next 30 years, a number of larger municipalities, under the provisions of the Public Health

Act of 1848, appointed physicians to such positions. Leeds appointed a Medical Officer of Health in 1866; Manchester in 1868; Birmingham in 1872; and Newcastle in 1873. Among these men were some of the leaders of public health, such as John Simon, during the latter part of the nineteenth century.

From the beginning, the activities of the Board of Health encountered the opposition of vested interests. Even its most elementary proposals for the improvement of drainage and water supplies were opposed in the sacred names of property and human freedom. Efforts were made to gain support for the activities of the Board, and Chadwick issued instructions to the field staff on how to win friends and influence people in local communities. As time went on, however, the Board became more and more unpopular. Too many toes were stepped on; individuals and groups whose interests were adversely affected became increasingly vigorous in their opposition. Fuel was added to the fire by the strong centralizing tendency of the board, due in large measure to Chadwick's influence. At a time when local government with its multiplicity of authorities was still widely entrenched, any attempt to diminish the freedom of local authority was bound to arouse antagonism.

In 1854, the tide of criticism rose so high that Parliament, despite the efforts of the Commissioners, refused to renew the Public Health Act and the first National Board of Health came to an end. Shaftesbury clearly describes the nature of the opposition and the reasons for this defeat. "The parliamentary agents are our sworn enemies," he wrote, "because we have reduced expenses, and, consequently, their fees, within reasonable limits. The civil engineers also, because we have selected able men, who have carried into effect new principles, and at a less salary. The College of Physicians, and all its dependencies, because of our independent action and singular success in dealing with the Cholera, when we maintained and proved that many a Poor Law medical officer knew more than all the flash and fashionable doctors of London. All the Boards of Guardians, for we exposed their selfishness, their cruelty, their reluctance to meet and relieve the suffering poor, in the days of epidemic. The Treasury besides [for the subalterns there hated Chadwick; it was an ancient grudge and paid when occasion served]. Then come the water companies, whom we laid bare and devised a method of supply, which altogether superseded them. The Commissioners of Sewers, for our plans and principles were the reverse of theirs; they hated us with a perfect hatred." Some idea of the point of view and temper of the opposition is evident in the comment of *The Times*, which had originally supported the Public Health Act and now led in condemning the Board. "Aesculapius and Chiron," it wrote, "in the form of Mr. Chadwick and Dr. Southwood Smith have been deposed, and we prefer to take our chance of cholera and the rest than be bullied into health." With the disappearance of the first General Board of Health, Chadwick was relegated to the sidelines. At the early age of 54, he was forced to give up an active career in public administration, and while he was able to see the realization of many of his ideas in the course of his long life, he took no active part in their development.

"HOW QUAINT THE WAYS OF PARADOX!" It is not our intention to examine in detail the further development of public health in England, although some of the more significant events will be considered later. Of basic importance is that the changes initiated in the 1830s and 1840s were underlined and carried further during the period after 1848. At the same time, there pushed into the foreground new currents of thought and practice, of which some were hitherto only latent, while others appeared in response to new problems. The two strains of laissez-faire and social regulations, which were present in Bentham's thinking and were applied by Chadwick to public assistance and public health, persisted both in theory and practice throughout the century, but the relative emphasis and significance given to these approaches shifted more and more to social regulation.

"How quaint the ways of Paradox!" observed Sir William Gilbert, and nowhere is this comment more apposite than in the development of social action in relation to public health. The paradox has two aspects, one medical, the other social and political. The former concerns the role of medicine in the development of public health. Objective analysis of the beginnings of the sanitary reform movement in England around the middle of the nineteenth century leads to the conclusion that medicine played a secondary part in this process. The impulse to sanitary reform did not come from the medical profession, even though some physicians played a significant part in calling attention to the community problem of ill-health. Furthermore, medicine had little real knowledge to contribute toward a solution of the major problem, which concerned the transmission of communicable disease. Contagionists fought anticontagionists, but the bitter controversy had little effect on the establishment of public health legislation and administration. Indeed, it is noteworthy that the program of the sanitary reformers was based to a large extent on a structure of erroneous theories, and, while they hit upon the right solution, it was mostly for the wrong reasons. Broadly speaking, what happened was that the founders of modern public health, accepting certain postulates of economic and social policy, established institutional forms that would serve later to implement more accurate and effective medical knowledge. Significant instances of such forms are the supervision of local health services by a central authority, and the position of the medical officer of health.

Consideration of these institutions, however, goes directly to the heart of the political and social paradox. It is indeed a striking phenomenon in modern history that the introduction of economic freedom, far from doing away with the need for governmental intervention, control, and regulation, eventually led to an enormous increase in the administrative functions of the state. The 1830s and 1840s saw an outburst of legislative activity abolishing restrictive regulations and social obligations prevalent before the Industrial Revolution; but even while certain forms of social regulation were being discarded, others were replacing them. While the Industrial Revolution was still in its infancy, Robert Owen had foreseen the need for state action to curb some of the consequences of economic freedom. "The general diffusion of manufactures throughout a country," he wrote in 1851, "generates a new character in its inhabitants; and as this character is formed upon a principle quite unfavorable to individual or general happiness, it will produce the most lamentable and permanent evils, unless its tendency be counteracted by legislative interference and direction." Owen's warning was soon realized, and, while the new Poor Law created a system of labor incentives for the new class of factory workers, health laws and factory laws were laying the foundation for centralized authority to promote human health and welfare.

In fact, the question of health serves as a focal point around which the doctrines of economic freedom and political liberalism can be seen in various stages of modification. This transformation did not occur simply because of the growth of humanitarian sentiment or of a social conscience. Legislation on health and sanitation resulted from a variety of forces within the social and economic order. It resulted less from a concern for the welfare of the poor than from a growing realization after 1850 that endemic and epidemic disease caused by defective sewerage or infected food was a problem of the entire community. Furthermore, there was an increasing awareness that the cost involved was a form of social waste that could be eliminated. "Sanitary neglect," declared John Simon in 1858, "is mistaken parsimony. Fever and cholera are costly items to count against the cheapness of filthy residence and ditch-drawn drinking-water: widowhood and orphanage make it expensive to sanction unventilated work-places and needlessly fatal occupations. . . . The physical strength of a nation is among the chief factors of national prosperity." No one did more to impress this lesson on his countrymen than William Farr (1807–1883), who had been appointed compiler of abstracts in the Registrar General's office in 1838, and whose statistical reports provided the ammunition used in the campaigns waged during the middle and late nineteenth century against disease in the home, in the factory, and in the community as a whole. That the lesson was learned eventually becomes evident from a letter written in the early 1880s by Joseph Chamberlain. Describing health progress in Birmingham, he wrote: ". . . what are the facts? A saving of seven per thousand in the death rate—2800 lives per annum in the town. And as five people are ill for everyone who dies, there must be a diminution of 14,000 cases of sickness, with all the loss of money, pain and grief they involve."

At the same time, while the organization of the labor market by the new Poor Law was maintained relatively intact, protective legislative action improved working conditions in mines and factories and mitigated the harshness of the early laissez-faire system. This legislation was not extensive enough to throw the system out of gear. In fact, as compared with the stigma of the Poor Law and its workhouses, factory life was a lesser evil. Nevertheless, these laws helped to undermine the prevailing social philosophy. Furthermore, the new class of industrial workers, taking seriously the democratic implications of liberalism in terms of human rights and human dignity, and recognizing the effectiveness of group solidarity, organized themselves in trade unions and political parties, refused to compete against one another, and took action to secure for themselves various kinds of social services, including the health services.

TWO STEPS FORWARD, ONE STEP BACK. Seen in retrospect these historical trends seem clear and straight, but the process out of which they are abstracted was not so smooth. What looks like a steady, even advance over several decades is seen under closer scrutiny to consist of hesitant piecemeal changes, ad hoc expedients, and compromises resulting from bitterly waged campaigns against specific evils. Communities undertook to remedy specific and glaring sanitary deficiencies without considering very far how these were related to other defects. Nevertheless, the thread of continuity is not an illusion, an artifact of the historian. It is a reality derived from the circumstance that throughout most of the nineteenth century health workers confronted substantially the same problems. The same undesirable characteristics that had been uncovered in urban communities by the classic investigations of the 1830s and 1840s were still being exposed 30 years later. While the experience and knowledge of health workers increased, they continued to preach the same reasons for reform and to urge similar remedies. In short, the fundamental doctrines of sanitary reform remained virtually unaltered because the conditions to which they applied remained fundamentally the same.

EPPUR SE MUOVE. Questions of sanitation and epidemic disease overshadowed all else in the minds of health workers during this period, but without effective administrative instruments it was difficult to apply even such knowledge as was then available. The Municipal Corporations Act of 1835 was intended to remedy the weakness of local government, but while the reformed boroughs were somewhat more democratic in their organization they were hardly more effectual than before in the improvement and sanitary regulations of the community. For one thing, the sanitary legislation enacted during this period was largely permissive. Powers were conferred on local authorities, but few carried any obligation for enforcement, nor were all authorities interested in enforcing them. Consequently, local improvements continued to be made on a piecemeal basis. As new needs made themselves felt, they were met most often by a succession of ad hoc expedients, which left untouched far more than they remedied. The general result of these developments in the middle and late nineteenth century was to produce a patchwork of authorities, each with a different set of local boundaries, and each responsible for a very limited number of functions.

While municipalities at this time never even came within sight of overtaking problems of community health, enough progressive change did take place to yield useful though moderate benefits. Several factors were responsible. One was the slow, hesitant, but nonetheless unceasing, evolution of a central health department. The three landmarks, which stand out in this process, are the establishment of the General Board of Health in 1848, the creation of the Local Government Board in 1871, and the passing of the Public Health Act in 1875.

Following the downfall of Chadwick and his colleagues in 1854, the General Board of Health was re-established on an annual basis and carried on its work until 1858 when its medical functions were transferred to the Privy Council by the Public Health Act of that year. During this period, the Board achieved several important advances. In 1855, John Simon was appointed medical officer to the Board on a salaried basis; he was thus the first of a long line of medical men who have served in this capactiy since that time, first with the Privy Council, then with the Local Government Board and finally in the Ministry of Health. In the same year the Board also secured the enactment of a bill that recognized for the first time that there were needs common to a large urban area, namely, metropolitan London. This measure set up the Metropolitan Board of Works as the agency to deal with them. In 1858, the General Board of Health was finally abolished, and the supervision of the public health was transferred to the Privy Council, where it remained until 1871.

The Privy Council was authorized to have its medical department investigate matters affecting the health of the community, and to prepare reports on such studies for Parliament. The post of medical officer was reaffirmed and John Simon was continued in this office. In this capacity, he prepared a series of annual reports for the years 1858 to 1871, which reflect with considerable accuracy the state of public health in Britain at this time. Among the problems with which Simon dealt were cholera, diarrhea, dysentery, diphtheria, tuberculosis, and occupational diseases of the lungs, diets of working-class families, hospital hygiene, and housing. Simon saw the health of the community from a broad social point of view, and he took account of such factors as congested housing, working conditions in factories and mines, employment of mothers, poor nutrition, indeed, the whole unfavorable complex of factors that characterized the urban industrial community of the nineteenth century. Limited though he was by lack of staff, Simon threw a searching light on the grim and gloomy picture of community health in Victorian England.

Finally, beginning in 1869, the next major steps were taken to deal with the administrative problems of public health. In that year, a Royal Commission was appointed to study the sanitary administration of England. Reporting in 1871, it recommended the creation of a government department combining the adminstration of the Poor Law and of public health, to which all health functions exercised by government agencies should be transferred. The first fruit of this report was the creation in the same year of the Local Government Board, under whose aegis were placed the Poor Law Board and the Medical Department of the Privy Council. The Commission also proposed the consolidation of all public health legislation, and that the local health agencies be made more uniform in character. These accommodations were implemented by the enactment of the Public Health Act of 1875, which first put some semblance of order into English public health administration on a nationwide basis. The Act divided the entire country into urban and rural sanitary districts, subject to the supervision of the Local Government Board. As far as practicable, the existing local authorities were fitted into the new pattern. Wherever there was a borough council, it became the local health authority, and the same was done with local boards of improvement commissioners. At the same time, it became mandatory for each district to have a medical officer of health. For the first time there was a reasonably coherent and adequate system of local administration capable of dealing with problems of community health.

Improvement during this period resulted not only from the creation of an adequate administrative apparatus. A second important factor was the existence of an alert and militant group of professional and lay people, who had recognized the nature of the various problems of urban life and were eager to see that they were corrected. For example, while the various Health of Towns Associations had rapidly faded into oblivion following the passage of the Public Health Act in 1848, they were soon revived in various places and endeavored to enlist public support for sanitary improvement. Thus, the Manchester and Salford Sanitary Association was founded in 1852.

To such groups may be added the first professional health workers, particularly the medical officers of health. Just over one hundred years ago, in 1856, the first health officers in London took steps to form a professional association. Under the Metropolis Management Act, passed in 1855, the appointment of medical officers of health had been made compulsory for the various London districts, and by 1856, 48 physicians had been appointed. In May 1856, the Metropolitan Association of Medical Officers of Health was formed. As the number of such officials outside London increased, they began to join the Association, which in 1873 became the Society of Medical Officers of Health. John Simon was the first president of the Association and remained in this position until 1861. Following the passage of the Public Health Act of 1875, there was a rapid increase in the numbers of medical officers of health. Among the first acts of the Metropolitan Association was to set up committees to inquire into drainage, the sale of unwholesome meat, adulteration of food, and the relation of meteorological phenomena to the state of the public health. The Association did not hesitate to let its voice be heard and was consulted by government departments.

As time went on, the effect of these influences became gradually apparent. A study made in 1879 showed, for instance, that most larger urban communities had obtained a constant water supply, adequate in quantity and possibly less in quality. Nevertheless, a great deal still remained to be done. By the end of the third quarter of the nineteenth century, however, the basic adminstrative work had been achieved, and with the enactment of the Public Health Act of 1875, sanitary legislation came to a virtual halt for many years. The succeeding period was one of consolidation in which public health workers concentrated on further improvement of sanitary conditions in areas where action was needed. The sanitary reform movement had sown the seeds and from 1875 to the end of the century the fruit ripened and began to be gathered.

URBANISM AND THE ORIGINS OF AMERICAN PUBLIC HEALTH IN THE NINE-TEENTH CENTURY. With the growth of the sanitary reform movement in England, and the creation of the General Board of Health in 1848, leadership in public health thought and practice passed into the hands of the British. The impact of these developments was felt in Europe and America. France, Belgium, Prussia, and other continental states were affected in varying degree, but nowhere was this influence more pervasive than in the United States.

As in other countries, epidemics were prominent among the situations that precipitated early action in the interest of community health in the United States. When these occurred, governmental authorities sought medical advice on the proper measures to be taken. Confusion regarding etiology and transmission prevailed, but control was based upon two procedures, quarantine and environmental sanitation. In 1795, for example, the Governor of New York appealed to the state medical society concerning an epidemic then prevailing in the upper part of New York City. A committee was appointed, and a report issued the following year. The recommendations contained in the report deal essentially with environmental sanitation, more specifically with such matters as "the accumulation of filth in the streets," obstructed water drains and drainage of low-lying areas, improvement of dock and river shores to prevent the collection of refuse, and the pollution of the air by such establishments as slaughter houses and soap factories. Effective implementation of these proposals was not possible, however, so long as there was no permanent health organization in the municipal government. Indeed, as in England, one of the basic problems involved in the genesis and development of public health in New York and other American cities during the nineteenth century was the need to create an effective administrative mechanism for the supervision and regulation of the health of the community.

During the first three decades of the nineteenth century, American cities grew steadily, if not spectacularly. Social conditions were generally favorable during this period, and problems, such as pauperism, were not acute. Reflecting this situation, public health administration was simple in organization and limited in scope. Between 1800 and 1830, only five major cities established boards of health. Even as late as 1875 many large urban communities had no health departments.

The character of public health organization at this time is well illustrated by New York City. In 1798, New York was struck by an epidemic of yellow fever in which there were 1600 deaths. Until then, the municipality had no authority to issue health regulations, but the need for power to meet such emergencies was recognized by the state legislature and the city was granted authority to pass its own health laws. The beginning of a permanent public health administration did not come into existence until the following decade. It may be said to date from March 26, 1804, when John Pintard was appointed City Inspector of Health. From 1810 to 1838, the health inspectors were a branch of the Police Department. The responsibility for dealing with health matters on a day-to-day basis, and for seeing that various laws and regulations were made effective, was shared by the City Inspector with two other officials, the Health Officer and the Resident Physician. The former, appointed by the state, was concerned with the application of quarantine laws to vessels entering the port. The latter was a municipal official whose function was to be on the alert for and to discover cases of communicable diseases within the city. Health administration, environmental sanitation, particularly in relation to the control of epidemics, and the collection of vital statistics were the areas within which the City Inspector performed his duties.

Some of these health officials were well qualified to deal with problems of community health. Successive City Inspectors recognized the value of accurate vital statistics, and Cornelius B. Archer, City Inspector in 1845 and 1846, secured the enactment of a law providing for birth registration. Thomas K. Downing, City Inspector from 1852 through 1854, succeeded in 1853 in having enacted an improved Birth, Marriage, and Death Registration Act. Nevertheless, the administrative machinery available was intolerably inefficient. For one thing, these positions were much sought after, and political machinations played a considerable part in the filling of the posts. As a result, the officials were often subject to political influence, and in numerous instances were highly incompetent. Furthermore, this situation was aggravated by the division of authority, for in addition to the three health officials there was also an advisory Board of Health, which recommended to the Common Council measures for dealing with health problems. Obviously, conditions of this kind did little to foster the growth of efficient public health administration. The resulting inefficiencies might be tolerated while social conditions were favorable, but the prolonged intrusion into such an unstable situation of profoundly disturbing elements was bound to throw into sharp focus the basic inadequacy of existing arrangements.

At this very time, profound changes in the political, economic, and social life of various European communities were setting in motion a stream of migration that was to upset with violent impact the situation that had obtained during the first three decades of the century. The terrific shock produced by the unexpected influx of swarms of impoverished immigrants was first felt in the seaboard cities like New York and Boston, where inadequate provision for the increasing complexity of such problems as housing, water supply, sewage disposal, and drainage soon brought into being a whole brood of evils that found their most characteristic expression in the urban slum.

As immigration and population increased, housing became a pressing problem. Cheap quarters were needed, and, as in Britain, the new arrivals found shelter in the older sections of the city in private houses, old warehouses, breweries, or any building with four walls and a roof. The development of cheap urban transportation facilitated this process as those with a higher income moved to new districts on the periphery. Within the old sections, no new housing was generally provided for the lower income groups until the 1850s and then came the tenement proper, which replaced converted dwellings and other makeshift housing in larger cities. The tenement was originally a multiple dwelling designed to provide cheap housing for the workers but soon became synonymous with slum dwelling. Throughout the nineteenth century, there was perpetual overcrowding. Such toilet facilities as existed were highly inadequate, and recreational arrangements except for the saloon were nonexistent. Small wonder that disease, crime, and immorality became problems of the slum districts. City life for a large number of people was sordid and unhealthy, and the significance of such conditions for the community as a whole could not be overlooked.

Meanwhile, contacts with Europe brought knowledge of what was going forward in other parts of the world. Facing slum conditions similar to those in Great Britain and France, Americans were influenced by points of view and methods already applied in those countries. The pioneer studies of Villermé in Paris, and the striking reports of Chadwick, Smith, and other sanitary reformers in England, were paralleled between 1830 and 1870 by a series of equally significant inquiries in America. As in England, the early public health movement was permeated with a spirit of social reform and was conceived in its broadest aspects. In 1837, the physician Benjamin W. McCready, in his pioneer essay on occupational medicine, had already called attention to the emergence of slums in New York. He was concerned not merely with working conditions in shops and factories, but also with the miserable living conditions of the workers. However, this was only at the beginning of the American industrial revolution and the rapid expansion of population. The population of New York was estimated at 75,770 in 1805. It was 123,000 in 1820 and rose to 515,000 in 1850. By that time, the situation was truly acute, and it is no accident that the first penetrating study of the health problems of the community was published by John C. Griscom in 1845. Griscom, a physician, had been City Inspector of the New York Board of Health, and to his formal report at the end of the year he appended "A Brief View of the Sanitary Condition of the City." Three years later, Griscom expanded this supplement into a small book entitled *The Sanitary Condition of the Laboring Population of New York*. Chadwick's influence is clearly manifest in the title of Griscom's inquiry; indeed, the latter's work was known to Southwood Smith and Chadwick. The breadth of Griscom's approach to community health problems is illustrated by his analysis of the slum economy of the 1840s, and its relation to the sanitary condition of the population. What is equally interesting is that the system described by Griscom is still to be found today, with only minor differences, in urban slum areas inhabited by underprivileged ethnic groups, such as Negroes or Puerto Ricans.

"The system of tenantage," wrote Griscom, "to which large numbers of the poor are subject, I think, must be regarded as one of the principal causes, of the helpless and noisome manner in which they live. The basis of these evils is the subjection of the tenantry to the merciless inflictions and extortions of the *sub-landlord*. A house, or a row, or court of houses is hired by some person of the owner, on a lease of several years, for a sum which yields a fair interest on the cost. The *owner* is then relieved of the great trouble incident to the changes of tenants, and the collection of rents . . . these slum properties, in order to admit a greater number of families, are divided into small apartments, as numerous as decency will admit. . . . These closets, for they deserve no other name, are then rented to the poor, from week to week, or month to month, the rent being almost invariably required in advance. . . ."

This study already contains in essence the principles and objectives that were to characterize the American sanitary reform movement for the next 30 years. Briefly, these were first, "that there is an immense amount of sickness, physical disability, and premature mortality, among the poorer classes"; second, "that these are, to a large extent, unnecessary, being in a great degree the results of causes which are removable"; third, "that these physical evils are productive of moral evils of great magnitude and number, and which, if considered only in a pecuniary point of view should arouse the government and individuals to a consideration of the best means for their relief and prevention"; and fourth, "to suggest the means of alleviating these evils and preventing their recurrence to so great an extent."

Central to this program is the concept of preventable death. It was by exploring the associations between living conditions and greater or lesser expectation of survival that the most notable successes in achieving sanitary reforms were won. In general, the miasmatic or filth theory of disease was accepted, but despite the absence of knowledge concerning microbial organisms as *materies morbi*, it was possible to make an effective attack on the health problems of the community just as the English were doing at the same time. Here, as well, the statistical approach provided an invaluable weapon, and vital statistics assumed a new social significance.

Catastrophe often precedes and brings into sharp focus the need for social change. In America during the nineteenth century, and especially during the period under consideration, this element was provided by recurrent epidemics of various communicable diseases—yellow fever, cholera, smallpox, typhoid fever, and typhus fever. While it was recognized that dire poverty, inadequate housing, and unsanitary surroundings took their toll in sickness and lives, this knowledge was dramatically impressed upon public opinion by every invasion or outbreak of epidemic disease, and the need for effective public health administration became a matter of terrifying urgency.

As urban communities grew and their sanitary condition deteriorated, it was increasingly evident that there was need for health reform. Efforts to change the situation were thwarted by those interested in maintaining the status quo. Clearly, if something concrete was to be achieved, the forces of the community would have to be mobilized for control of disease and improvement of health. This necessity led to the establishment after 1845 of a number of voluntary health associations, patterned in considerable degree after organizations that had been found effective in Great Britain. By bringing together physicians, public officials, and civic-minded laymen, such organizations were able to create a broad base for the mobilization of the forces of the community. Imbued with a high moral purpose, the members of these associations regarded themselves as "enlisted in a crusade against a gigantic and growing evil." These voluntary groups undertook to educate the public to the advantages of public and private hygiene, to press for administrative reform, and to take action for the elimination of crowded, poorly ventilated, and filthy tenements, impure water supplies, inadequate sewerage, and unwholesome food.

A BOOKSELLER TURNS CRUSADER. From the 1840s onward, there was constant agitation to tackle community health problems and to improve urban living conditions. As in Great Britain, the sanitary survey proved the most useful tool for the purpose. In 1845, the year in which Griscom published his investigation of New York City, steps were taken in other parts of the United States to carry out sanitary surveys of urban communities. One of the most interesting of these endeavors was stimulated by the National Institute, a distinguished scientific body in Washington, D.C. In 1845, the medical department of the Institute endeavored to survey the nation's health, but with small success. When the American Medical Association was founded in 1847, the Institute urged that it establish a hygiene committee, which could undertake sanitary surveys and endeavor to secure a uniform system for the collection of vital statistics. Such a committee was formed by the American Medical Association in 1848, and it actively attempted to secure sanitary surveys from various sections of the country. Among the first critical discussions of the unwholesome nature of slums in American cities are those of this committee based on the information that it collected. While the surveys that were made were inadequate in many respects, they did show collectively the great need for better public health organization. This lesson was further driven home by the cholera epidemic, which broke out in 1849 and continued to harass different parts of the United States for some two years.

Concurrently, events were moving along similar lines in Massachusetts to produce the most famous of the early public health documents in the United States, the Shattuck *Report*. Published in 1850 by the Massachusetts Sanitary Commission, the report was the work of Lemuel Shattuck (1793–1859) of Boston, a bookseller and publisher. Originally a teacher in Detroit, he had become interested in community affairs; and later, when a member of the school committee in Concord, Massachusetts, he reorganized the public school system of the town. Through an interest in genealogy, he recognized the need for accurate vital statistics, and he implemented this recognition by stimulating the organization of the American Statistical Society in 1839 and by securing in 1842 the passage of a law in Massachusetts initiating statewide registration of vital statistics. This law became a model for other states. In 1845, Shattuck issued a *Census of Boston*, which was not only a prelude to his more famous *Report* of 1850 but is worthy of consideration in its own right because it provided a solid foundation for the accurate recording of statistics in the United States.

The census revealed a high general mortality and a shocking infant and maternal mortality. Communicable diseases, scarlet fever, typhus and typhoid fevers, diphtheria, tuberculosis, were widely prevalent. Living conditions for the lower income groups were grossly unsatisfactory. Finally, there was no concept that the community had any responsibility to cope with problems of public health. Stimulated by these findings, as well as by the activities and ideas of the contemporary British and French sanitary reformers, Shattuck engineered the appointment of a commission to make a sanitary survey of Massachusetts. Shattuck was chairman and wrote the report of the Commission.

The Shattuck *Report* has had an excellent press in our day and has recently been reprinted. Upon its appearance in 1850, however, it had practically no effect. Indeed, as Henry I. Bowditch later remarked: "It fell still-born from the State printer's hand." One of its major recommendations that a state board of health be established to deal with the urgent and distressing health conditions revealed by the *Report* was not implemented until 19 years later. Nevertheless, the *Report* is an important landmark in the evolution of community health action. It outlined a basis for sound public health organization and made recommendations that to a large extent have been realized in the intervening hundred years. Shattuck recommended the establishment of a state health department, and local boards of health in each town. In addition, he urged sanitary surveys of particular urban communities and other localities. Considering Shattuck's interest in vital statistics, it is not surprising to find detailed recommendations on this subject. These include a decennial census, uniform nomenclature for causes of disease and death, and collection of data by age, sex, race, occupation, economic status, and locality. Environmental sanitation, control of food and drugs, and communicable disease control are considered at length. Stress is laid on vaccination against smallpox. Well-child care, the health of school children, and mental health are all touched on. Health education is given a great deal of attention. The far-sighted character of the report is indicated by Shattuck's proposals on smoke control, alcoholism, town planning, and the teaching of preventive medicine in medical schools.

The appeal of Lemuel Shattuck and his *Report* to the modern public health worker is easily understandable. In large measure, he previsaged the pattern of public health organization and practice that developed and has endured in the United States over the past hundred years. As a result, it is tempting to remove him from the context of his time and place and to turn him into a myth. Lemuel Shattuck was a man of his time and generation, and in practice was limited by contemporary political and social trends. As John Blake has recently shown, he played an equivocal role in providing Boston with a new water supply. What his plan would have looked like in practice, we do not know, for it was not implemented. Shattuck endeavored to have the major recommendations of the *Report* enacted into law, but he was unsuccessful. He died in 1859, and it was left to others to take effective action. The great achievement of Shattuck was to take ideas and practices of his predecessors and contempories, to adapt them to the American scene within a broad and coherent pattern of organization, and in essence to formulate a complete health policy.

THE NEW YORK SANITARY SURVEY OF 1864. Meanwhile, other groups and individuals continued to study the health problems of urban communities, to expose the seriousness of the high sickness and death rates of cities, and to urge remedial action. Between 1857 and 1860, four National Quarantine and Sanitary Conventions were held in Philadelphia, Baltimore, New York, and

Boston, respectively. The fifth convention was to have met in Cincinnati in 1861 but was never held owing to the outbreak of the Civil War. These meetings were stimulated by Wilson Jewell, a medical member of the Philadelphia Board of Health. International Sanitary Conferences held at Paris in 1851 and 1852 suggested to him the value of such meetings. The National Conventions were concerned with quarantine on the one hand, and the sanitary organization and regulations of communty health on the other, and many participated who were later to be in the forefront of American public health, among them Drs. Stephen Smith, Elisha Harris, A. N. Bell, and E. M. Snow. Furthermore, the Conventions prepared the way for the American Public Health Association, which was organized in 1872.

However, the most effective study in terms of results was made in New York City. A committee of the New York State Senate, appointed in 1858, had taken evidence and reported the need for reorganization of the municipal health administration. It attributed the high rate of mortality prevaling in New York to the "overcrowded condition of tenement houses, the want of practical knowledge of the proper mode of constructing such houses, deficiency of light, imperfect ventilation, impurities in domestic economy, unwholesome food and beverages, insufficient sewage [*sic*], want of cleanliness in the streets and at the wharves and piers, to a general disregard of sanitary precautions, and finally, to the imperfect execution of existing ordinances and the total absence of a regularly organized sanitary police." Nevertheless, basic reform was not initiated until after the publication in 1865 of a detailed report by the Council of Hygiene and Public Health on the unsanitary conditions prevailing in the city. The Council had been formed in 1864 by the Citizens Association, a group organized in the early 1860s to clean up the city government, and comprised a group of prominent physicians, among whom may be mentioned Willard Parker, Valentine Mott, Edward Delafield, Alonzo Clark, Gurdon Buck, Stephen Smith, Elisha Harris, and Henry D. Buckley. This group undertook to carry out a sanitary survey of the city, and they enlisted the aid of a number of young physicians. For the purpose of the survey, the city was divided into 29 districts and one physician was assigned to each district as a sanitary inspector. A survey schedule was drawn up, and the investigation was carried out during the summer of 1864. Elisha Harris edited the findings and the material was published in 1865 under the title *Report of the Council of Hygiene and Public Health of the Citizens' Association of New York Upon the Sanitary Condition of the City.* The total cost of this enterprise was $22,000, but the money was well spent. The conditions that were uncovered were even more shocking than had been suspected. Widespread public interest was aroused, the aid of community leaders, such as ministers, was enlisted, and eventually the matter became a significant political issue.

While the Council of Hygiene had been carrying out its survey, another department of the Citizens' Association, the Council of Law, had drafted a public health law. It was prepared under the judicious direction of Dorman B. Eaton, a New York lawyer, who had become interested in community health problems in 1859, and who in 1864 had endeavored unsuccessfully to have the state legislature pass a bill reorganizing the health administration of the municipality. Eaton was later to be active in the creation of the National Board of Health. The bill was introduced into the state legislature in 1865. After an initial setback, it was passed early in 1866, and on March 5, 1866, the Metropolitan Board of Health came into being. In passing, it is worth noting that the Council of Hygiene was modeled after the French *conseil de salubrité*, and the Metropolitan Board of Health was based on the English sanitary system.

As organized under the new law, the health administration of the city was turned over to a Board of Health empowered to act within the Metropolitan Sanitary District of New York State. This area included the counties of New York, Kings, Richmond, and Westchester, as well as the towns of Flushing, Jamaica, and Newtown in Queens County. Extensive power was conferred upon the Board, which was empowered to create ordinances, to execute them, and to sit in judgment on its own acts. The Board consisted of a president appointed by the Mayor, four physicians who were sanitary commissioners, the health officer of the port, and four police commissioners. In 1870, the administrative organization was altered, and the nucleus of the present New York City Health Department was created. Its jurisdiction included only the actual City of New York as then constituted, that is, the present boroughs of Manhattan and the Bronx. The department comprised four bureaus: Sanitary, Sanitary Permits, Street Cleaning, and Vital Statistics.

The activities of the New York City Health Department during the succeeding two decades reflect the evolution of the modern public health program. It must be kept in mind that until the 1880s and even later there was firmly implanted in both the lay and the medical mind the idea that disease was caused by dirt. Translation of this idea into practical consequence took the form of specific measures intended essentially to eliminate filth and to improve the physical environment, especially of the poorer classes. This activity is reflected in the varied duties performed by the sanitary inspectors, most of whom were physicians. They investigated outbreaks of such communicable diseases as smallpox, typhus fever, typhoid and scarlet fevers, inspected tenement houses, reported on defective plumbing or ventilation, vaccinated against smallpox, and conducted sanitary surveys. In 1874, an effort was made to stem the wastage of infant life, especially in tenement houses. A simple leaflet on infant care was prepared and widely distributed. In the same year, leaflets describing the means by which diphtheria spreads, its symptoms, and the precautions to be taken were also issued by the Health Department. These efforts may be considered the beginning of public health education in New York by an official agency. In 1874, a corps of vaccinators was likewise organized, and a laboratory for the preparation of vaccine virus was established. The development of medical bacteriology brought with it a major shift of emphasis in the program of community health action. From the control of man's environment attention was turned to the control of specific communicable diseases. However, that is already the story of the most recent period in the evolution of public health, to which we will turn in the next chapter.

The enactment of the New York Metropolitan Health Bill of 1866 was a major triumph and marks a turning point in the history of public health not only in New York City, but in the United States as a whole. One of the basic problems with which the pioneer public health workers were concerned was the lack of adequate administrative machinery. The civil service during the early nineteenth century was small in numbers, limited in function, and recruited almost wholly by patronage. A change from a haphazard to an efficient administration was as essential to the development of a complicated urban industrial society as the provision of new scientific knowledge. In fact it was the provision of a stable administrative foundation, which made it easier to incorporate new scientific knowledge into public health practice. It was in New York City that such a foundation was created for the first time in the United States, and an example was set for others to follow. According to Stephen Smith, it was "declared officially and judicially to be the most complete piece of health legislation ever placed on the statute books," and it led to the creation of new and effective health departments in various municipalities and states. The first state health department had been established by Louisiana in 1855, but it was not effective. In was in 1869 that Massachusetts finally adopted the ideas of Lemuel Shattuck and organized a suitable state health department. Other states followed in rapid succession: California, 1870; District of Columbia, 1871; Minnesota, 1872; Virginia, 1872; Michigan, 1873; Maryland, 1874; Alabama, 1875; Wisconsin, 1876; and Illinois, 1877.

A PREMATURE NATIONAL HEALTH DEPARTMENT. As state and municipal health departments began to appear, the idea of a national health organization seemed to be the logical next step. At the Sanitary Conventions held between 1857 and 1860, the subject of a nationwide quarantine service had been broached. The idea of a unified, coordinated health service for the United States was again discussed at the first meeting of the American Public Health Association in 1872. Three years later a meeting was held in Washington, D.C., to consider plans for a Federal health department, but it achieved nothing owing to the rivalry of the medical departments of the Army, Navy, and the Marine Hospital Service. At this point, Dorman E. Eaton of New York was asked to draft a bill that would create a National Board of Health, but his proposal to place the medical departments of the three services on an equal footing proved unacceptable. Once again an epidemic brought the issue to a head. A severe outbreak of yellow fever ravaged the Mississippi Valley in 1878, causing great loss of life and creating economic havoc. At this point, there was public demand for action.

It must be remembered that until 1872 when the Marine Hospital Service was reorganized the Federal government had no interest in public health matters. Organization and action for the protection of community health was considered a local responsibility to be carried out by the state or the locality. Quarantine was generally a state function. The doctrine of state sovereignty continued to hold sway in the health field and was to handicap national public health action for many years. Under such circumstances, there could hardly be a concept of a national health policy, nor of an organization to implement it. Ideas along these lines were truly ahead of the time, and it was not until the twentieth century that they were realized. Nevertheless, in 1878, a first small and hesitant step was taken in this direction with the passage of the National Quarantine Act, which empowered the Surgeon General of the Marine Hospital Service to enforce port quarantine as long as he did not interfere with the laws and procedures of the states. Nor was he given any appropriation to carry out this objective.

Obviously, this symbolic gesture could not satisfy those who demanded effective action against future epidemic outbreaks. At its next session, in 1879, Congress finally adopted a bill, drawn by Dorman Eaton and sponsored by the American Public Health Association, creating a National Board of Health. The Board comprised seven physicians as well as one representative each from the Army, the Navy, the Marine Hospital Service, and the Justice Department. Its duties were to collect information on public health matters, to advise Federal government departments and state governments, and to report to Congress a plan for a national health organization with special attention to quarantine. The National Board of Health carried on its work until 1883, when appropriations for it were terminated, and it soon disappeared. It failed because of an unwieldy administrative structure, and because it aroused the antagonism of the states, who felt that their rights were being encroached on. Nevertheless, during its short life the National Board of Health showed how a Federal agency could further community health action on a nationwide basis. Furthermore, it pointed to the need for solving the problem of Federal-State relations if public health action on a national basis was to be effective.

Clearly, by the last quarter of the nineteenth century, a sound basis had been created for the further development of public health in the United States. Much still remained to be done, but the more extensive cultivation of the community health program and the rich rewards that have been garnered in our century were made possible because basic organizational problems had already been solved. Within the American political framework, action on a national basis could not take place until it was realized that many problems of health and welfare could not be handled locally. Meanwhile, the future direction of community health action was being determined abroad in Germany and France. At this point, therefore, let us turn to these countries and examine the state of public health as well as some of the problems that gave rise to the epoch-making discoveries that initiated a new era in public health.

SOCIAL REVOLUTION, INDUSTRIALISM, AND PUBLIC HYGIENE IN FRANCE. The Revolution and the needs of the Napoleonic regime had gradually begun to transform France from an agricultural to an industrial country. But it was only after the Restoration, and particularly during the reign of Louis Philippe (1830–1848), that the French economy created its first heavy industries and railroads. This economic process imposed strains and stresses, which were prolonged until the 1870s and which were reflected in the evolution of French public health. During this period, France faced many of the health problems already encountered in England, which were being met contemporaneously in the United States, Germany, and Belgium. As in England, the result of introducing steam power and machinery was to throw craftsmen out of work and to attract them to urban industrial centers by prospects of work and wages. The French urban population increased from 15 per cent of the total in 1830 to 25 per cent in 1846. Lack of proper housing, overcrowding, and the effects of periodic unemployment combined to make the life of the worker and his family a living death. The crowded cellars and attics of Manchester and Liverpool were duplicated at Lille and Rouen, and the baneful consequences of the industrial slum forced themselves upon the attention of physicians, writers, economists, and public officials. "How can anyone," asked Baudelaire, "whatever party one may belong to and whatever prejudices one may have been brought up on, fail to be touched at the sight of this sickly multitude breathing the dust of the factories, swallowing cotton-floss, their systems saturated with white lead, mercury and all the poisons necessary to the creation of works of art, sleeping amid vermin in quarters where the greatest and simplest of human virtues nestle by the side of the most hardened vices and the vomit of the penitentiary?"

These terrible conditions existed throughout the July Monarchy, and it was not until the 1840s that the French government took any remedial action on a national basis. The first piece of labor legislation in French history, a law regulating child labor in factories, was passed in 1841. Meanwhile, a vigorous group of public health workers had been carrying out a number of surveys and statistical studies of actual living conditions among workers in urban communities. The main impulses of this French public health group came from native problems and thinkers. Practical experience, both at home and abroad, acquired during the Revolutionary and Napoleonic Wars, had made many French physicians alert to public health problems, especially those of the community. This orientation was further reinforced by the fact that during the first half of the nineteenth century France was the most advanced country in political and social theory. After all, this was the time of Fourier, Saint-Simon, Comte, Cabet, Buchez, Considérant, Blanc, and Proudhon; and there was a considerable amount of cross fertilization between social science and public health. As a result, the French public health movement was permeated through and through with a spirit of social reform, or even revolution. Utopian socialists, such as Cabet and the followers of Saint-Simon, dealt with community health problems in their writings and in a few cases ventured to act on their theories. The appearance of cholera at Paris in 1831 led the Saint-Simonians to establish a free medical service staffed by physicians who belonged to the group. Then, in 1832, the *Globe*, a newspaper of Saint-Simonian persuasion, proposed that the city be provided with an adequate supply of good water, a proper sewerage system, as well as other facilities calculated to improve sanitary conditions and the health of the people.

The outstanding figure in the French public health movement of this period was Louis René Villermé (1782–1863), who has already been mentioned on several occasions. He is best known for his study of the health conditions of textile workers. This report, published in 1840 under the title *Tableau de l'état physique et moral des ouvriers employés dans les manufactures de coton, de laine, et de soie* (*Survey of the Physical and Moral Condition of Workers Employed in Cotton, Wool and Silk Factories*) aroused public opinion and led to the law of 1841 limiting child labor. Despite other investigations and reports by contemporaries of Villermé, no further action was taken until 1848. In August of that year, the Second Republic brought into being a public health advisory committee attached to the Ministry of Agriculture and Commerce. Consisting of seven members, its function was to advise the Minister on all matters relating to the public health. In December, 1848, another law created a network of local public health councils. In 1836, the government of Louis Phillippe had requested the Academy of Medicine to prepare a plan for the organization of health councils (*conseils de salubrité*) for all of France. Basically, this was the plan followed in 1848. There was a council for each *départment* and each *arrondissement*. The members of these bodies were named by the chief administrative officers of the department for a period of four years from among physicians, pharmacists, and veterinarians. The council was to meet every three months or whenever adjudged necessary. Their function was essentially advisory; they were consulted by the prefect whenever necessary, but they could not carry out any action themselves. This system was continued under Napoleon

III and was maintained by the Third Republic. It was generally recognized that it was relatively inefficient, and by the end of the nineteenth century, numerous proposals were offered to bring French public health organization up to the level of other western European countries in this regard. During this period, however, the greatest French contribution to public health was in another area, namely, in the application of science to the diagnosis, treatment, and control of communicable disease.

NATIONAL UNIFICATION AND HEALTH REFORM IN GERMANY. The development of public health activity and organization in Germany parallels in many respects the experience of England and France. Industrialism and urban expansion appeared later in Germany, but when they did, similar problems were created. Yet there was a significant difference. There was no united Germany, only a conglomerate group of German States of which Prussia was the most important and the largest. Unification of the German States was a major aim of German patriots and liberals during the nineteenth century, and to this objective was linked the question of health organization.

From Paris, the fountainhead of advanced thought, liberal ideas spread to Germany. As we have seen, industrialization and its attendant social problems led various investigators in England and France to study the influence of poverty, occupation, housing, and other factors on health. These currents of thought and action influenced German medical men and during the revolutionary year of 1848 they joined forces to secure overdue health reforms. Prominent in this group were Rudolf Virchow, Solomon Neumann, and Rudolf Leubuscher. These men held to certain principles on which they developed a program of action in the interest of the public health. The first of these principles is that the health of the people is a matter of direct social concern. Society has an obligation to protect and insure the health of its members. The second is that social and economic conditions have an important effect on health and disease, and that these relations must be subjected to scientific investigation. Virchow, for example, conceived the scope of public health as broadly as possible, indicating that one of its major functions was to study the conditions under which various social groups lived and to determine the effects of these conditions on their health. On the basis of this knowledge, it would then be possible to take appropriate action. Finally, the principle that follows from this is that steps taken to promote health and to combat disease must be social as well as medical.

The broad outlines of the program of action proposed on the basis of these principles are probably represented best by a draft for a Public Health Law prepared by Neumann and submitted to the Berlin Society of Physicians and Surgeons on March 30, 1849. According to this document, public health has as its objectives: (1) The healthy mental and physical development of the citizen;

(2) the prevention of all dangers to health; and (3) the control of disease. Public Health must care for society as a whole by considering the general physical and social conditions that may adversely affect health, such as soil, industry, food, and housing; and it must protect each individual by considering those conditions that prevent him from caring for his health. These may be considered in two major categories: conditions, such as poverty and infirmity, in which the individual has the right to request assistance from the state; and conditions in which the state has the right and the obligation to interfere with the personal liberty of the individual, for example, in cases of transmissible disease and mental illness. Public Health can fulfill these duties by supplying well trained medical personnel in sufficient numbers and adequate organization of medical personnel, and by establishing appropriate institutions for public health.

During the 1848 revolution, voices were raised for governmental action, and many specific measures were proposed, all of which fall within the broad program drafted by Neumann. An important problem was the provision of medical care for the indigent, and proposals were put forth by Virchow and others for public medical services for the poor, including free choice of physicians. It was realized, however, that provision of medical care was not enough, that it must go hand in hand with social prophylaxis. In consequence, Virchow proclaimed the right of the citizen to work, as a fundamental principle to be included in the constitution of a democratic state. (Here Virchow was no doubt influenced by the action of the French Provisional Government of 1848 in recognizing the right to work, the doctrine of the *droit au travail* that Louis Blanc had been preaching since 1839.)

The problem of the industrial worker also demanded attention. Although industrialization in Germany began later than in England and France, and proceeded at a slower pace during the first half of the nineteenth century, by 1848 the existence of a wage-earning class, an industrial proletariat, could no longer be overlooked. As in England and France, industrialization was ushered in by a slaughter of the innocents. Those that survived the cradle were given over to the tender mercies of the factory and the mine. To deal with this problem, Leubuscher proposed a program of industrial hygiene, with emphasis on the legislative regulation of working conditions. Particularly important was the question of limiting the working day. Leubuscher advocated the prohibition of child labor before the age of 14 years, reduction of the working day in dangerous occupations, protection of pregnant women, the establishment of standards for ventilation of work rooms, and the prevention of industrial poisoning through the use of nontoxic materials.

Demands were also made for uniform licensure of medical practitioners entitling them to practice in every German State; appointment of physicians to official positions on the basis of competitive examinations; and the establishment of a National Ministry of Health. Very important was the recognition that for investigation of the causal relations between social conditions and health problems it was necessary to have reliable statistics. Neumann was most active in agitating for the collection of accurate statistics.

The revolution of 1848 was defeated, but what the liberals could not achieve Bismarck did. It is within the framework of the process of unification carried out by Bismarck that later developments in health organization took place. The views of Virchow and the other reformers did not mature until later in the century. The leaders of 1848, Virchow and Neumann, remained active in politics and loyal to their principles. During the decades that followed 1848, the broad program of health reform was transformed into a more limited program of sanitary reform that was practically attainable. Action was taken to improve working conditions, particularly for women and children, and efforts were made to improve health administration. For example, in 1867, Lorenz von Stein, jurist and administrator, in a treatise on public administration dealt with the administrative aspects of public health. Stein pointed out that the health of individuals becomes a matter of public concern to the extent that individuals are subjected to noxious conditions over which they have no control, and to the extent that such persons become a burden on society. In these circumstances, he insisted, it is the duty of government to establish and to maintain conditions that would protect the individual, and to re-establish and promote his health in a positive manner. Stein was considerably influenced by English health legislation, and cited the English experience in support of his thesis.

During the 1860s and 1870s agitation for public health reform again became prominent. Physicians and laymen organized associations to work for this purpose; various cities improved their water supplies and sewerage systems; and the North German Confederation and later the Reichstag of the German Empire occupied themselves with health problems. With creation of the Second Reich following the Franco-Prussian War, it became possible to consider realistically the creation of a central public health unit. Finally, in 1873, a Reich Health Office was set up and in 1876 it began to function. This was the beginning of a unified public health organization for Germany as a whole.

It was around this period that Virchow occupied himself with problems of sewage disposal, especially in Berlin. The cesspool and the outdoor privy still dominated the scene. Furthermore, the majority of people in Berlin had no central water supply and obtained their water from wells. Through the efforts of Virchow, a good water supply and a proper sewerage system were introduced, and the largest German city was successfully cleaned up. At the same time, similar efforts were being made in Munich by the great German hygienist Max von Pettenkofer (1818–1901). In 1873, he addressed the Society for Popular Education on the value of health to a city. The purpose of these lectures was to urge the need for thoroughgoing sanitary reform in order to improve health conditions. It was Pettenkofer who made hygiene an experimental, laboratory science, but he was fully aware that man's health is influenced not only by his physical environment but also by the social world in which he lives. Health is a resultant of the combined action of a number of factors, and all of these would have to be taken into account. Pettenkofer pointed out that public health is a matter of community concern, and that any measures taken to help those in need react to the benefit of all.

Pettenkofer made Munich a healthy city, as Virchow did Berlin. However, the significance of his work extends beyond this laudable achievement. A trained physiologist and chemist, Pettenkofer was the first to submit all aspects of hygiene to laboratory analysis. He initiated pioneer work on the hygiene of nutrition, clothing, ventilation, water, and sewage. In 1865, he was given the first chair of experimental hygiene at Munich. With Pettenkofer, science entered the field of hygiene and public health, just as it was doing contemporaneously in clinical medicine, and a new dimension was added to the study of community health problems.

AN ERA OF STATISTICAL ENTHUSIASM. Throughout this period, the methods available for the study of community health problems were limited essentially to rational empiricism, critical observation, the survey, and, from the late 1820s onward, to statistical analysis. As yet the public health worker was largely without tools and techniques comparable to those that in clinical medicine were beginning to yield important discoveries. The worker in the public health field was without autopsies, a microscope, or a laboratory, and without experiments except those that nature might chance to produce. In consequence statistical methods were seized upon eagerly by many and applied with considerable vigor.

From a political, economic, and social point of view, the decades from 1830 to 1850 were the opening period of the era in which we still find ourselves. Like all such seminal periods, it was marked by exaltations and enthusiasms, and it is no surprise to find these characteristics evident in the statistical study of health problems. Westergaard aptly characterized this period as an era of enthusiasm.

Around 1830, studies of health problems based on numerical data began to appear in increasing numbers. Concerned with questions of community health and clinical medicine, these investigations soon attracted wide professional and public attention. In fact, the decades from 1830 to 1870 represent the flood tide of such studies on the continent of Europe, in Great Britain, and in the United States. With great zeal, numerous investigators studied the problems of health under a wide variety of circumstances. Some studies were undertaken in the course of official inquiries, others by private citizens whose interest was attracted to a specific social or health problem. Many were concerned with the question of differential mortality and the effect on health of such factors as economic and social class, occupation, race, imprisonment, intemperance, or lack of proper sanitation. It is patently impossible to list and to discuss all such studies here. For our purpose, a few representative samples will suffice.

In France, Parent-Duchatelet and D'Arcet studied the effect of tobacco on the health of workers handling it. Benoiston de Chateauneuf examined the differential mortality of rich and poor. Villermé's studies of differential mortality in various districts of Paris have been mentioned, as well as his survey of the health of textile workers. He also studied the mean duration of illness at different ages so as to apply this knowledge to the organization of mutual aid societies.

Among English contributors, William Farr and William A. Guy may be mentioned. The former has already been introduced. Throughout his long and fruitful career, Farr made numerous contributions to the statistical study of health problems. Particular attention may perhaps be called to his numerous studies of occupational mortality. While Guy cannot be considered on the same level as Farr, he deserves to be better known. Professor of Forensic Medicine at the University of London, he was also an indefatigable student of statistical problems, a frequent contributor to the *Journal of the Statistical Society of London* (which started publication in 1838), and an active participant in the English public health movement. Guy was especially interested in the influence of occupation on health, and in his testimony before the Health of Towns Commission introduced evidence of the disabling effect of occupational hazards. He studied bakers, scavengers, printers, tailors, and many other groups of workers. In addition, he examined the causes leading to the choice of an occupation, the effects of season and weather on mortality, and the duration of life among the gentry, the aristocracy, the clergy, and the professions.

While many of the studies of this period were highly effective in furthering the cause of sanitary reform, there were certain defects common to all of them. Many studies were carried out on institutional populations, for example, patients in hospitals, prisoners, and asylum inmates. As a result, the samples with which they dealt were in most cases too small or not representative. Despite these shortcomings, however, there is evidence that the question of precision in statistical results was attracting increasing attention. For the most part, however, the question was handled by rule of thumb. One aspect of the problem was to decide when the number of observations was large enough to avoid error. Different authors employed different practical rules. Thus, in his study of textile workers, Villermé calculated the probable duration of life only where more than 100 deaths had been observed.

While medical statisticians were still groping for solutions to the problem of precision, mathematicians had developed tools for dealing with it. Laplace's great work on probability, the *Théorie analytique des probabilités*, had appeared in 1812. In this work, he called attention to the significance of probability theory for medical investigations but had not pursued the matter further. Then, in 1837, Poisson published his important *Recherches sur la probabilités des jugements* in which he showed how to calculate the mean error of a difference between two observed frequencies, an operation directly applicable to the statistical handling of public health problems. Three years later, Jules Gavarret, a student of Poisson, published his *Principes généraux de statistique médicale* in which he applied his teacher's work. Despite its merits, however, Gavarret's treatise did not receive the attention it deserved. Ten years after the appearance of this book, for example, Guy still expressed the opinion that "the formulae of the mathematician have a very limited application to the results of observation; and that if incautiously applied they may lead to very great errors."

This pattern of uneven advance, of hesitating and uncertain development, was not peculiar to the health field. It is one aspect of a general process that characterizes the state of development of various biological and social sciences toward the middle of the nineteenth century. Joseph A. Schumpeter in his *History of Economic Analysis* gives a similar picture of the relations during this period between economics and statistical analysis. Yet it was at this time that the first major step was successfully taken to bring mathematical analysis to bear on the data of community health compiled by observation and enumeration. This was the achievement of Adolphe Quetelet (1796–1874), Belgian astronomer and mathematician.

What did Quetelet do? He gathered together the statistical tendencies and developments of his time, built them into a systematic structure in terms of a guiding theoretical concept, and undertook to show how it could be applied in practice. Quetelet recognized that variation is a characteristic of all biological and social phenomena, and that such variation occurred around the mean of a number of observations. Based on this recognition, he developed a methodology that comprised the determination of statistical averages, the establishment of the limits of variation around an average, and investigation of the conditions under which variation would occur. Furthermore, he showed that the distribution of observations around a mean corresponded to the distribution of probabilities on a probability curve. The theoretical expression of this methodology was Quetelet's concept of the average man (*l'homme moyen*). The germ of his contribution is to be found in his work *Sur l'homme*, which appeared in 1835, and it was fully developed in the book *Du systéme social* published in 1848.

Quetelet was peculiarly well suited to make his important contribution. During a visit at Paris in 1823 and 1824, he had come into close contact with French mathematicians interested in the theory of probability, among them

Laplace, Fourier, and Poisson. Later he also entered into friendly relations with French physicians concerned with the statistical study of health problems, of whom the most important were Villermé and Benoiston de Chateauneuf. Through these contacts and influences, and because of his connection with the handling of official statistics, Quetelet had an abundance of data at his disposal. Also, as an active organizer of and participant in numerous statistical congresses, he was able to spread widely his ideas and work. Finally, because he stated the results of his mathematical analysis clearly and lucidly, Quetelet was able to reach a large public with his writings. His numerous publications thus facilitated a general appreciation and adoption of his ideas.

The statistical treatment of public health problems continued into the second half of the nineteenth century when Francis Galton and Karl Pearson began to attack the problems of correlated variations and the asymmetry of frequency distributions, thus opening up the most recent period in the statistical analysis of health problems.

WOMEN AND CHILDREN FIRST. Closely related to the movement for the betterment of urban health was the demand for amelioration of working conditions. Some of the evils found in the early factories were extremely long hours of work under wretched and unsanitary conditions, the general employment of the cheap labor of women and children, frequent accidents due to unprotected machines, and lack of ventilation and insufficient time for meals. Factory reform may be considered as beginning in England in 1802 with the enactment of the Health and Morals of Apprentices Act. This measure forbade night work for pauper apprentices in cotton and woolen factories, and in a strict sense it was not a Factory Act, but merely an extension of the Elizabethan Poor Law relating to parish apprentices. As the government was responsible for these children, it found itself compelled, when circumstances warranted, to regulate their working conditions. Additional measures were passed during the following decades. By 1831, night work for employees less than 21 years of age was prohibited, and the 69-hour week was extended to all workers younger than 18 years of age. It should be remembered that these measures applied only to cotton mills.

Not until 1833 was the first effective Factory Act passed, and then only as a by-product of the bitter conflict between the industrial and agricultural interests and the continuing agitation of the workers themselves. During the 1830s and 1840s, the movement for factory reform became part of the broader struggle between the two chief divisions of the British ruling group, the landowners and the manufacturers. At the same time, the factory workers linked their agitation for parliamentary reform with demands for shorter hours, better working conditions, and prohibition of child labor. The fight for a 10-hour day began, and after a savage political struggle, the Factory Act of 1833 was enacted.

However, to the profound disappointment of the workers, only child labor was protected. Indeed, the commissioners who framed the act denounced the committees that were agitating for the 10-hour day on the ground that they "seem scarcely ever to have considered the law of supply and demand as applicable to the working classes." They favored protective legislation for children but regarded it as unsound for adult women and men.

The act applied to all textile factories, excepting lace. It prohibited completely the employment of children younger than 9 years of age, and provided that children between 9 and 13 years were not to be employed longer than nine hours a day or 48 hours a week. For persons between 13 and 16, the working day was limited to 12 hours per day, 69 hours in a week. The cleaning of machinery while in motion was prohibited, and every factory owner was required to provide two hours schooling daily for all children employed in his plant. Finally, and this is most important, provision was made for enforcement of the law by appointing four inspectors. They were empowered to enter any factory at all times, call upon witnesses for information, and even to pass minor regulations whenever it seemed necessary. The information gathered was to be used to draw up annual reports on conditions in factories. In these reports, the inspectors did not simply confine themselves to their statutory duties but concerned themselves in the broadest sense with the social life and well-being of the workers.

It was owing to these activities, as well as to a number of mine catastrophes, that public attention was drawn to conditions in the mines. It appears probable also that the recognition of the need for a study of conditions in mines was a result of suspicions that children, prohibited from working in factories, were being sent to the coal mines. In 1840, on a motion of Lord Ashley, a commission was set up to investigate child labor in mines and factories. The commission consisted of four members, two of whom, Southwood Smith, the physician who was active in sanitary reform, and Thomas Tooke, an economist, had participated in the Factory Commission of 1833. The two other members, Leonard Horner and R. J. Saunders, were factory inspectors. Some 20 subcommissioners were appointed to serve under them. In 1842, the Commission published its first report dealing with mines. The evidence of the report was strikingly emphasized by a number of vivid drawings of women and children at work in the mines. This feature had been included by Southwood Smith so that "members of Parliament, who might think themselves too busy to read the text of the report would turn over its pages to glance at the illustrations."

The report disclosed a picture of social evil in the coal fields, which made an extremely profound impression on public opinion. With the exception of North Staffordshire, where the needs of the potteries for juvenile labor were paramount, the employment of young children was common in all coal fields.

The employment of female labor was prevalent only in certain districts. Women were used mainly to haul or push coal carts along narrow passages, often no more than 18 inches high; and also to convey the coal to the surface in baskets carried on their backs. It was clear from the report that work in the mines was not conducive to long life or good health. The incidence of accidents, resulting in disabling injuries or death, was high, and a comparison of the statistics of infant and adolescent mortality in the mine fields with those in other districts of England and Wales reveals a death rate four or five times greater than in the agricultural districts. Nevertheless, the labor of women and children was cheap and plentiful, an almost irresistible argument for outweighing any considerations of safety or health.

The Commission's disclosures shocked the English public. Victorian England was even more shocked by the total absence of religious education among the mine children, and the revelation that women, almost completely naked, worked side by side with men in the pits under conditions conducive to immorality, than it was indignant over the injurious effects of their labor on the health of these mine workers. A month after the appearance of the report, Ashley introduced a Mines Bill into Parliament. After vigorous opposition and a number of compromises, the Mines and Collieries Act of 1842 was passed. The Act prohibited the employment underground of women and of boys younger than 10 years of age. No person younger than 15 years of age was to tend a steam engine. However, there were no other restrictions on the hours of work. Very important for the future was the creation of a mine inspectorate. This Act was far from satisfactory, and no real effort was made at first to render its provisions effective. Nevertheless, the first step toward the regulation of conditions in mines had been taken, and a valuable precedent established for future action. The Act of 1842 was the first of a series of legislative measures, which at the beginning indirectly and later directly affected the health of workers in the British mining industry.

The early factory and mine acts are not only of intrinsic interest, but also because the manner in which they came into being is more or less typical of the entire body of nineteenth-century legislation for the protection of workers in Britain. All the important acts were preceded by agitation and public inquiries and were enacted into law in the face of determined opposition. On the whole, the development of factory and mine legislation between 1830 and the end of the century reflects little credit on the coal owners, the manufacturers, and their spokesmen.

Early in 1846, the indefatigable Lord Ashley introduced a Ten Hours Bill in Parliament. After a vigorous debate during which the historian Macaulay declared that it was the duty of legislators to protect humanity against the demands of industry, the bill became law in 1847. The Act stipulated that after

May, 1848, when it was to become effective, there would be a 58-hour week for all women and for young persons 13 to 18 years old. Then, in 1850, a subsequent Factory Act established a statutory working day for women and young persons from 6 a.m. to 6 p.m., with one and a half hours for meals.

Thus, by the middle of the nineteenth century, certain important although limited steps had been taken to regulate conditions of work in factories and mines. The principal achievements were the appointment of inspectors, the restriction of the hours of work for women and children in a limited number of industries, chiefly textiles, and the establishment of certain safety regulations particularly for the fencing of machinery. Most of the industrial population was not covered by the Act described, and many years elapsed before other industries were brought within the scope of factory legislation.

The protection of the law began to be extended to workers in nontextile industries in the 1860s. The picture of ill-health among industrial and domestic workers disclosed by John Simon's reports of 1860 to 1862 and the findings of Children's Employment Commission of 1861 resulted in the passage of the Factory Act of 1864. This law placed the manufacture of pottery, matches, hosiery and lace, paper staining, and a number of other industries under the provisions of the factory acts already in operation. The Factory Act of 1867 brought under regulation a number of other industries, including iron foundries, copper and brass foundries, blast furnaces, and in general any plant employing 50 or more persons in manufacturing. The same year saw the enactment of the Workshops Regulation Act applying to manufacturing establishments employing fewer than 50 people. In 1860, a consolidating Coal Mines Act was passed which made the mine inspectorate a permanent institution, extended inspection to the ironstone mines connected with the coal pits, added new safety provisions, and raised the age of employment for boys underground to 12 years of age and for engine tenders to 18 years. There was as yet no legislative action to remedy or ameliorate the social and economic consequences of occupational disease.

With the rise of modern industry in Germany during the 1830s, especially in the newer industrial districts on the Rhine, the need for rectification of certain evils in factories and mines became apparent. In 1839, a Prussian royal decree restricted the use of children in industry. Employment of children younger than 9 years was prohibited; night work was forbidden for those between 9 and 16 years; and the maximum working day for employed children was fixed at 10 hours. Characteristically enough, this law was the result of reports by military surgeons on the decline in military fitness of the inhabitants of the Rhenish industrial districts. Local officials, teachers, and clergymen were made responsible for the administration of the law. In 1840, similar measures were promulgated in Bavaria and Baden. A Prussian law of 1853 prohibited the employment of children younger than 12 years, and inspection to see whether the law was being obeyed was made optional. On June 24, 1865, a General Mining Law was passed in Prussia requiring inspectors to investigate the safety of mines and to report any circumstance endangering the life and health of the miners. This law was later (1869) incorporated in the Industrial Code of the North German Confederation. This code also prohibited the employment of children younger than 12 years, and limited the work day of children younger than 14 years to six hours. Night work was prohibited for all young persons. This code was adopted by Württemberg and Baden in 1872 and by Bavaria in 1873. Factory inspection was not made obligatory in the German Empire until 1878.

Regulatory industrial legislation in France and Belgium dates from 1813 when an imperial decree prohibited the employment of children younger than 10 in mines, instituted a number of protective measures, and assigned the duty of inspection to the mine engineers. With the dissolution of the Napoleonic Empire and the establishment of the Belgian kingdom, this law seems to have been repealed, for child labor was quite common in Belgian mines during the nineteenth century. Various attempts to prohibit this evil failed, and it was not until 1884 that legislative action was taken to eradicate it and to regulate the labor of women and children. Aside from the 1813 law mentioned, the first piece of labor legislation in France was the Act of 1841 regulating child labor. This law forbade the employment of children younger than 8 years in factories. Between the ages of 8 and 12, they were permitted to work an eight hour day, and between 12 and 16 not more than 12 hours a day. However, the law was observed in the breach. Throughout the July Monarchy, the working conditions of men, women, and children in factories and mines continued to be appalling. The revolution of 1848 set forth important principles of social legislation and summed up its health program under the concept of social medicine. Indeed, the health situation of the masses was so poor that Louis Napoleon in his bid for power endeavored to ingratiate himself with the workers by means of a program of social legislation, including old-age pensions, free medical care for the indigent, and a compensation scheme for injured workers. Practical results of these hopes and plans were meager, however, and it was not until the Roussel law of 1874 that women and children younger than 12 years of age were protected in any way in factories and mines. Legislation did not concern itself with the working conditions of adult men nor was attention given in general to the maintenance of their health.

Concern for the health of American factory and mine workers followed closely the pattern described for England and the Continent. The coming of industrialism in the early nineteenth century was accompanied by the exploitation of the labor of women and children in dismal, unsanitary mills. During the 50 years between 1830 and 1880, efforts to improve the lot of factory labor were concerned primarily with the imposition of the most elementary regulations curtailing the length of the working day, limiting the age of employment, and introducing safety regulations. Attention was given primarily to the lot of women and children. Child labor legislation was inaugurated by Pennsylvania in 1848. The following year New York passed a law prohibiting the employment of children younger than 10 years. By 1860, a number of industrial states of the north had enacted some sort of child labor legislation. The effect of such laws was limited, however, for factory inspection was still nonexistent. Furthermore, there were no laws as yet to deal with unsatisfactory working conditions. Massachusetts was one of the first states to deal constructively with the latter problem. Beginning in 1852, Massachusetts over the following three decades enacted a body of legislation concerned with safety devices for steam boilers, dust removal in textile mills, safeguards for industrial machinery, and proper lighting, heating, and ventilation of factories. Finally, in 1888, general factory inspection was introduced.

Throughout most of the nineteenth century, efforts to improve the condition of factory and mine workers were concerned primarily with women and children. Ameliorative action was initiated as a reaction to the horrible conditions under which children worked, then to the underground employment of women and children, and it was not until the end of the nineteenth century and during the twentieth century that measures were taken to deal with the condition of adult workers. Furthermore, much of this had little direct connection with contemporary medical study of occupational disease. Medical testimony on the poor health of industrial workers was used to support the cause of reform, but as yet the study of occupational health was carried on in large measure apart from the agencies and groups concerned with regulation of the industrial environment.

Nevertheless, during this period, a number of studies were carried out which developed in very creditable fashion the basis established by Ramazzini and others in the eighteenth century. During the early nineteenth century and even later, the French led in the scientific study of occupational health. As late as 1822, Patissier offered physicians a French translation of Ramazzini, albeit enriched by his own observations. At this very time, however, other physicians were making original studies in this field. Obviously, it is impossible to discuss all of them, and a few have already been mentioned. Most important is Villermé to whom reference has been made at several points. The other great French hygienist of this period, A. Parent-Duchatelet (1790–1836), who is best known today for his treatise on prostitution in Paris, was concerned chiefly with the problem of sewerage and dealt with the health problems of sewer workers. In 1838, L. Tanquerel des Planches (1809–1862) published his classic treatise on lead poisoning. L. F. Benoiston de Chateauneuf (1776–1862) and H. C. Lombard (1803–1895) dealt with the influence of different occupations on pulmonary tuberculosis. Not only physicians occupied themselves with such problems of occupational health. The chemist J. B. A. Chevallier (1793–1879) studied industrial poisons. In 1846, the physician Th. V. J. Roussel (1816–1903) published a treatise on the diseases of workers in match factories, which was a pioneer study of occupational phosphorous necrosis. Occupational stigmas were studied by Ambroise Tardieu, who published his monograph in 1849 and who contributed greatly to occupational medicine during the middle nineteenth century.

By this time, the subject of occupational health had begun to receive increasing attention in Britain. The first original English work to deal with the influence of occupation on health was the book by the Leeds surgeon Thackrah, published in 1831. Slowly interest in the medical aspects of occupation increased and more articles began to appear in the professional journals of the period. Some of the best investigations in England were the statistical analyses of William Farr and the reports prepared under the direction of John Simon. Most significant was the work of E. H. Greenhow who in the 1860s studied the prevalence of industrial disease in manufacturing districts of England. Greenhow paid particular attention to dust diseases of the lungs. Other reports dealt with necrosis of the jaw (phossy jaw) suffered by workers in the match industry. The full effect of such studies was not to be felt, however, until the twentieth century.

In the United States, the medical study of occupational health did not really exist prior to the nineteenth century. To be sure, scholars and scientists like Cotton Mather and Benjamin Franklin were aware of certain hazards. For example, the latter knew of lead poisoning among typesetters and others who worked with lead. The influence of Ramazzini and other European authors is still to be felt in publications of the early nineteenth century, such as the anonymous *Remarks on the Disorders of Literary Men . . .* (1825) and G. Hayward's *A Lecture on Some of the Diseases of a Literary Life* (1833). The pioneer American work in this field, however, is generally considered to be Benjamin W. McCready's prize essay written in 1837 for the Medical Society of the State of New York. This monograph, entitled *On the Influence of Trades, Professions and Occupations in the United States in the Production of Disease*, reflects the influence of Thackrah and exhibits the first impact of growing urbanism and industrialization. A number of publications that appeared between 1837 and the 1870s are indicative of the problems that attracted the attention of physicians and others. Among these may be mentioned Johnson: Colica pictonum. . ., *St. Louis med. surg. J.* 1847–1848; Skeel: Lead colic, or mine sickness, *St. Louis med. surg. J.* 1848–1849; Gardner: Hygiene of the sewing machine, *Am. med. Times,* 1860; Wyman, Observations on dust, *Boston med. surg. J.,* 1862; Carpenter: Mining considered with regard to its effects upon health and life, *Tr. med. Soc. Penn.,*

1869; and Walker: Occupations of the People, *Atlantic Monthly,* 1869. Further-more, the development of mining in the West (California and Nevada) pro-duced a considerable literature on mine hygiene by physicians, engineers, and laymen. The literature on this subject as well as on other aspects of industrial health increased even further during the 1880s and particularly the 1890s.

Throughout this period, knowledge on industrial health was slowly being accumulated, and it was to be the accomplishment of the twentieth century to unite medical research, administrative action, and social reform for the com-mon goal of improving the health of the worker.

A PERIOD OF GREAT EPIDEMICS. While the working man's environment in factory and mine was slowly being brought under control, outbreaks of infec-tious disease and the problem of general sanitation continued to be the main concern of those occupied with the health of the community, for this was a pe-riod of great epidemics. On four occasions during the nineteenth century, Eu-rope and America were scourged by severe invasions of Asiatic cholera resulting from world pandemics. Yellow fever was dreaded even more than cholera in the United States. Beginning with the dreadful attack of yellow fever on Philadel-phia in 1793, a series of great epidemics recurred periodically until almost the end of the nineteenth century. While cholera and yellow fever caused conster-nation and panic when they appeared, other infectious diseases were continu-ally present in urban communities during the whole of the nineteenth century, appearing from time to time in the form of severe outbreaks and taking a heavy toll of lives. Most important were smallpox, typhus, typhoid, dysentery, diph-theria, and scarlet fever.

While the biological element in the causation of these epidemics cannot be disregarded, they were due in considerable measure to economic and social fac-tors. The railroad and the steamship revolutionized transportation during this period. With steam, shipping was no longer dependent on the uncertainties of the weather. Ships and trains arrived on schedule; perishable goods could be carried; and more people traveled. The world began to grow smaller. Distant places could be reached with comparative ease and in relatively short time. As a result, trading communities having extensive contacts with countries whose sanitary and health conditions were much poorer were continually exposed to the importation of cases of communicable disease. When communities with unfavorable environmental conditions, such as polluted water supplies, grossly inadequate sewerage, and congested housing, were invaded, the development of epidemics is hardly surprising. Communicable diseases arising in the intestine, such as cholera, typhoid, and dysentery, are transmitted through contaminated water, food, utensils, or through the patient directly. Other diseases, such as diphtheria, scarlet fever, and smallpox, are generally communicated from per-son to person by droplets from the mouth. In either case, the conditions prevailing in urban communities throughout most of the nineteenth century facilitated the spread and flare-up of infectious diseases.

The great cholera pandemics of 1831 and 1832, 1848 and 1849, and 1853 and 1854 originated in India, where the disease had been epidemic since 1816, and spread from Asia into Europe. The swift incubation period of cholera and its rapid course help to explain why the disease had not spread beyond Asia during earlier centuries when transportation was slow and difficult. Furthermore, the propagation of such a disease requires a rapid movement of large numbers of people, and this condition was provided in the nineteenth century, for this was also a period of great migrations. War, political unrest, famine, and, most important of all, economic conditions set large masses of people in motion, many of whom moved westward toward America creating what Marcus Hansen called the Atlantic Migration.

Thus Asiatic cholera did not invade America until 1832. It was brought to Quebec in Canada by immigrants from Ireland and then spread rapidly down the newly developed Erie Canal through New York State and westward into the Mississippi Valley. Cholera also entered the cities of New York and New Orleans, whence it spread along the Atlantic seaboard and into the interior. The epidemic of 1849 followed a similar course. Coming from Asia as before, it invaded Europe in 1847. Russia, Germany, France, and Great Britain were all attacked. The disease was again brought to the United States, this time by German immigrants. From New Orleans, it spread up the Mississippi Valley, arriving just in time to accompany the "Forty-niners" to California. There was another invasion of cholera in 1866, and the last epidemic occurred in 1873. Thereafter, with better understanding of the cause and mode of transmission of cholera, and with more effective methods of control available, the disease receded and has not reinvaded the United States since then.

The great epidemics invaded Europe at a time when many regarded such outbreaks of disease as a thing of the past. England had been free of the plague since 1665. True, the epidemic of 1720 at Marseilles was still remembered, but there, too, the disease had not returned. Minor local epidemics of plague or yellow fever had occurred in southern Europe. Having suffered repeatedly from yellow fever, Americans were somewhat more aware of the problem of epidemic disease. Wherever cholera struck, however, it was soon realized that energetic control measures had to be taken to stop this new scourge. But what measures? For those who believed in the theory of a specific contagion, the proper thing to do was to carry out a strict quarantine. More widely held at this time, however, was the miasmatic theory. According to this theory, communicable diseases arose from effluvia produced by decaying organic matter. When these emanations were brought forth under certain meteorological conditions, epidemics developed. From this theoretical position, it followed ineluctably that what was needed was to clean up the community, not to quarantine people and goods. Furthermore, this view was more congenial to commercial nations and communities for whom any hindrance in the free transit of goods and people was highly disadvantageous. Nor should it be forgotten that the practices of quarantine was much more rigid and severe than it is today when the conditions of disease transmission are better understood. As a result, the origin, transmission, and control of communicable diseases became burning political and public health issues in the nineteenth century. At the same time, the great epidemics acted as stimuli toward practical action. The need for controlling the spread of epidemics raised the question of international cooperation for this purpose, and eventually led to the foundation of an international public health organization. In England, the propaganda value of the cholera epidemic of 1848 cannot be discounted in the creation of the General Board of Health. Similarly, in the United States, port quarantine on a national basis was established in 1878 as a direct result of the 1873 epidemic. The power to enforce this measure was given to the Surgeon General of the Marine Hospital Service, thus creating the nucleus that eventually became the United States Public Health Service. Finally, it was through a study of cholera that John Snow developed a sound epidemiological basis for the development of the modern theory of contagion.

—AND SOME SMALLER ONES. Cholera and yellow fever were terrifying disasters, but other endemic diseases were equally if not more effective in taking a heavy toll of life. Smallpox was present in American and European urban communities during the nineteenth century, appearing from time to time in epidemic waves. The struggle to control this dangerous and disfiguring disease lasted for many years, and it was not until the twentieth century that it was actually controlled in the United States. While vaccination was available and had been shown to be effective, a certain proportion of the population remained unvaccinated. Popular suspicion kept many from being vaccinated, and in some degree this attitude was justified. The method of vaccinating from arm to arm did have its dangers. Erysipelas, syphilis, and other infectious diseases were sometimes spread this way. After the middle of the century, however, the danger of disease transmission was eliminated. In 1845, Negri of Naples began to propagate virus in cows, thus eliminating the dangers inherent in the use of humanized virus. The practice spread from Italy to France in 1866 and then to Germany and other parts of Europe. Virus obtained from France was introduced into a herd of cows near Boston in 1870, and this was the beginning of the use of calf lymph in the United States. The use of sterilized glycerine for the preservation of lymph was first recommended by Robert Koch.

Important causes of death among children were scarlet fever and diphtheria. By the end of eighteenth century, a clinical concept of scarlet fever had been generally recognized by physicians. Clinicians were clear about Scarlatina simplex, that is, mild scarlet fever without complications. There was some confusion with diphtheria, but then shortly after the turn of the century, scarlet fever declined in virulence, and for about the first quarter of the nineteenth century, there was small interest in a more precise understanding of the disease. In the 1830s, however, there was a change for the worse. Scarlet fever began to increase in virulence, culminating in a period of some 40 years (1840–1880) during which there were frequent and severe epidemics in Europe and America.

In 1831, an outbreak of a very malignant type occurred in Dublin, and in 1834, Ireland was ravaged by the disease, which caused as many deaths as cholera had in 1832. The first great epidemic covering all of England occurred in 1840, a second came in 1844, and a third in 1848. The worst English epidemics occurred during the period 1850 to 1890. The United States experienced similar outbreaks. In New York City, for example, scarlet fever was very rarely encountered between 1805 and 1822. During those 18 years, there were only 43 reported deaths from scarlet fever. After 1822, the disease gradually assumed an epidemic character, and by the end of 1847, there were 4874 deaths. Thereafter, there was a progressive decline until 1845, when a second epidemic wave began to build up, which reached its culmination in 1857 with 1325 deaths. In 1865, when the Council of Hygiene reported on the sanitary condition of New York, scarlet fever was noted as prevalent and often fatal. Similar trends may be observed in Chicago and other localities.

There is no question that a change occurred after 1830, and scarlet fever became, as Charles Creighton noted, "the leading cause of death among the infectious diseases of childhood." It remained so in Europe, in Great Britain, and in the United States until the last decades of the nineteenth century. After 1880, the severity of scarlet fever diminished, and at present it is probably milder than at any period in its history.

The transmissible nature of scarlet fever was in large measure accepted during the nineteenth century. However, it was in the study of diphtheria that a significant forward step was taken to establish the specific nature of the disease and its transmissibility. The method, which put diphtheria and other communicable diseases on a sound clinical foundation, thus making possible their further investigation, was developed from two directions. In the seventeenth century, Thomas Sydenham had developed the concept of a disease as an entity, an objective thing in itself, that might be observed at the bedside, and then described and classified. This clinical trend was paralleled by an anatomical approach to the study of disease. Anatomical investigation had been sedulously cultivated for centuries, and in the course of innumerable dissections and autopsies, a mass of pathological observations was collected. Gradually, the view gained ground that the reactions observed in human beings under the stress of disease are related to the lesions found after death. This idea was first given effective expression by G. B. Morgagni (1682–1771) in his work *De sedibus et causis morborum* (*On the Seats and Causes of Disease*), which appeared in 1761 at Venice. The fusion of the clinical and anatomical trends and their systematic application was the great contribution of the Paris school of clinical pathologists from 1800 to 1850. In their work, there emerged from the confusion of the eighteenth century a relatively clear and critical picture of diseases based upon the idea that there was a definite connection between the clinical findings at the bedside and the anatomical lesions observed at autopsy.

Application of this method to the problem of diphtheria, or "angina maligna," as it was then called, produced a fundamental contribution toward an understanding of the disease and gave it its present name. Down to about 1860, angina maligna was most prevalent in France, and it was there that this advance was made by Pierre-Fidèle Bretonneau (1778–1862), chief physician to the Hospice Général at Tours. In 1818, an epidemic designated as "scorbutic gangrene" of the mouth and throat appeared among soldiers in garrison at Tours. Shortly thereafter the civilian population near the barracks was attacked by angina maligna. Bretonneau studied the epidemic, which prevailed from 1818 to 1820, with scrupulous care, maintaining accurate records of his clinical observations and postmortem studies. These observations, augmented by a great deal of additional material, were then published in 1826 under the title *Des inflammations spéciales du tissu muqueux, et en particulier de la diphthérite, ou inflamation pelliculaire* (*On Specific Inflammations of Mucous Tissue, and Particularly on Diphtheritis, or Membranous Inflammation*). This classic work swept away the earlier unclear concepts of malignant angina, throat distemper, and croup, establishing in their place the doctrine of *diphthérite* as a specific disease. Bretonneau coined the term *diphthérite* from the Greek word *diphthera* (a piece of leather, a prepared hide); in 1855, in his final memoir on the subject, he dropped it for the term *diphthérie* (diphtheria), which we use today.

Bretonneau had a clear concept that communicable diseases are specific and that this specificity is determined in large measure by the nature of the disease cause. Based on his investigations, he concluded that diphtheria was a disease in which the characteristic anatomical feature, the false membrane, resulted from some unknown special agent acting on the body. He knew that in man diphtheria was communicable, having traced the disease from family to family in several deadly epidemics. Although Bretonneau's concept was remarkably clear and accurate, the problem of diphtheria was still not completely solved. Nor could it be until the postulated causative agent was discovered and its etiologic relationship to the disease demonstrated. Bretonneau did not attempt to relate the communicable principle of *diphthérite* to microscopic organisms that were already known and were being discussed in his time. It was not until the close of the nineteenth century that this essential aim in the investigation of diphtheria was finally achieved.

Bretonneau's concept of diphtheria left the problem of transmission unresolved. If the disease were transmissible, was this due to a specific microorganism? A number of investigators undertook to study experimentally this and related problems. An important factor in furthering these researches was the pandemic of diphtheria that broke out at various points in Europe and North America between 1856 and 1858 and soon spread to almost every part of the globe. During the earlier part of the nineteenth century, France, Denmark, and Norway had been the only countries severely affected by epidemics of diphtheria, but after the fifth decade of the century, the disease was to be found in all civilized communities of the temperate zone. The incidence and severity of diphtheria varied widely during this period, but it was overwhelmingly a disease of childhood, not of adult life. A second epidemic wave appeared in Europe around 1890, which then declined steadily over the next 30 years. While the spread of diphtheria gave great impetus to research, the results were generally confusing. Apart from the work of Friedrich Trendelenburg and Max Joseph Oertel, pathological anatomists and experimental investigators contributed little to establish Bretonneau's concept on a firmer foundation. Trendelenburg in 1869 reported the successful inoculation of diphtheritic material in animals, and his results were confirmed and extended by Oertel in 1871. The solution of the problem was to come, however, from another direction—from studies intended to elucidate the cause of disease in terms of specific microorganisms.

Meanwhile, evidence pointing in this direction was being gathered by other students of epidemics. Much that we know about the epidemiology of measles derives from the classic study made by Peter Ludwig Panum (1820–1885) during an epidemic on the Faroe Islands in 1846. After an epidemic prevalence in 1781, measles disappeared completely from the islands for 65 years. Reintroduced in 1846, the disease soon became epidemic, attacking a majority of the population. Panum, then 26 years old and just out of medical school, was sent to the islands by the Danish government as a member of a medical commission to provide necessary aid to the inhabitants and to make a careful study of the epidemic. His report, published in 1847, established the fundamental epidemiological features of measles. (Parenthetically, it may be noted that his report took the form of a medical topography and clearly illustrates the transition from the earlier generalized approach to community health problems to the more specifically epidemiological point of view that was being developed and applied.) Panum showed that the incubation period was generally 13 to 14 days, the rash appearing at that time after previous exposure. He found all ages susceptible to the disease, and he also noted that one attack conferred immunity. Furthermore, Panum showed that the disease is most communicable during the eruption and flourishing of the rash and that it may also be transmitted during the prodromal period, but he found no evidence of transmission in the desquamation state. Finally, he concluded that measles is a purely contagious disease, and therefore that isolation is the surest means of arresting its progress. Many other interesting topics are considered by Panum in his report. In the light of current concern with the question whether simpler societies have less mental illness than highly complex ones, it is interesting to read Panum's discussion of this problem more than a century ago and his conclusion that "there is hardly any country, hardly, indeed, any metropolis, in which mental diseases are so frequent in proportion to the number of people as on the Faroes." One further fact in connection with the Faroe Islands is worth noting. Another epidemic appeared in 1875, and on this occasion, it was shown that only persons younger than 30 years, who therefore had not been affected by the previous epidemic, were susceptible. By the latter part of the nineteenth century, it was generally accepted that measles was caused by some microscopic *materies morbi*, "that this poison reproduces itself within the diseased organism, and that the spread of the disease from person to person and from place to place takes place solely by the conveyance of the poison."

Two other names stand out as having made significant contributions to the principle that specific infection, by some agency resembling a living organism, is the sole source of communicable disease. They are John Snow (1813–1858) and William Budd (1811–1880), who must be counted among the great epidemiologists. John Snow was a medical practitioner in London and was in his own day far better known as an anesthetist than as one of the most brilliant epidemiologists of all time. Indeed, his reputation was such that in 1853 and again in 1857 he administered chloroform to Queen Victoria when she was delivered. Snow had seen cases of cholera at Newcastle-on-Tyne during the epidemic of 1831 and 1832, when the disease recurred in 1848 he began actively to study it. He was then in London, and his first communication appeared there in 1849 as a pamphlet entitled *On the Mode of Communication of Cholera*. During the epidemic of 1854, Snow carried out a more systematic investigation, which involved also the consumers of water from the Broad Street pump. In the course of his study, he examined the distribution of deaths from cholera in the southern sections of London where drinking water was supplied by several private water companies. Snow showed that the number of deaths in each area corresponded to the degree of pollution of the part of the Thames River from which each company obtained its water. In 1855, Snow published a second, enlarged edition of his 1849 pamphlet in which he set forth his definitive views on the etiology and spread of cholera. The clinical features of the disease led him to infer that the poison of cholera enters the alimentary canal directly by mouth, and that this poison is probably a specific living being derived from the excreta of a cholera patient. Furthermore, he showed that cholera can be transmitted from person to person through soiling of the hands or through contaminated food and water. Finally, Snow pointed out that defective sewerage made it possible for the dangerous wastes from cholera patients to permeate the ground and to pollute wells or other supplies of water used by the community. Snow showed conclusively that the agent of cholera infection could be carried in water, but he, too, did not identify the infecting agent. These views were not immediately accepted, although John Simon, William Farr, and other health workers were aware of them. Not until 1883 when Koch isolated and cultivated *Vibrio cholerae* was the essential correctness of Snow's teaching proved.

Simultaneous discovery is by no means uncommon in the field of science; it is not surprising therefore to find that the views formulated by Snow had been developed independently by his countryman and contemporary, William Budd. In 1849, the year in which Snow's first communication appeared, Budd also published a pamphlet on *Malignant Cholera: Its Mode of Propagation and its Prevention* in which he advanced similar conclusions. Cholera in his view was caused by a specific living organism, breeding in the human intestinal tract and disseminated by contaminated drinking water. Budd recognized that these views also applied to typhoid fever, which he studied for more than 30 years. His contributions to the epidemiology of typhoid appeared in the *Lancet* and the *British Medical Journal,* and it was not until 1873 that these studies were summed up in a volume entitled *Typhoid Fever, its Nature, Mode of Spreading and Prevention.* Based on his observations and theoretical inferences, Budd advised that the excreta of typhoid patients be disinfected so as to reduce the incidence of the disease. As a provincial practitioner, however, his views aroused no great interest and remained without much influence on official public health practice.

Nonetheless, the cumulative effect of investigations and researches, such as those of Bretonneau, Panum, Snow, and Budd, cannot be denied. Epidemiologically, they marked an important advance in understanding the nature of communicable diseases, and they all pointed in the same direction—toward the theory of an animate contagion, a living organism able to reproduce itself. What, then, prevented the acceptance of this view?

MIASMA VERSUS CONTAGION—AN EPIDEMIOLOGICAL CONUNDRUM. As a matter of fact, by the early nineteenth century, both contagionist and noncontagionist explanations of the origin and spread of infectious diseases were quite old. Both theories derived from a fusion of ancient concepts and empirical observations, and their history throughout the centuries had been a series of ups and downs, of ascendancy and devaluation. As might be expected from such a process, in the course of time the two viewpoints merged in some degree to produce an intermediate position.

Consequently, for most of the nineteenth century, three theoretical positions may be distinguished. First, there was the miasmatic theory that epidemic outbreaks of infectious disease were caused by the state of the atmosphere. During the nineteenth century, this was held generally in the modified version that poor sanitary conditions produced a local atmospheric state that caused such diseases. Many of the sanitary reformers, among them Edwin Chadwick and Southwood Smith, held this view, which abundantly justified their endeavors for sanitary improvement. Then, there was the view that specific contagia are the sole causes of infections and epidemic diseases. This was the strict contagionist position taken by Budd and Snow, and the one with which health workers today are most familiar because of the great impact of the bacteriological discoveries at the end of the nineteenth century. The third position was adopted by those who endeavored to conciliate or to compromise the miasmatic and contagionist theories, and may be called limited or contingent contagionism. While admitting that infectious diseases are due to contagia, either specific or nonspecific, the proponents of this view held that the latter could not act except in conjunction with other elements, such as the state of the atmosphere, condition of the soil, or social factors. This was the most widely field theoretical position, and among its advocates were John Simon and Max von Pettenkofer. Its popularity was due in large measure to its portmanteau character. Able to accommodate a variety of elements, some of them mutually inconsistent, this view persisted into the last decades of the nineteenth century. As late as 1888, for instance, Dr. J. Lewis Smith, at that time Clinical Professor of Children's Diseases at Bellevue Hospital Medical College in New York, held the opinion that the virus of diphtheria grew in foul, damp places and that the sewer systems of large cities were infected. He believed that most children developed diphtheria by inhaling infected sewer gas. Practically, limited contagionists tended more often than not to oppose the consequence of contagionism, such as isolation and quarantine.

In the contest between the miasmatic and contagionist theories, the former was dominant until the latter part of the nineteenth century. Erwin H. Ackerknecht, in an excellent study of anticontagionism, has pointed out that, curiously enough, it was "shortly before their final and overwhelming victory, that the theories of contagion and the contagium vivum experienced the deepest depression and devaluation in their long and stormy career, and it was shortly before its disappearance that 'anticontagionism' reached its highest peak of elaboration, acceptance, and scientific respectability." Scientifically, the miasmatist and contagionist theories were too evenly balanced for any clear-cut decisions to be made on the basis of the existing evidence. The positions of both parties contained a number of weak spots. Both sides made use of unreliable information and biased observations as a basis for reasoning. Frequently, the dangerous intellectual procedure of reasoning by analogy was employed, and there was still an inadequate appreciation and application of experimental methods. Finally, neither group had any knowledge of certain important links in the chain of infection, such as the human carrier and the insect host. The scientific standpoint taken was frequently related to nonscientific, that is, political, economic, and social, factors.

A clue to an understanding of the ascendancy of anticontagionism during this period is provided by the observation that it coincides with the rise of liberalism. Anticontagionists in many instances were liberal reformers who fought for individual freedom against despotism and reaction. This group numbered among its leaders Virchow, Southwood Smith, Magendie, Chervin—all known as liberals or radicals. Contagionism found its concrete expression in the institution of quarantine and its officialdom. The economic implications of quarantine have been pointed out, but it must be emphasized that to merchants and industrialists quarantine meant financial loss and intolerable shackles to business expansion. Thus, an attack against contagionism was a blow against bureaucracy and for freedom, against reaction and for progress. This is not to suggest that anticontagionist leaders consciously let themselves be influenced by prevailing commercial interests. Nevertheless, since many physicians were liberal and belonged to the middle class, it is not surprising to have this coincidence of outlook.

FIRST STEPS TOWARD INTERNATIONAL HEALTH ORGANIZATION. The controversy concerning the origin and transmission of infectious diseases made itself felt not only within various countries but in the international sphere as well. As commerce and transportation developed and distances shrank during the nineteenth century, it was no longer a matter of indifference what kind of health conditions prevailed in different parts of the world. International cooperation for the prevention of transmissible diseases became a matter of the greatest importance, and in 1851, the first step was taken toward the creation of an international health organization with the opening of the first international sanitary conference at Paris.

While this meeting is generally regarded as the beginning of international public health, attention must be called to several earlier efforts in this direction. The problem of sanitary organization was apparently treated from an international point of view for the first time by Johann Peter Frank. In 1776, when he set about collecting material for the work that eventually became the great *System*, he wrote a brochure explaining his intentions and inviting colleagues to help him by sending material. This "Letter of Invitation to Scholars . . ." (*Epis-*

tola Invitatoria ad Eruditos . . .) was addressed to learned men in the German States and other countries. In this work, Frank discusses the need for regulation of medical licensure on an international basis and stresses the need for exchange of information on health. The result of his appeal was disappointing, and Frank remained unheeded by his contemporaries.

The first significant practical steps toward controlling the spread of epidemics on an international basis was taken in the early nineteenth century. In 1833, Mehemet Ali, ruler of Egypt, set up a sanitary board headed by a Consular Commission of Health, representing various European countries. This Commission stressed the importance of protecting European countries, and undertook to deal with problems of quarantine and international hygiene. The body soon grew too powerful for the taste of the Egyptian ruler, and in 1839, he dissolved it. A new sanitary board was created in January 1840, in which the foreign powers had no representation. In 1843, however, Mehemet Ali agreed to have certain European countries represented without a vote. This was the state of affairs at the time of the Paris conference.

International cooperation had also begun in one other instance. In 1839, a meeting took place in Constantinople between the Health Committee of the Sublime Porte and the representatives of the foreign powers accredited to the Turkish Empire. At this meeting, it was attempted to reach an understanding with regard to the quarantine system. In particular, the delicate problem of interference with trade had to be adjusted and a number of regulations were laid down. The purpose was to promote free intercourse between Turkey and the European countries in the absence of plague. While the quarantine system was an extensive one, it was not efficient.

The first proposal for an international sanitary conference was made in 1834 by Segur de Peyron, an inspector in the French sanitary service. A similar suggestion was made in 1843 by the British government, but it was opposed by Austria as premature, as there was no foundation on which to develop a set of regulations that would be acceptable to the different powers. The idea was taken up in 1845 by the Frenchman Melier, on whose urging the French Government finally took the initiative for the first international sanitary conference, which opened in Paris on August 5, 1851. The countries represented were Austria-Hungary, the Two Sicilies, Spain, the Papal States, Great Britain, Greece, Portugal, France, Russia, Sardinia, Tuscany, and Turkey. Each state was represented by two delegates, a diplomat and a physician, since it was recognized that the conference had to deal with technical and medical problems as well as administrative and diplomatic ones. The object of the conference was to remove all unnecessary delays to international commerce while safeguarding the general health.

Obviously, the delegates who gathered at Paris, early in August, faced a difficult task. From the preceding discussion, it is clear that a group of medical men gathered from all parts of Europe were not likely to find it easy to agree. While the intentions of the delegates were good, the long discussions and controversies among the medical members led nowhere. Indeed, the proceedings of their conference read in part like a text in the epidemiological theories of the period. Nevertheless, the importance of this first venture in international collaboration in the interest of world health was clear to all, and, with immense patience, a convention and a series of regulations were worked out. These regulations represent a first attempt at an international sanitary code; they dealt with problems of quarantine and the reporting of cholera, plague, and yellow fever. At the same time, it was agreed that nothing could be considered that might in any way be regarded as interfering with the sovereignty of each country.

The immediate result of the conference was meager indeed. The convention was ratified only by France, Portugal, and Sardinia, and both Portugal and Sardinia withdrew from the convention in 1865. Nevertheless, the seed of international cooperation in health matters had been sown and in time would produce an effective organization. The importance of international health problems was underlined during this period by the cholera pandemic that started in 1863, and by the opening of the Suez Canal on November 17, 1869. Further conferences were held at Paris in 1859, at Constantinople in 1866, and at Vienna in 1874. None of these conferences produced any practical results. Yet these meetings kept alive the idea of international collaboration, and much later work had its origin in their discussions. However, it was not until the end of the century that agreement was finally reached on practical action in the interest of international health. Before this could happen, however, a greater degree of understanding and agreement on the origin and transmission of infectious diseases had to be achieved. This achievement was accomplished through the development of bacteriology and immunology, the sciences that have exercised the most profound influence on community health action from the end of the nineteenth century to the present day.

-VII-
The Bacteriological Era and Its Aftermath (1875–1950)

THE SPECIFIC ELEMENT IN DISEASE. A sniffling, coughing New Yorker who turns to a friend in the subway and says, "Gee, have I got a virus!" is expressing colloquially a theory of infection that has had momentous, even revolutionary, and certainly unanticipated consequences through its application over the past half century. Outstanding among these consequences is the virtual eradication or the effective control in many areas of communicable diseases spread by water, milk, and food, or transmitted by insects, rodents, and man himself, so that in countries like the United States once-dreaded diseases, such as yellow fever, typhoid fever, diphtheria, and malaria, are a thing of the past. As an immediate result, decades have been added to the average life span, but in turn this development has led to a drastic alteration in the age structure of the population, since many more people than ever before survive into the middle and older years.

These effects stem directly from the incontrovertible demonstration toward the end of the nineteenth century that specific microscopic creatures rather than vague chemical miasmas produce infectious diseases. That infectious diseases can have a living particulate cause was not exactly new in the middle of the nineteenth century. From remote antiquity, the idea had been advanced by thoughtful and penetrating observers that infectious diseases were transmitted by contagion and caused by "seeds," "animalculae," or "worms." This idea had its start without benefit of bacteriology, and some material progress was made even before germs were discovered. Yet it was not until the second half of the nineteenth century that medical opinion slowly began to change and to veer toward this view. In some degree this change was a reaction to the ineffectiveness of the miasmatic theory, but even more significant was the rapidly accumulating evidence in support of the idea that specific microorganisms caused contagious, epidemic diseases.

"A MORE RATIONAL ACCOUNT OF THE ITCH." As far back as the seventeenth century, scabies had been shown to be due to the itch mite, *Acarus scabiei*. The mite was seen by August Hauptmann (1657), Michael Ettmüller (1682), and G. C. Bonomo who described it fully in his letter to Francesco Redi in 1687. Bonomo relates how he had seen poor women extract with the point of a pin little "bladders of water" from the "scabby skin" of children who had the itch, and cracked "them like fleas upon their nails," and how "scabby slaves in the Bagno at Leghorn" often performed the same service for each other. Thereupon, he "quickly found an Itchy person and asking him where he felt the greatest . . . itching, he pointed to a great many little Pustules not yet Scabb'd over," from one of which he took out a very small white globule. Then, Bonomo continues, "observing this with a microscope, I found it to be a very minute Living Creature in shape resembling a tortoise. . . ." He then goes on to make a very significant comment. "From this Discovery," Bonomo says, "it may be no difficult matter to give a more Rational account of the Itch, than Authors have hitherto delivered us. It being very probable that this contagious Disease owes its origin neither to the Melancholy Humour of Galen, nor the corrosive acid of Sylvius, nor the particular Ferment of Van Helmont, nor the Irritating Salts in the Serum of Lympha of the Moderns, but is no other than the continual biting of these Animalcules in the Skin."

Bonomo's description and his sagacious inference from his observations remained without influence. The discoveries and reports of Leeuwenhoek aroused some interest in the theory of an animate contagion, but without any tangible results in support of the doctrine. Sporadic comments on the subject are to be found in the eighteenth century. In 1757, for example, Nyander, a pupil of Linnaeus, asserted that the itch mite and the cheese mite were identical, and that mites caused plague, smallpox, syphilis, and dysentery. Nevertheless, the first influential demonstration of a specific organism responsible for a specific disease was not made until the nineteenth century.

A DISEASE OF SILKWORMS. Bretonneau had postulated that a specific disease, such as diphtheria, developed "under the influence of a contagious principle, a reproductive agent," but he did not endeavor to link this agent with microscopic animalcules. The actual demonstration of the truth of this hypothesis was provided by Agostino Bassi (1773–1856), a civil servant of Lodi. In Bassi's time, the dreaded disease of silkworms called *muscardine* by the French and *mal del segno* or *calcinaccio* by the Italians, had caused great damage to the silk industry of Lombardy. On the basis of studies carried out over many years, he reached the conclusion that the disease was communicable and that the silkworm was contagious long before its death. By means of the microscope, Bassi recognized that the causative agent of muscardine was a cryptogamic parasitic fungus. He realized that the disease was transmitted by contact and infected food, and developed methods for its prevention in silkworm nurseries.

After carrying on his studies for nearly 20 years, Bassi in 1834 finally presented his theory of contagion to the medical and philosophical faculties of Pavia, and over the next two years published his great work *Del mal del segno, calcinaccio o moscardino*. A second edition of the entire work appeared in 1837. At the same time Bassi's work was confirmed by Balsamo-Crivelli (1835) and Audouin (1836). The former showed that the fungus seen by Bassi was *Botrytis paradoxa*, and renamed it *B. bassiana* in honor of its discoverer. From his discoveries, Bassi drew far-reaching conclusions as to the nature of contagious diseases, attributing smallpox, typhus fever, plague, syphilis, cholera, and pellagra to living parasites. Furthermore, in the case of cholera he advocated strict isolation of the patient as well as disinfection of the excreta and clothes.

Observations along similar lines were also reported at this time from France and Germany. The French microscopist, Alfred Donné, in 1837, published his microscopic investigations of pathological discharges, especially of the human genital organs. In this work he first drew attention to and described the flagellate protozoon *Trichomonas vaginalis*. Then, in 1839, J. L. Schoenlein discovered a fungus in the condition known as favus; Robert Remak in 1840 named it *Achorion schoenleinii* after him and demonstrated its contagiosity.

A REVOLUTIONARY ANATOMIST FIGHTS A REARGUARD ACTION. In 1840 there appeared at Berlin a slim volume entitled *Pathologische Untersuchungen*, whose author, Jacob Henle (1809–1885), then 31 years old, had just entered on his duties as professor of anatomy at Zürich. This book is today regarded as a landmark in the history of bacteriology and of communicable diseases because of its first section, which deals with "miasmata and contagia and miasmatic-contagious diseases." Unlike other important medical contributions, however, this essay does not contain a single new discovery. Its contribution was of another order; based on deductive considerations from the observations of others and through logical and cogent arguments, Henle formulated a theory that living microscopic organisms were the cause of contagious and infectious diseases.

Jacob Henle believed that freedom of thought and exact methods of observation and investigation were essential for the advancement of biological and medical knowledge. His political liberalism—he had been imprisoned in 1835 for his political connections—reinforced the rational cast of his scientific thought. In fact, the volume in which the essay on miasmas and contagia appeared was a preliminary study for Henle's future work which bears the significant title, *Handbuch der rationellen Pathologie*, i.e., a textbook of rational pathology.

The main object that Henle had in view in this essay was to bring some order into the confused welter of ideas on the origin of communicable diseases, which existed around the middle of the nineteenth century. His reasoning was based on facts collected by his predecessors and contemporaries, and it is noteworthy that Henle was very catholic in his choice of data, ranging from veterinary medicine to fetal pathology. His argument and conclusions may be summarized as follows: In cases of infectious disease, the morbid matter apparently increases from the moment it enters the body, leading to the conclusion that it must be organic in nature, since only living organisms have this faculty. Furthermore, the quantity of morbid matter is out of proportion to the effects it produces. The fact that a period of incubation usually precedes the outbreak of the disease also supports this conclusion. Having made it logically plausible that the causative factor in infectious diseases is a living organism, Henle considered the nature of the unknown parasite and, basing his views on the observations of Bassi and Audouin, concluded that it is very likely a member of the plant kingdom. This conclusion was also supported by the work of Cagniard-Latour and Schwann, who in 1837 showed that fermentation was due to the action of small organisms—yeasts.

Henle saw clearly that only by accurate observation and experiment would the problem of contagious disease be solved. As a guide for workers in this field, he laid down the postulates of proof that would have to be met in order to demonstrate conclusively that a specific organism was the cause of a specific disease. The conditions that Henle postulated—constant presence of the parasite, isolation from foreign admixtures, and reproduction of the disease by means of the isolated parasite—created problems that were difficult to solve, and it was not until more than 30 years later that one of his students, Robert Koch, was able to fulfill the conditions and furnish definitive proof that Henle's theory was correct.

The work of Bassi, Cagniard-Latour, Schwann, and Schönlein, reinforced by the theoretical analysis of Henle, stimulated the investigation of numerous disease products, and in the next few decades the presence of many microscopic organisms was recorded in diseases of man and animals. The fungus *Microsporon audouini,* which causes ringworm, was described in 1843 by David Gruby (1810–1898), a Hungarian Jew who worked in Paris for many years. Between 1843 and 1846, he conducted a remarkable series of studies on the etiology of ringworm, and with the rather crude microscope available to him foreshadowed modern work on trichophytons. He described the collection of fungi around the hair shaft in ringworm of the beard, and the presence of the fungus in the hair shaft in tinea tonsurans. Then, in 1850, bacteria were added to the list of possible pathogenic microorganisms. In a communication to the Société de biologie of Paris, Casimir Davaine and Pierre Rayer reported the transmission of anthrax by inoculating healthy sheep with the blood of animals dying of the disease, and the finding in the blood of dead sheep of micro-scopic rod-shaped bodies. Five years later, F. A. A. Pollender, a West-phalian physician, published a report on the microscopic examination of blood from an animal with anthrax. As early as 1849, he had observed the bodies described by Davaine and Rayer, and he gave a much more precise and detailed account of the rods. Pollender was inclined to consider them as of vegetable nature, but he could not say how they were related to the disease. These findings were con-firmed in 1857 by F. A. Brauell, a professor of veterinary medicine at Dorpat, who also carried out a long series of experiments on the transmission of an-thrax in animals. Further facts were added during the 1860s, but it was chiefly through the work of Davaine that attention remained centered on anthrax and its rod-shaped bodies.

Meanwhile, the theory that infectious diseases were due to the growth of germs in the body remained unacceptable to many capable physicians and others in the scientific world. Truly, between 1834 and 1850, the fungoid cause of certain diseases had been established, but, for many known communicable diseases, such an origin could not be substantiated, and the germ theory of dis-ease was rejected as a dead hypothesis. The intellectual climate of the period, as it relates to this doctrine and Henle's thought, is well described by Hip-polyte Bernheim, who is best known for his part in the development of psy-chotherapy. Writing in 1877, he pointed out that "serious observers recognized the emptiness of these fantastic concepts. Toward the middle of the century, this doctrine [of an animate contagion] was generally abandoned as an artifi-cial elaboration of the mind, without any scientific basis. Among medical lead-ers, Henle was perhaps the last who in 1853 still defended the doctrine of a *con-tagium verum* with the same determined conviction as when he had defended it with great logical vigor in 1840. In the last ten years, however, the parasitary doctrine has regained considerable credit in public opinion because of new in-vestigations and more positive findings." Obviously, in the opinion of Henle's contemporaries around the middle of the century, he was fighting a gallant rearguard action in defense of an obsolete idea. Yet, as Bernheim clearly indi-cates, it was at this very time that the germ theory began to recover from a state of comparative extinction. The impulses for this recrudescence came from a number of different directions, some of which had no immediate connection with the problem of contagious disease.

FERMENTS AND MICROBES. Of these impulses, probably none was ulti-mately of greater import than the questions concerning fermentation and spon-taneous generation. Historically, these problems were intertwined, and it was the knowledge gained in endeavoring to solve them that finally led to a fruit-ful understanding of the nature of contagious disease. Fermentation and pu-trefaction have been known to man for thousands of years, and he has used the processes involved to make bread and wine, to brew beer, to mature cheese, or to tan hides. Empirical observation and traditional practice remained the essential basis of these technologies until the early decades of the nineteenth century when the enormous expansion of demand created by the new urban populations made it necessary to acquire a more rational understanding on which to develop large-scale production. Here, as frequently happens, scientific and philosophic interests of almost equal antiquity, which had been pursued independently, impinged on technological problems.

Man has always been profoundly interested in the question of the origin of life and various speculations were entertained by the peoples of antiquity. The thought of ancient science was most completely summed up by Aristotle, who developed a theory that living creatures arise not only from other living things but also from lifeless matter. By the overwhelming authority given to his views, Aristotle's theory dominated the minds of men until the seventeenth century, when three Italian physician-naturalists, Francesco Redi, Antonio Vallisnieri, and Marcello Malpighi, struck the first important blows at the doctrine of spontaneous generation. Redi showed experimentally that maggots do not arise spontaneously in decaying meat, but develop from eggs deposited by flies. Similarly, Vallisineri and Malpighi explained that worms arose from eggs laid by other worms, how insect eggs were introduced into fruits and plants, and how maggots got into the frontal sinuses of sheep. Thus, it seemed that the question of spontaneous generation had been settled, but as is common in the history of science, new circumstances revitalized a theory that had apparently been disproved.

Leeuwenhoek's discovery of bacteria revived the question: Were these minute creatures spontaneously generated or did they arise from pre-existing seeds? Investigators soon found that these minute organisms were intimately associated with the familiar processes of fermentation and putrefaction. They were present in sour milk, rotting meat, or spoiled bouillon, wherever decay or fermentation took place. Furthermore, all that was required to have swarms of organisms appear where there had been none previously was to put easily spoiled organic matter in a warm place for a short time. In the light of such observations the idea was easily established that microscopic creatures were actually being produced from lifeless matter. Experiments to disprove this view were undertaken in the eighteenth century by the great Italian scientist, Lazzaro Spallanzani (1729–1799). From his investigations he concluded that such organisms were carried into infusions by the air, and that when flasks containing organic matter were hermetically sealed, the air excluded, and heat applied long enough, no organisms developed. Spallanzani's results were applied practically by Nicolas Appert, a retired distiller and confectioner of Paris. He devised a method of preserving food and wine by sealing them in flasks, which were then heated to boiling for a time. Nevertheless, this experience in food preservation remained restricted to the food industry and had no effect on the scientific world.

Despite the work of Spallanzani, the theory that organisms could arise spontaneously in organic infusions continued to be widely held and debated far into the nineteenth century. During this period, the question of spontaneous generation became involved with the problems of fermentation and putrefaction. These phenomena were generally considered to be the result of chemical changes in organic matter. For many years, these changes were believed due to some influence of the air, and a number of investigators attacked this problem. Experiments of great value were carried out by Franz Schultze (1836), Theodor Schwann (1836–39), and H. Schröder and T. von Dusch (1854). Of the largest significance, however, were the studies of Schwann. These led him to conclude that putrefaction in a meat extract was due not to air as such, but rather to some element in the air that was destroyed by heat. Schwann inferred that putrefaction occurred when germs or seeds of molds and infusoria from the air had access to organic matter and developed by deriving their nutrition from the latter. Finally, he expressed the view that putrefaction and fermentation were probably essentially similar processes due to the action of living organisms. It was in the course of this work that Schwann described the yeast plant and the way it reproduces by budding. Owing to inadequacies of technique, however, Schwann and other workers sometimes met with inconsistent results for which they could not account, with the consequence that many scientists remained unconvinced and the controversy over spontaneous generation and fermentation continued unabated.

THE SILKWORM DISEASE AND THE GERM THEORY. On December 7, 1854, in an opening address to his students, Louis Pasteur (1822–1895), then newly appointed as professor of chemistry and dean of the Faculty of Science at Lille, remarked that in the fields of observation "chance favors only the mind which is prepared." Certainly, it is no mere coincidence that this revealing comment so aptly describes the element in Pasteur's own work, which enabled him to explain the mysteries of fermentation, spontaneous generation, and ultimately of contagious disease.

A glance at the work with which Pasteur began his brilliant scientific career is necessary in order to understand what he achieved and how he did it. He made his first important discovery as a chemist in 1848 by demonstrating the true nature of tartaric acid and establishing the existence of molecular asymmetry. And it is this phenomenon of molecular asymmetry which provides the key to all of Pasteur's later work. He found that tartaric acid existed in two crystalline forms that were chemically similar, but that the crystals differed from each other as mirror images, or as a right-handed glove differs from a left-handed one. Furthermore, he demonstrated that this difference can be detected by the optical activity of these crystalline forms when in solution, one solution rotating the plane of polarized light to the right, the other to the left.

Pasteur extended these studies to other organic compounds, showing that many substances exhibited optical activity. For this work Pasteur received the Rumford medal of the Royal Society in 1856.

These borderline studies between chemistry and crystallography seem remote indeed from the problem of contagious disease, but they ultimately led Pasteur into his fundamental discoveries in the realm of microbiology. It was in 1854 that Pasteur began to study fermentation, a subject that was to occupy him for more than 20 years. Initially, he investigated lactic fermentation because it produces amyl alcohol, which exhibits rotatory powers. Before long, in 1856, this interest was reinforced by another stimulus, an appeal for help on a practical problem from M. Bigo, the father of one of his students. Lille at this period was "the richest center of industrial activity in the north of France," and the center of the French brewing and distilling industry. From time to time, beer would spoil or wine would sour without any discernible cause. M. Bigo was a manufacturer of beetroot alcohol and wanted advice on how to prevent his product from spoiling while it was fermenting. Using the microscope, Pasteur noted the presence of round globules when fermentation was proceeding properly, and that these were supplanted by long vibrios when fermentation became lactic. This was a very simple, practical test any brewer could use to avoid failures in fermentation. As he continued with his study of fermentation, Pasteur also discovered that in the fermentation of tartaric acid a small mold, probably *Penicillium glaucum,* attacked the right-handed form of the acid, leaving the left-handed form untouched. From this finding, he concluded that vital processes operate asymmetrically and that fermentation, since it operates on asymmetrical molecules of sugar, must be produced by living organisms.

Continuing into the 1860s, Pasteur investigated various kinds of fermentation: butyric, acetic, alcoholic, and others. He was able to show in each case that the process depended on the presence and activity of a certain organism. In his studies on beer and wine, Pasteur demonstrated that when fermentation went astray it was due to contamination with foreign organisms that produced substances other than the desired alcohol. Then he went further than this. He not only revealed why the fermentation process became "abnormal," but also how to prevent this condition. He showed how to suppress the activities of all organisms other than those of the desired specific ones by simply heating wine for a short period at a certain temperature. As a result, the undesirable ferments would be killed off. This process is of course the familiar method of *pasteurization,* now generally applied to milk and to other food products. While studying fermentation, Pasteur also discovered the existence of anaerobic life, that is, that certain organisms grow not in the presence of air, but only in its absence; and it was he who in 1863 first used the terms "aerobic" and "anaerobic." This observation was of immense import, for it led Pasteur to the investigation of putrefaction and to the view that this process is a kind of fermentation due to microbial activity, a view that in turn produced a deep impression on Joseph Lister who at once saw its significance for surgery.

Intimately connected with these questions was that of spontaneous generation. If Pasteur's position that specific organisms were responsible for particular fermentative changes was correct, and he could show that the exclusion of these organisms effectively prevented the occurrence of fermentation, then the doctrine of spontaneous generation became untenable. In a now historic controversy with F. A. Pouchet, Director of the Natural History Museum at Rouen, he was able to show that microbes are universally present in the atmosphere. Furthermore, being particulate and subject to gravity, they can settle on liquids or solids and initiate the changes of fermentation or decay. However, if air is filtered through cotton wool, for example, it is incapable of starting these processes. In short, Pasteur demonstrated experimentally the fictive character of the theory of spontaneous generation.

His researches on fermentation were interrupted in May 1856, by an urgent appeal from his teacher and friend, J. B. Dumas, the celebrated chemist. A mysterious and protracted epidemic had been ravaging the French silkworm nurseries, and the result was an industrial calamity for the stricken districts. Although Pasteur had never seen a silkworm in his life, he was asked to study the problem. To it he came with one inestimable advantage—a prepared mind. Pasteur's scientific career contains instance after instance of the interaction of technical need and scientific discovery. He worked on problems of immediate economic interest, but his concern went beyond the specific problem, no matter how important it might be, to its broader ramifications. Thus, while studying fermentation, he had already considered the possibility of a causal relation between germs and disease. If fermentation is due to minute living creatures, why should not such organisms be capable of producing the changes that occur in putrid and suppurative diseases. In 1862, in a note to the Minister of Public Instruction, after discussing the presence of germs in the atmosphere, Pasteur remarked: "How wide and useful to pursue is the field of these studies which bear such a close relationship to the various illnesses of animals and plants, and which certainly provide a first step along the desirable path of serious research into putrid and contagious diseases." Then in 1863, in an interview with Napoleon III, Pasteur informed the Emperor that his "ambition was to arrive at the knowledge of the causes of putrid and contagious diseases."

So in 1865 Pasteur dropped his work on fermentation and set up a laboratory at Alais where he was to work on the silkworm problem over the next five years.

After two years of hard work, he was convinced that silkworms were affected by two distinct communicable diseases, *pébrine* and *flâcherie,* each caused by different parasitic microorganisms. By 1868, he was in a position to indicate the causes of these conditions and how to control them, thus saving another of the great industries of France. At the same time, these researches also gave a great impetus to the germ theory of disease.

A BOTANIST PLAYS HOST TO AN UNKNOWN DOCTOR. Pasteur suffered a stroke in 1868, and for a time the state of his health, as well as the conditions resulting from the Franco-Prussian War and its aftermath, limited his activities. It was not until 1877 that he returned to the study of infectious disease in animals and man. Meanwhile, important contributions to a final solution of the problem set by Henle in 1840 were coming from other directions. In 1865, Joseph Lister undertook the first brilliant application of Pasteur's researches to the control of disease in human beings. (This will be considered in detail later.) In the same year Jean-Antoine Villemin, a French army surgeon, reported to the Academy of Medicine a series of experiments which showed that tuberculosis could be transmitted by inoculation from one infected animal to another. His work was developed further in his important book, *Études sur la Tuberculose,* published in 1868. Villemin's further studies led to the conclusion that tuberculosis does not originate spontaneously in man or animals because of atmospheric alterations, heredity, or poor environmental conditions, but it is caused by some organized virulent principle, presumably a microscopic germ, capable of multiplying in the affected organism and of being transmitted by direct contact or through the air. However, he was not able to demonstrate the germ, and his work did not have the impact it merited. It was during this period also that Casimir Davaine was carrying on his studies of anthrax, which attracted the interest of scientific and medical circles and helped to strengthen the germ theory of disease.

By the 1870s, the investigations of Pasteur and others had led to a partial solution of the problem concerning the connection between microbes and disease, but the final and clinching proof was not yet in hand. Such proof, however, had to await the invention of techniques that would permit rigorously controlled experiments, and particularly techniques for the isolation and handling of microscopic organisms. Thinking about microorganisms and disease was confused because knowledge concerning the biology of microbes was confused. Various investigators claimed to have seen or even to have demonstrated that one kind of organism could be converted into another. The famous Austrian surgeon, Theodore Billroth, maintained that there was only one organism capable of undergoing infinite variation. Obviously, such thinking could hardly lead to clarity. Opposed to this doctrine of pleomorphism was another view, due mainly to the labors of Pasteur on fermentation, which asserted the existence of specific organisms, constant in form and recognizable morphologically. Pasteur endeavored to obtain such organisms in a pure state, but owing to the methods he used, particularly because he worked with fluid cultures, his success was limited. Other investigators also tried to obtain pure cultures using fluid media, but the difficulties were almost insuperable.

A period characterized by solid advances in techniques and consequently in knowledge began in the 1870s. It was due in large measure to Ferdinand Cohn (1828–1898), professor of botany at the University of Breslau, who was the foremost student of bacteria at the time and who contributed greatly to the establishment of bacteriology as a science. Cohn's studies on bacteria began with his recognition of their plant nature. Bacteria had been included in the vegetable kingdom in 1849 by Joseph Leidy, but it was Cohn who firmly established their identity with plants. Beginning in 1851, his systematic investigations carried on over more than two decades were largely responsible for bringing some order into the confusion that characterized the knowledge of bacteria and their place in nature. Cohn recognized the need for an accurate classification of bacteria according to genera and species, but he also saw clearly that morphology alone was an inadequate basis. He was fully aware that morphologically similar organisms could differ greatly from each other in their physiological characteristics, and that the latter might be used as taxonomic criteria. An extremely important advance along this line was made by Cohn's student and co-worker Joseph Schroeter (1835–1894) in his researches on pigment production by chromogenic bacteria. He grew the organisms on solid media, such as potato, flour paste, meat, or egg albumen, and found specific pigmented colonies. The bacteria differed from colony to colony but were constant in one and the same colony. There is no doubt that Schroeter obtained pure cultures of the organisms with which he was working, or that essentially he had developed a technique for obtaining pure cultures. However, the far-reaching applications of this technique were to be developed by other hands.

At the end of April 1876, Cohn played host in his laboratory to an unknown country doctor who claimed to have discovered the life history of the *Bacillus* that causes anthrax. Davaine's experimental studies had rendered it highly probable that anthrax was due to the rod-shaped organisms found in the blood, which he called bacteridia. While this view was shared by other investigators, there were still gaps in the natural history of the disease. At this point, Robert Koch (1843–1910), the country practitioner, threw a flood of light on the obscurities of anthrax and cleared up the mystery. Koch lived in Wollstein, a small town in Posen, near Breslau, where he practiced and served as district medical officer. Impelled by a desire to study disease experimentally, he set up a laboratory in his home and found time between patients to investigate anthrax. Using mice as experimental animals, he inoculated them with blood from sick cattle and soon found the rods described by Davaine. Koch showed that the disease was transmissible and reproducible in a series of mice for more than 20 generations. He then went on to study the life cycle of the rods, and for this purpose devised a hanging-drop preparation in which the organism could be grown and observed. In the course of his studies, Koch discovered the spore stage of the anthrax bacilli, thus confirming Cohn's prediction of a resistant phase in its life cycle, and then showed that the spores again developed into typical rods. The epidemiological significance of these phenomena was not lost upon him. Finally, Koch demonstrated that the isolated anthrax *Bacillus* and no other microorganism would produce the disease in a susceptible animal. He had unequivocally proved the validity of the conditions laid down by Henle, his teacher at Göttingen, and medical bacteriology was ready to be born.

Since Ferdinand Cohn was considered one of the foremost investigators of bacteria of his time, it was only natural for Koch to turn to the eminent professor in nearby Breslau to demonstrate his findings. The historic demonstration began in Cohn's institute on April 30, 1876, and lasted three days. Among those present were the pathologists Julius Cohnheim and Carl Weigert, the anatomist L. Auerbach, and the chemist Moritz Traube. Koch completely convinced them of his discovery, and his classical paper, which appeared in 1876 under Cohn's aegis, was immediately recognized as a fundamental contribution. For the first time, the microbial origin of a disease had been incontrovertibly demonstrated and its natural history elucidated.

By the middle of the 1870s, a decisive basis of knowledge and technique had been achieved for the further study of bacteria and the diseases they produce. The advances that followed during the next two decades occurred with almost explosive rapidity, but in general they followed two distinct lines of development. One trend, characteristic of the work of Koch, led to the development of technical methods for the cultivation and study of bacteria. Pasteur and his co-workers took another direction, turning their attention to the mechanisms of infection, and developing the consequences of this knowledge for the prevention and treatment of contagious diseases.

Koch devoted himself to the development of techniques for handling bacteria so as to obtain pure cultures. Most significant were his use of solid nutrient media to grow organisms, and the introduction of methods for fixing and staining them. At first he tried gelatin, but soon replaced it by agar-agar at the suggestion of Frau Hesse, the wife of one of his co-workers. The superiority of this substance over gelatin eventually established it throughout the world as the standard medium in bacteriological culture technique. The study of bacteria by means of dyes grew out of staining methods used in histology. An attempt to stain bacteria, using carmine and fuchsin in watery solutions, had been made in 1869 by Hermann Hoffmann, professor of botany at Giessen. As a practi-

TABLE 3
Discovery of Pathogenic Organisms

Year	Disease Organism	Investigator
1880	Typhoid (bacillus found in tissues)	Eberth
	Leprosy	Hansen
	Malaria	Laveran
1882	Tuberculosis	Koch
	Glanders	Loeifler and Schutz
1883	Cholera	Koch
	Streptococcus (erysipelas)	Fehleisen
1884	Diphtheria	Klebs and Loeifler
	Typhoid (bacillus isolated)	Gaffky
	Staphylococcus ⎱ Streptococcus ⎰	Rosenbach
	Tetanus	Nicolaier
1885	Coli	Escherich
1886	Pneumococcus	A. Fraenkel
1887	Malta fever	Bruce
	Soft chancre	Ducrey
1892	Gas gangrene	Welch and Nuttall
1894	Plague	Yersin, Kitasato
	Botulism	van Ermengem
1898	Dysentery bacillus	Shiga

cal technique, however, bacterial staining stems from the work of Carl Weigert (1845–1904) in 1875, when he showed that cocci in tissues could be demonstrated by staining them with methyl violet. The methods of staining were greatly improved by Koch from 1877 onward, and progress in this field was very rapid over the succeeding decades. Much of this was due to the fundamental contributions of Paul Ehrlich (1854–1915) on the staining of white blood cells by aniline dyes.

Armed with the methods devised by Koch, it became possible to attack, more or less systematically, various problems of infectious disease. Within a few years, largely between 1877 and 1897, the microbial causes of numerous human and animal diseases were revealed for the first time, a harvest garnered overwhelmingly by German investigators. Until the 1880s, microbes had been shown to be the probable or certain etiological agents in only a few diseases. Obermeier (1868–1873) had shown that a spiral organism was consistently present in cases of relapsing fever and that the disease was transmissible; Koch in 1876 had demonstrated the causal role of the anthrax bacillus; and in 1879 Neisser discovered the gonococcus. Then with the 1880s the golden age of bacteriological discovery was ushered in. Retrospectively, it is clear that the situation was ripe by that time. As if a dam had burst, causative organisms of various diseases were demonstrated in rapid succession, often several in one year. The explosive character of this process is clearly seen from Table 3.

As these organisms were brought to light and their pathogenic role confirmed, questions arose concerning the mechanisms of microbial action. How is bacterial infection produced? How can it be prevented or its consequences treated? After 1877, French bacteriology in the hands of Pasteur and his coworkers began to apply itself to these questions. Resistance to infection was recognized as an important problem, and Pasteur directed attention to the practical and theoretical questions connected with it. Laboratory experiments on anthrax provided tantalizing hints that susceptibility to infection could be modified. Pasteur found, for example, that by lowering the body temperature of hens their resistance to anthrax was diminished. He observed furthermore that the virulence of pathogenic microbes could be modified under various conditions. Thus, between 1880 and 1888, Pasteur began to investigate the modification of virulence in disease-producing germs. Following the lead provided by Jennerian vaccination, he conceived the idea of preventing infectious diseases by means of vaccines prepared from such attenuated strains. Of the greatest import were the results of Pasteur's work on chicken cholera, swine erysipelas, and rabies, researches that led to the development of immunology and that were to have a profound and practical impact on the creation of a scientific public health program at the beginning of the twentieth century.

ANTISEPSIS AND ASEPSIS IN SURGERY. While Pasteur, Cohn, Koch, and other investigators were creating a firm basis for the study of contagious diseases by demonstrating the causative microbes, on the other side of the English Channel a young surgeon provided further support for the germ theory of disease by applying it to the prevention of wound infection. Until the middle of the nineteenth century, surgery was seriously limited in two ways. Most important was the almost inevitable occurrence of wound infection, which frequently ended in fatal sepsis. This complication was especially common in hospitals where patients mysteriously succumbed to "hospital gangrene," or to an even vaguer "hospitalism." Inadequate means for the control of pain was the other limiting factor. This restricted the scope of surgical intervention, since speed was essential to reduce shock. The introduction of ether anesthesia in 1846 rendered surgery painless, but the terrible scourge of sepsis remained. If anything, the so-called hospital diseases became even more rampant, assuming epidemic proportions in many places. The authorities in Nürnberg considered the demolition of the General Hospital, and a like radical decision was accepted by the governors and staff of the Lincoln County Hospital in England. Sir James Simpson summed up the situation when he asserted that "the man laid on the operating-table in one of our surgical hospitals is exposed to more chances of death than the English soldier on the field of Waterloo." This was the situation when the surgeon Joseph Lister (1827–1912) introduced antiseptic surgery.

Early in his career, Lister had begun to study inflammation, and his investigations led him to suspect that infection and pus formation in wounds were due to putrefaction of the tissues. Furthermore, he felt that this process was due to something carried by the air, a belief reinforced by the striking difference in mortality between patients with simple fractures and those who had sustained compound fractures. The major difference between these conditions is that in the latter the skin is torn and the underlying tissues come into contact with the air. In 1865, Lister's colleague, Thomas Anderson, professor of chemistry at Edinburgh, drew his attention to the work of Pasteur, who had just shown the ubiquity of bacteria in the air, and that fermentation, of which putrefaction was a variety, was due to contamination with such organisms. Lister immediately grasped the possible connection between Pasteur's findings and the problem of wound infection. Here certainly is a striking instance of the "prepared mind" at work. Furthermore, it occurred to Lister as a logical consequence that "decomposition in the injured part might be avoided without excluding the air, by applying as a dressing some material capable of destroying the life of the floating particles." A chemical seemed most suitable and Lister thought of carbolic acid, which had been used for the disinfection of sewage at Carlisle. (Although he was unaware of the fact, the French pharmaceutical chemist Jules Lemaire had recommended carbolic acid as a disinfectant as early as 1860.) The "antiseptic principle," as Lister termed it, was first applied on August 12, 1865, and his report of the results appeared in the *Lancet* between March and July 1867.

The antiseptic method of treating wounds produced astonishing results, but Lister's views at first had a checkered career. While his initial publication received a cordial reception in some quarters, acceptance of his technique and the principle underlying it was neither rapid nor widespread. For the most part, his colleagues responded with disparagement, sharp criticism, and outright condemnation. Lister's experience in this respect hardly differed from that of Holmes and Semmelweis, his predecessors in solving the mystery of wound infection. Oliver Wendell Holmes (1809–1865), in 1847, independently had discovered the clue to puerperal fever. As the latter put it, "Puerperal fever is caused by conveyance to the pregnant woman of putrid particles derived from living organisms, through the agency of the examining fingers." Both were met by opposition, abuse, and, in the case of Semmelweis, malicious persecution as well. The result was that Holmes retreated to his professorial settee to seek solace in the arms of literature; while Semmelweis, after years of unequal struggle, was driven mad and died, several days after having been committed to an asylum, of a septic wound of the finger, ironically enough a victim of the very disease he had striven so passionately to prevent.

Lister, however, was in a more favorable position to overcome opposition. Indeed, he might have described the situation as Holmes did a decade later by saying that "a little army of microbes was marched up to support my position." Bacteriological research was now being brought to bear on the problem. Through the work of Davaine on experimental septicemia of rabbits (1872), of Klebs on the pathology of gunshot wounds (1871 and 1872), and, finally, the decisive investigations of Koch (1878) and Ogston (1880–83) on the etiology of traumatic infective diseases, it was incontrovertibly shown that wound sepsis is due to specific pathogenic bacteria.

Furthermore, Lister soon acquired a number of disciples on the European continent. Most of these were Germans (Thiersch, von Volkmann, Stromeyer, Saxtorph, von Bergmann), but there were also a few French surgeons among them (Lucas-Championnière was most active). Through their influence as well as the efforts of Lister himself, the antiseptic principle of treatment was finally adopted even in Great Britain. Lister's methods had been relatively crude, and in the 1880s they were gradually replaced by techniques based on the principle of asepsis. These techniques developed chiefly by von Bergmann in Berlin endeavored to ensure freedom from bacteria in the field of operation by disinfecting as far as possible anything that would enter the area—hands, instruments, linen—through heat, chemical, and physical means. Ultimately, these methods derived from those developed to achieve sterilization in bacteriological technique. Such methods, developed especially out of bacteriological work, have also had important applications in public health practice, especially in the detection and control of communicable diseases.

BACTERIOLOGY AND THE PUBLIC HEALTH. By the last decade of the nineteenth century, some of the pertinent questions concerning contagious diseases had been answered by demonstrating specific causative organisms in numerous instances and showing how infection might be prevented. Nonetheless, certain observations remained unexplained and mysterious. In some diseases, such as typhoid fever and cholera, new cases did occur in persons who had had no direct contact with individuals affected by the disease in question. In other diseases, however, people who had been exposed to contact with sick individuals remained unaffected. Additional knowledge was clearly essential for a full understanding of the sources and modes of microbial infection. Light was finally thrown upon these obscurities in the germ theory of disease during the closing decade of the nineteenth century and the first decade of the twentieth by a number of brilliant investigations that revealed the part played by vectors, or intermediaries, in the transmission of communicable diseases.

The discovery was made that human beings in apparent good health could themselves serve as carriers of pathogenic organisms. As early as 1855, Pettenkofer had suggested that healthy human carriers could transmit cholera, but this hypothesis was not substantiated until the end of the century. Friedrich Loeffler (1884) and Émile Roux and Alexandre Yersin (1889) noted the presence of virulent diphtheria bacilli in the throats of healthy individuals, as well as the persistence of infecting organisms during convalescence. These were isolated observations, however, and led to no generalization. It was in connection with the cholera epidemic of 1892 and 1893 that the significance of the human carrier was first realized. In 1893, Koch emphasized the importance of the convalescent carrier, but while he recognized the role of the well carrier, he did not regard such individuals as important. In the same year, however, William Hallock Park (1863–1939) and Alfred L. Beebe, his assistant, in the bacteriological laboratory of the New York City Health Department, carried out a series of investigations in which they definitely established the concept of the carrier in diphtheria and demonstrated the value of routine bacteriological examination in the diagnosis of the disease. Park and Beebe examined 48 well family contacts to diphtheria cases and demonstrated the bacillus in 24 cases. They concluded "that the members of a household in which a case of diphtheria exists should be regarded as sources of danger unless cultures from their throats show the absence of diphtheria bacilli." The last important piece of knowledge was thus provided for an understanding of the process by which a contagious disease could be transmitted within a community. Typhoid fever was the third disease in which the importance of the carrier was demonstrated. This was first pointed out by Reed, Vaughan, and Shakespeare in 1900 in their study of typhoid fever in army camps during the Spanish-American War, and two years later by Robert Koch, whose influence led to the acceptance of the concept. During the first decade of the twentieth century, the significance of the carrier was also demonstrated for epidemic cerebrospinal meningitis and poliomyelitis, and by 1910, when C. V. Chapin published his classic book *The Sources and Modes of Infection,* the role of the human carrier was well established.

Paralleling these contributions was the equally important demonstration of the role of the animal vector, thus closing the last important gap in the germ theory of disease. Actually, the solution to the problem of the intermediate host did not appear suddenly; as in other areas of scientific endeavor, it was only the culmination of a long series of observations, theories, and experiments. As early as 1790, the Danish physician and veterinarian, Peter Christian Abildgaard (1740–1801), seems to have observed that animal parasites may pass the various stages of their life cycle in different animal hosts. However, this phenomenon, known as metaxeny, was not related to disease transmission until the latter half of the nineteenth century. The phenomenon was demonstrated experimentally in cestodes by F. Küchenmeister in 1851. More knowledge of the biology of parasitism was needed, however, for further advance, and this was provided at this time by a number of zoologists, among whom Rudolf Leuckart (1822–1898) was outstanding. In fact, his work on the human parasites is the foundation on which all subsequent research in this field has been based. On Leuckart's suggestion, the Russian naturalist Fedschenko, in 1858, discovered the life cycle of *Filaria medinensis* (the Guinea worm of man) and showed that a small arthropod, *Cyclops*, the water flea, transmitted the worm. Then, in 1868, Leuckart and Melnikoff demonstrated that the dog tapeworm was transmitted by the dog louse and showed that a parasite feeding on an animal could be an intermediate host and transmit a disease. In 1877, Patrick Manson (1844–1922), then medical officer to the Chinese Imperial Customs at Amoy, illuminated the life-history of *Filaria bancrofti,* the parasitic worm that causes filariasis. He showed that the young parasites were sucked up by mosquitoes with the blood on which they feed and they develop in the insects, and he concluded that the latter transmit the worms to new victims, although the mechanism he postulated turned out to be incorrect. Manson's work had little influence on general epidemiological thinking, but it is important because it led directly to the work of Ross on malaria, which finally made the animal vector a matter of worldwide interest.

Despite these researches, however, the real significance of the animal vector was not fully appreciated until the last decade of the nineteenth century. The report of Theobald Smith (1859–1934) and F. L. Kilborne on Texas cattle fever in 1893 finally drew general attention to this problem. In a series of brilliant and conclusive experiments, they proved that the disease was due to a protozoan parasite, *Piroplasma bigeminum,* which attacked the red blood cells, that ticks feeding on infected cattle passed the pathogenic microorganism on to their offspring, and that this second generation was then able to infect susceptible cattle.

The animal carrier could no longer be overlooked, and in the next few years, this type of transmission was demonstrated in other important communicable diseases. David Bruce (1855–1931) in 1894 and 1895 worked out the etiology of nagana, a disease of cattle and horses in Zululand, and he showed that it was due to a trypanosome transmitted by the tsetse fly. Then in 1897, Ronald Ross (1857–1932), an army surgeon in the Indian Medical Service, revealed the secret of malaria. Alphonse Laveran (1845–1922), a French army surgeon, had discovered the malarial parasite, now called *Plasmodium,* in 1880, but the mode of infection remained completely unknown. In 1894, Patrick Manson, proposed the theory that malaria was transmitted by mosquitoes. This hypothesis was certainly not new. Older writers like Lancisi had connected the mosquito with malaria, and during the nineteenth century, a number of students of the malaria riddle suggested that mosquitoes might transmit malarial fever. This idea was most clearly expressed in 1853 by Louis Beauperthuy (1803–1871) of Venezuela, and in 1882 by A. F. A. King (1841–1914) in the United States. Laveran (1884), Flügge (1889), and Koch (1892) also expressed the view that the malarial parasite was transmitted by mosquitoes.

Ross became interested in malaria in India, and while he was on leave in

1894, he sought out Manson in London, from whom he learned of the mosquito theory. Immensely impressed, Ross determined to test the hypothesis on his return to India. After two years of unrelenting effort, on August 20, 1897 ("Mosquito Day"), he found the human malaria parasite in the stomach wall of a "dapple-winged" (*Anopheles*) mosquito. The consequences of this momentous discovery were perhaps nowhere better envisaged than in the last stanza of the noble poem composed by Ross several days later. He wrote:

I know this little thing
A myriad men will save
O Death, where is thy sting?
Thy victory, O Grave?

Unfortunately, bureaucratic machinations prevented Ross from following up his discovery, and it was not till the following year that he was able to resume his research. He was now compelled to work with avian malaria because human subjects were unavailable; but finally, in the summer of 1898, having traced the development of the *Plasmodium* in the mosquito, Ross provided the clincher when he infected healthy birds by the bite of mosquitoes fed on malarious birds. The mystery of malaria was solved! Again administrative callousness interfered, denying Ross the final triumph of demonstrating the transmission of human malaria. This demonstration was provided in the same year (1898) by the Italian zoologist G. B. Grassi (1854–1925) and his collaborators, G. Bastianelli (1865–) and A. Bignami (1862–1929), of the Hospital of the Holy Spirit in Rome. To be sure, not all the problems connected with malaria had been solved, and there was still a great deal to learn, but the basic work was done.

At the very time when the malaria mystery was being solved, light was also cast upon the secrets of one of the gravest of all pestilences: bubonic plague. The plague bacillus was described by A. Yersin and S. Kitasato working independently in 1894 during the Hong Kong epidemic. Then, in 1897, M. Ogata of the Hygiene Institute of Tokyo observed plague bacilli in rat fleas and first offered the suggestion that fleas from plague rats could not only contain the pathogenic organisms but might also transmit the infection to man. By the end of 1897, close students of plague were convinced that the disease was transmitted to man from the rat. But how was this accomplished? How was the rat infected? The answers to these and other questions were provided by P. L. Simond (1858–1947), the pioneer French epidemiologist, in 1898. Based on observations as well as on experimental evidence, he took the position that plague was primarily a disease of rats spread by rat fleas. This work has withstood the test of time and is basic to all later work on the epidemiology of plague.

From the end of the eighteenth through the nineteenth centuries, the problem of yellow fever and its causation provided one of the major fields on which opposing epidemiological armies clashed in battle in an unending war for the greater glory of miasma or contagion. Proponents of the factor of contagion vigorously urged quarantine precautions and opposed those who with equal force insisted on the significance of local insanitary conditions. But all to no avail, for both were partially correct and the linking element capable of producing a synthesis of these opposing truths remained unknown. Then, in the last year of the nineteenth century, a dramatic series of events revealed the crucial role of the mosquito and made possible the control, if not the eradication, of yellow fever.

The mosquito as a possible agent in the transmission of the disease had been suggested by Beauperthuy in 1853, but this hypothesis was given its classic formulation in 1881 by Carlos J. Finlay (1833–1915), a Cuban physician. He maintained that yellow fever was transmitted by *Stegomyia fasciata,* the mosquito now known as *Aedes aegypti,* but the experimental evidence offered in support of this theory was inconclusive. This was the situation when the United States occupied Cuba following the Spanish-American War. Compelled to face the problem of yellow fever, an army commission was dispatched in 1900 to study the disease. Walter Reed (1851–1902) headed the commission as chairman, with James Carroll (1854–1907), Jesse W. Lazear (1866–1900), and Aristides Agramonte (1869–1931) as his associates. Based on Finlay's theory, a series of experiments was conducted on human subjects, since lower animals susceptible to yellow fever were unknown at the time. Members of the commission as well as volunteers from among the soldiers and civilian employees of the army took part in these experiments. (In the course of the investigation, Lazear, a member of the commission, contracted yellow fever following an accidental bite and succumbed to the disease.) In October 1900, the commission was able to report to the American Public Health Association that "the mosquito acts as the intermediate host for the parasite of yellow fever"; and by the following year, experiments carried out at Camp Lazear confirmed this beyond any doubt. Furthermore, the commission demonstrated that while the specific cause of yellow fever was present in the blood of patients, it was able to pass through a porcelain filter capable of preventing the passage of the smallest known bacteria. Loeffler and Frosch, in 1898, had shown that hoof-and-mouth disease in cattle was due to a filterable virus; and Reed and Carroll demonstrated this for yellow fever in 1901 by infecting nonimmune persons through injection with filtered and diluted serum from yellow fever patients. Thus, for the first time, a specific human disease was proved to be caused by a filterable virus. Finally, Reed and his co-workers showed that while yellow fever was definitely transmissible, it was not contagious; in short, there was no transfer of the disease by contact. A clear and definite course of action emerged from these investigations: yellow fever could be most effectively controlled by eliminating mosqui-

TABLE 4
Arthropods Responsible for the Transmission of Human Disease

Disease	Vector	Investigator	Year
Dengue	Mosquito	Bancroft	1906
Rocky Mountain spotted fever	Wood tick	Ricketts, King	1906
Typhus, epidemic	Body louse	Nicolle	1909
Sandfly fever	Sandfly	Doerr, Franz, and Taussig	1909
Typhus, murine	Rat louse	Mooser	1931
	Rat flea	Dyer	1931
Colorado tick fever	Wood tick	Topping, Cullyford, and Davis	1940
Rickettsialpox	Mite	Huebner, Jellison, and Pomerantz	1946

toes and by protecting the sick from their bites. This conclusion of the Yellow Fever Commission was at once accepted and in February 1901, measures along the lines it proposed were put into effect in Havana. The results were dramatic indeed. By September of that year, yellow fever had been wiped out in the city; nor has it reappeared.

Since then, arthropods have been proved responsible for the transmission of other human diseases. Some of these are given in Table 4.

The pioneers of medical entomology share with bacteriologists the credit for the far-reaching achievements of modern public health and preventive medicine. However, bacteriology profoundly affected public health in still another important respect, through the development and application of immunology. Artificial production of immunity had been known for more than a hundred years, having been established for the prevention of smallpox, first through the introduction of variolation and later by the discovery of Jennerian vaccination. The essential principle that a mild case of the disease protected the individual from further attacks even when the infection was potent was employed empirically without any understanding of the mechanism underlying the phenomenon. Efforts were made to achieve similar results by direct inoculation with other disease. Francis Home, in 1758, endeavored to emulate the success of variolation by inoculating 12 children, varying in age from 7 months to 13 years with fresh blood from patients in the acute stage of measles. This method of *morbillisation*, intended to produce a mild form of the disease that would confer permanent immunity, aroused great interest and hope among Home's contemporaries. William Buchan wrote in 1761 that "no greater boon has ever been discovered for the health of infants than small-pox inoculation; and it is greatly to be hoped that measles, a disease akin to it, may be treated in same way." In 1793, Charles Buxton in a medical dissertation mentioned the practice as a "most powerful means of alleviating the common sequences of measles."

Success was claimed for such experiments in 1841 in Hungary. In France, a long series of experiments with syphilis led, about the same time, to a serious proposal to inoculate the youth of the nation with this disease. Fortunately, this proposal was not acted on, but logically it seemed justified and certainly offered a prospect as alluring as the Venusberg. In this way the idea of immunization was kept alive, but it was not until Pasteur's studies on chicken cholera and anthrax in the early 1880s that a rational basis was provided on which to build a real knowledge of the immunizing process.

Pasteur was greatly impressed by the observation that in some diseases, such as smallpox, a single attack sufficed to produce lasting immunity. Apparently, he suspected that protection against certain infectious diseases might be obtained by a method like vaccination, and while studying chicken cholera he found this to be true. In the course of his experiments, Pasteur observed that the causative organism of chicken cholera tends to vary in virulence and that the virulence may be attenuated. Having inocculated hens with attenuated cultures, he then had the happy inspiration to inject them with virulent organisms and found that they were immune. Thus, in 1881, Pasteur established the principle of prophylactic inoculation, a principle that he demonstrated almost at the same time for anthrax and somewhat later for swine erysipelas (1883) and rabies (1884 and 1885).

The development of protective vaccines stimulated interest in the phenomenon of immunity and led investigators to look for the mechanisms that inoculation appeared to set in motion. It was not long, however, before it was discovered that there was no simple answer to the problem of immunity. Metchnikoff, in 1883, described phagocytosis, that is, the process by which cells in the blood surround and destroy bacteria, but other investigators soon showed that the blood serum alone was also capable of destroying bacteria. These observations led to a long period of research in which the bactericidal and immunological properties of the blood have been thoroughly studied, and a number of effective substances for the prevention and treatment of communicable diseases have been developed.

The first important line of investigation on these problems was initiated in a series of papers published between 1888 and 1890 by Emile Roux (1853–1933) and Alexandre Yersin (1863–1943), two French bacteriologists, co-workers of Pasteur, who have already been mentioned. On the basis of his finding that in diphtheria bacilli were present at the site of the membrane but could not be recovered from internal organs, Loeffler had suggested that the disease was due to a poison elaborated by a microbe. Roux and Yersin proved that the bacilli produced such a poison, which can be separated from the bacterial cells themselves and when inoculated into animals is capable of producing the symptoms and type of death characteristic of infection with the diphtheria bacilli. Finally, stressing the importance of demonstrating the diphtheria organism in the diagnosis of the disease, they developed a technique that essentially has been employed by all subsequent investigators.

The work of Roux and Yersin was fundamental not only in clarifying the mechanism of diphtheria and in developing a suitable diagnostic technique, but equally in providing a point of departure for investigations that led eventually to effective methods for treatment and control not only of diphtheria but of a number of other communicable diseases as well. Their investigations aroused intense interest, and efforts were made to create an artificial immunity to diphtheria. On December 3, 1890, Karl Fraenkel (1861–1915) published in the *Berliner klinische Wochenschrift* the results of his studies showing that it was possible to establish an artificial immunity in guinea pigs by injecting them with attenuated cultures of diphtheria bacilli. The following day Emil von Behring (1854–1917) and his Japanese co-worker Shibasaburo Kitasato (1852–1931) published in the *Deutsche medizinische Wochenschrift* an account of the immunity to tetanus. In this brief but fundamental paper, they pointed out that the immunity of rabbits and mice that had been treated with tetanus cultures depends on the capacity of the cell-free blood serum to render innocuous the toxic substances elaborated by the tetanus bacilli. A week later (December 11, 1890) Behring alone published a paper on immunization against diphtheria, in which the essential facts reported in the earlier communication on tetanus were confirmed as well for this disease. The foundation was thus laid for the specific serum therapy and prophylaxis of diphtheria as well as of other infectious diseases. A year later, on Christmas night 1891, a child in von Bergmann's clinic in Berlin became the first person to be treated with diphtheria antitoxin. It was not, however, until after Roux, on September 4, 1894, read his classic paper at the Eighth International Congress of Hygiene and Demography at Budapest that diphtheria antitoxin began to be employed generally.

By the end of the nineteenth century, it had become evident that a high degree of resistance to the causative organisms of certain communicable diseases could be produced by the injection of these germs in an attenuated live state, or when dead, or by inoculation with extracts from such organisms. This became known as the principle of active immunization. At the same time, it was found that the blood of such immunized animals contained substances, known an antibodies, that not only destroyed invading organisms but also had unusual therapeutic and prophylactic powers when injected into sick persons. Immunity could thus also be transmitted passively. Paul Ehrlich (1854–1915) was the first to differentiate between active and passive immunization (1892). Pasteur's discovery of prophylactic vaccines was soon followed by the development of others for cholera and plague (Haffkine) and for typhoid (Pfeiffer and Kolle; Wright). More recently, vaccines have been prepared for tuberculosis (Calmette), yellow fever (Theiler and Smith), and poliomyelitis (Salk). Immune sera were also developed for diphtheria (as described), tetanus, snake bite poisoning, and botulism.

The fact that pathogenic microbes stimulated antibody production in the blood had other important consequences. Richard Pfeiffer, a German bacteriologist, noted that cholera and typhoid organisms clumped together and even disintegrated when placed in serum containing appropriate antibodies. This agglutination phenomenon was first used in 1896 by Fernand Widal, a French clinician and bacteriologist, for the diagnosis of typhoid fever. This was the beginning of serum diagnosis, which has since been employed in diagnosing a number of different communicable diseases. The value of the method is due to the specificity that in general characterizes immunity reactions. It was by this means that Schottmüller in 1900 separated paratyphoid fever as a distinct entity within the group of enteric fevers. Another important development in this field was the complement fixation test, of which the principle was discovered in 1901 by Bordet and Gengou, and Wassermann's modification of it as a test for syphilis in 1906. Despite modifications introduced since, this test is still basic. From 1917 on, a group of flocculation tests—Meinicke, Kahn, and others— have rivaled the Wassermann but have not replaced it. A complement fixation test was also developed for the diagnosis of glanders.

It is almost impossible to overemphasize the consequences for the health of the community of the development of microbiology and immunology. Action in the interest of community health today comprises an intricate maze of activities involving the services and energies of a wide variety of professional and lay people. Much of this work stems from the application of bacteriological and immunological knowledge to the actual problems of disease control. As set up in the nineteenth century, health departments were concerned essentially with contagious disease control through environmental sanitation. Prevention was a natural corollary of refuse and sewage removal according to the miasmatic theory of contagion. The real objective of public health administration in abating sanitary nuisances was to prevent outbreaks of contagious disease. However, as bacteriologists identified the microorganisms responsible for specific diseases and uncovered their mode of action, the way was open for the control of infectious diseases on a more rational, accurate, and specific basis. Such activity by public health authorities became possible on an unprecedented scale.

The new science of bacteriology was brought to the United States in the 1880s by a small group of pioneer workers, among whom were T. Mitchell Prudden of New York, George M. Sternberg of the U.S. Army, William H. Welch of Johns Hopkins University, and D. E. Salmon of the Bureau of Animal Husbandry. While Americans contributed only in a limited degree to the growth of microbiological knowledge, they were more alert than their European confreres to its practical implications. Out of this awareness there developed a new public health institution, namely, the diagnostic laboratory for the application of bacteriology.

One of the earliest bacteriological laboratories in the United States was set up in 1887 by Joseph J. Kinyoun, of the Marine Hospital Service, in one room of the Marine Hospital on Staten Island, New York. Its purpose was to carry on research. In 1892 it was moved to Washington, where 10 years later this unit became the Hygienic Laboratory. At this time a Biologies Control Division was established to test and to guarantee the safety and effectiveness of the various serums, vaccines, and related biological products that were being developed. Public health laboratories were also established in 1888 by Charles V. Chapin in Providence, Rhode Island, and by Victor C. Vaughan for the state health department of Michigan. The primary purpose of these units was analysis of water and food.

It was in New York City, however, that the new knowledge of bacteriology was first really applied in public health practice. In 1892, as a result of the cholera epidemic in Hamburg, a division of bacteriology and disinfection was established in the City Health Department to guard against entry of the disease. Owing to the initiative of Hermann M. Biggs (1859–1923), who was to become one of the great leaders of American public health, a small diagnostic laboratory was included in the division. After the cholera scare was over, the laboratory, instead of being discontinued, began to employ bacteriological procedures for the control of diphtheria. In 1893, the young physician, William H. Park, was placed in charge of this work as bacteriological diagnostician and inspector of diphtheria.

In this laboratory, the discoveries of Pasteur, Koch, and others were systematically applied to the protection and improvement of the community's health. Park's work on diphtheria was the outstanding achievement of his life, and millions of children living today owe their existence to him. The production of the first diphtheria antitoxin ever made outside of Europe was begun by Park in late summer of 1894. There is scarcely an area of public health, however, which has not been affected by the bacteriological laboratory. Before long it became what amounted to a research institute, and work was being done not only on diphtheria, but also on tuberculosis, dysentery, pneumonia, typhoid fever, scarlet fever, and the role of milk in disease.

Establishment of public health laboratories by other local and state health departments followed rapidly after New York City had set an example. It was clear that the application of microbiology held rich promise of usefulness in the control of communicable disease. In 1894, Henry P. Walcott, Health Commissioner of Massachusetts, organized a laboratory to produce diphtheria antitoxin for the citizens of the state. Early in 1895 a laboratory for the diagnosis and control of diphtheria was also established in Philadelphia. Within a few years, almost every state and practically all large cities in the United States had established a diagnostic bacteriological laboratory. Through these laboratories, health departments to a considerable extent took over the task of diagnosing communicable diseases, and in order to control these diseases provided free biological products to doctors in practice and to public health officers.

Other countries lagged behind the United States in the acceptance and development of the public health laboratory. In Great Britain, for example, the establishment of such units was slow during the first quarter of the present century. Until after the end of the nineteenth century, laboratory work related to the public health was performed in hospital or university laboratories. While it was recognized that bacteriological investigations were essential in modern public health work, arrangements to provide such services were primitive in many parts of the country. Several areas lacked completely any laboratory facilities, in others they were quite inadequate, and commercial laboratories developed in many places to fill the need. A fairly widespread system of "postal pathology" developed, in which laboratories agreed to examine specimens sent to them by mail from places situated at a considerable distance. In 1897, Rupert Boyce had been appointed as the first municipal bacteriologist at Liverpool, and in succeeding years some of the wealthier local authorities put up laboratories of their own. However, these were few in number. In many localities, voluntary hospitals found public health laboratory work a lucrative source of additional income, and provided routine services. This remained the situation until shortly before World War II.

Despite differences in the rate of development of the public health laboratory service, its enormous value to the community cannot be exaggerated. The responsibility of government to protect the health of the people is concretely exemplified in the public health laboratory. Furthermore, the laboratory represented the practical outcome of the microbiological period, just as the organization of the health department had been a product of the earlier sanitary reform movement. Just as the health department provided an appropriate administrative mechanism for dealing with community health problems, so the public health laboratory provided a suitable scientific tool for the implementation of the public health program.

The way was now clear for the development of public health administration along more rational lines than had ever been possible before. A scientific understanding of the elements involved in the transmission of communicable diseases led health authorities to act with greater discrimination in quarantine and environmental sanitation. The empirical shotgun methods of an earlier day could now be made more precise and definite. Thus, quarantine regulations were modified in the light of bacteriological discoveries. By establishing the incubation period in a given disease, the number of days required for quarantine could be set more exactly. Similarly, by showing how water or food transmitted disease under given conditions, control of such conditions could be undertaken more effectively.

THE VANISHING DISEASES. The first decade of the twentieth century had a solid basis for the control of a number of infectious diseases, and throughout succeeding decades up to the present advances along this line have continued with increasing tempo. The meaning of this trend is clearly evident in the case of diphtheria. By 1900, diphtheria could be diagnosed by precise bacteriological methods, the sick person could be treated with diphtheria antitoxin, and well carriers could be detected, thus making possible really effective control. The next important step was to be made in the direct prevention of the disease.

This was achieved eventually by active mass immunization, a method developed logically from earlier knowledge on the use of diphtheria antitoxin as a passive immunizing agent as well as a therapeutic agent. In 1902, Dzierzgowsky showed that immunization in a human being could be achieved by increasing doses of diluted toxin. The use of toxin neutralized by antitoxin was then suggested by Theobald Smith in 1909. Von Behring in 1913 substituted such a mixture for the diluted toxin and demonstrated that it induced immunity safely in animals and man. At the same time, it was necessary to know the natural history of diphtheria within the community: How many children of different ages had already acquired immunity, how many were well carriers, and what children were highly susceptible? A simple test for immunity by injecting minute amounts of toxin into the skin was developed by Bela Schick (1877–) in 1913. This test made it possible to define more accurately the need for active immunization, as well as the results obtained thereby. Finally, in 1923 G. Ramon showed that toxin treated with formalin (anatoxin) had advantages as an immunizing agent over the earlier toxin-antitoxin mixture. (Anatoxin is now known as toxoid.) Later, alumprecipitated toxoid was found to have still greater antigenic potency.

Knowledge and tools thus became available for a full-scale mass attack on diphtheria. Such an endeavor was first attempted for the protection of children by W. H. Park and Abraham Zingher (1885–1927) in New York City. In 1920 active immunization of school children began, and by 1928 some 500,000 had been immunized. Attention was then concentrated on the preschool children, and in 1940 it was estimated that no less than 60 per cent of this group were protected. By this date, the disease had been virtually eliminated as a cause of death, with the mortality rate at 1.1 per 100,000. This was in striking contrast to a rate of 785 per 100,000 in 1894. With the adoption of immunization in New York and other large cities, such as Toronto, and then progressively in other countries, proof of its efficacy became increasingly evident. During

World War II, there was a sharp rise in the incidence and severity of diphtheria in Germany as well as in certain countries occupied by the Germans, particularly Norway and the Netherlands. Since 1945, however, diphtheria immunization has been largely accepted in European public health practice, and the incidence of diphtheria has declined sharply.

That the drop in diphtheria morbidity and mortality is not wholly due to preventive immunization appears to be indicated by the fact that this decline set in actually in the nineteenth century before diphtheria antitoxin began to be used generally, and continued progressively even before preventive immunization became widespread. The death rate among children up to 10 years of age in New York City was 785 per 100,000 in 1894, declining to less than 300 in 1900; and in 1920, when active immunization of school children began, it fell below 100. This decline is related to the fact that certain communicable diseases, among them diphtheria, occur in waves with intervening periods during which the disease is either absent or at least significantly rare. Consequently, it is more difficult to evaluate the effectiveness of therapeutic or preventive measures if they are instituted during the waning of an epidemic wave. Nevertheless, whatever the relative weight of the factors that have brought about an almost complete disappearance of diphtheria, it is certain that the experience of the disease in large communities like New York or Toronto or London has been significantly better in the postimmunization period than might have been expected from the trend of either morbidity or mortality in the preimmunization period. Certainly, the downward course of diphtheria morbidity and mortality has at least been accelerated by preventive immunization.

The decline of diphtheria was not an isolated case. Many other important infectious diseases had begun to wane before the full effects of the bacteriological discoveries made themselves felt. Beginning about 1870, there was a continuing downward trend in mortality due to a decline in the frequency of certain diseases, chiefly yellow fever, smallpox, typhoid and typhus fevers, malaria, and tuberculosis. For example, in America, those great epidemic terrors—cholera and yellow fever—disappeared, never to return, before the specific causes of these infections were discovered and before exact knowledge of their transmission became known. These trends were roughly the same in the most progressive areas, particularly the municipalities, of western Europe and America. This is indicated in the general mortality rates for England and Wales and for France from 1841 to 1910 (Table 5).

These trends undoubtedly reflect in part the impact of the earlier sanitary reform movement. Acting on the theory that "a clean city is a healthy city," housing was improved, the physical environment was cleaned up, efforts were made to provide unadulterated food and clean water; in short, action was taken to provide decent living conditions. The English experience with typhus fever

TABLE 5
Death Rates in England and Wales and in France per 1000 Inhabitants

Years	England and Wales	France
1841–1850	22.4	23.3
1861–1870	21.3	23.6
1881–1885	19.4	22.2
1891–1895	18.7	22.3
1896–1900	17.7	20.7
1901–1905	16.0	19.6
1906–1910	14.7	19.2

TABLE 6
Average Annual Death Rate from Typhoid Fever (per Million Persons) in England and Wales

1871–1880	1881–1890	1891–1900	1901–1910	1911–1920	1921–1925
332	198	174	91	35	25

is an excellent case in point. Until 1870, there was very little variation in the death rate from "fever" in London. For the decade 1861 to 1870, the rate was 904 per million, but in the succeeding decade (1871 to 1880), it declined to 374. During this period, typhus fever was officially separated from other "fevers," and in the next two decades, its decline was nothing short of spectacular. In 1906, three years before Nicolle's discovery that the body louse transmitted typhus, the annual report of the London County Council stated that there were no more deaths from the disease that year. Slum clearance, regulation of lodging houses, increased use of cotton clothing, especially underwear, and consequent improvement in personal cleanliness played their part in reducing the prevalence of typhus fever.

The course of typhoid fever during this period was almost as dramatic as the experience with typhus. Its decline in England and Wales is clearly shown in Table 6 by the death rates from 1871 to 1925.

The trend in the United States was equally phenomenal, so that by 1947, the death rate was 0.2 per 100,000 persons for both typhoid and paratyphoid fevers. The initial decline in typhoid fever coincided with the introduction of proper sewerage systems and even more of protected water supplies. Later, further improvements in sanitary engineering, specifically protection of water through purification and of milk through pasteurization, fly control, detection of well carriers, isolation of patients and bacteriological diagnosis continued and intensified the earlier trend. Vaccination against typhoid was significant in specific groups, such as armies. In the case of typhoid fever, the influence of the bacteriological era in extending the work of the sanitary reformers is clearly apparent.

Syphilis, a major social disease, also underwent a dramatic change. The death rate declined from 18 per 100,000 persons from 1920 to 1924 to 8 per 100,000 persons in 1948. In the past decade, it has been reduced even more. This improvement has been due to many things. Significant among these have been the blood tests for couples about to be married and for pregnant women, mass screening surveys, the control measures instituted during World War II, and the health education campaigns. Most important, however, was the introduction in 1946 of penicillin for the treatment of syphilis by John F. Mahoney.

This account of the decline in specific infectious diseases cannot be pursued further in any detail owing to limitations of space. One cannot omit to note, however, that children were the chief beneficiaries from the victories won in the battle against communicable diseases. The degree of benefit obtained from measures for the improvement of milk and water is clearly shown by the trend of infant mortality in New York City. In 1885 the infant death rate was 273 per 1000 live births; by 1915 it had dropped sharply to 94 per 1000. Similarly, in New Haven the death rate for infant diarrhea dropped from 205 per 200,000 in 1881 to 19 in 1926. Equally beneficial results were obtained through the widespread adoption of smallpox vaccination after 1870.

Children also benefited from a decline in the virulence of scarlet fever. After 1880 the severity of the disease diminished. A review of the experience of Providence, Rhode Island, with regard to scarlet fever from 1865 to 1924 shows that the death rate of children aged 2 to 4 years decreased during this period from 691 to 28.3 per 100,000. Since the attack rate does not present a corresponding decrease, the decline in the number of deaths cannot be attributed to a lower prevalence or to changes in the population, but must have been due to a diminution in the severity of the disease. From 1886 to 1888, 1 in 5 patients died, while from 1923 to 1924 only 1 in every 114 cases ended fatally. A similar trend has been demonstrated for England and Wales. The late 1930s witnessed an accelerated decline in the case fatality rate. To some extent, this probably reflected an improvement in medical care, since it coincided with the introduction of the sulfonamides for the treatment of scarlet fever and its complications.

This great gain in child life has had considerable impact on the development of community health problems and action over the past 50 years. What this meant in simple quantitative terms can be seen from the following estimates. According to W. S. Thompson, the probable number of survivors to age 65 from 1000 births in the United States increased from 325 in 1875 to 695 in 1940. For Europe, an estimate by M. Pascua is illuminating. Based on the death rates of 1900, he calculated the number of deaths that would have occurred in Europe in 1947, and he showed a theoretical saving of one and three quarter million lives for that year. There is no doubt that the decline in mortality, and especially in infant deaths, has been an important element in the aging of the population, which has been so characteristic in recent decades of the United States and of other economically advanced countries.

Infant mortality is a sensitive indicator of community health because it reflects the influences exerted by various social factors. It is particularly sensitive to environmental conditions, such as housing, sanitation, and pure food and water. Housing is important, for example, because overcrowding favors the spread of respiratory infections and lack of adequate washing facilities increases gastrointestinal infection. The level of infant mortality varies as well with the availability of medical care and proper knowledge of infant nutrition. Reduction of mortality in general, and of infant mortality specifically, went hand in hand with improvements in living conditions and health services. However, the benefits of these improvements did not fall equally everywhere. Global figures for infant mortality conceal marked differences between various classes of the community, and such differences are just as great between various peoples of the earth.

The solid and enduring advances in community health action in western Europe and the United States over the past 75 years were not attained in a vacuum. These achievements are intimately related to the evolution of technology and industry, which made possible the accumulated wealth from which the funds needed for profitable investment in the improvement of community health could be obtained. The appalling inequalities in health conditions that exist throughout the world today are directly and intimately connected with the fundamental problems of wealth and poverty. Improvements in living conditions, health services, and consequently in reduction of preventable disease and death have not been uniform throughout the world or even within the economically advanced countries. In the United States, for example, a comparison of infant and maternal mortality between various states shows in general that the poorer states have higher rates. In 1946, the per capita income in Massachusetts was more than 1300 dollars while in South Carolina it was 729 dollars. At the same time, infant mortality in South Carolina was 30 per cent higher than in Massachusetts and maternal mortality was more than double. Therefore, before proceeding to examine the problems with which public health has concerned itself during the past four or five decades, it is essential to look at their economic and social context, the framework within which we must deal with the present-day challenges of community health.

-VIII-
The Bacteriological Era and Its Aftermath (Concluded)

ECONOMIC AND SOCIAL TRENDS IN A CHANGING SOCIETY. Protection of the community against communicable diseases and sanitation of the environment have been and still are major aspects of the public health program. As a result of community action along these lines arising from the sanitary reform movement and the bacteriological discoveries, the crude death rate had markedly declined by the first decade of the twentieth century. During this period, however, new developments occurred which vastly broadened the horizons of public health workers and turned their attention to new tasks. Surveying the community with a critical eye, some of those engaged in health and social work were not entirely satisfied with what they saw. It became evident, for instance, that steps taken to clear up the environment of urban areas, while of great value, were of little avail in dealing with problems of maternal and child welfare, of tuberculosis, or with a number of other health problems found among the poorer classes of the community. This trend appeared in the United States and in a number of countries of western Europe around the turn of the century.

The economic and social world within which this development took place was that of advancing industrialization accompanied by an expansion of urban communities. The world that Great Britain had helped to industrialize was catching up with her, and her earlier industrial honeymoon was ending. Other countries like the United States and Germany were forging abreast or even ahead of her, but as they did so similar social and health problems began to emerge in all of them. In the sprawling cities, the impact of poverty and unemployment threw into sharp relief the wastage of human resources. As we have seen, in the nineteenth century, the dire social condition of the masses in England had stirred ardent reformers to constructive activity in the field of community health. Yet, after 50 years of public health work, there were clear indications that the health of the community was still in many ways deplorable.

Charles Booth, who surveyed the working-class districts of London from 1889 to 1902, felt that the general level of living had improved. The real purchasing power of the worker had risen, but these were gains only by comparison with the extremely low wage levels of the mid-nineteenth century. Booth's investigations in London and Rowntree's study of York in 1899 showed that a substantial portion of the laboring population was living on incomes beneath a subsistence level. The more the condition of the poorer classes in the community was investigated, the more unsatisfactory their health and social situation was found to be. Malnutrition was rife and the health and physical fitness of the more poorly paid members of the working class was defective. Maternal mortality was high. While infant mortality had declined, the condition of children attending school as well as that of preschool children was found to be extremely poor.

Similar evils were present in the great cities of the United States. When America laid aside its arms after Appomattox and turned to the pursuits of peace, it stood on the threshold of an unparalleled industrial expansion. The following 50 years saw a tremendous, unrestrained growth of industry and a phenomenal growth of congested urban communities. Slum areas were not new in American cities; at the end of the nineteenth century, however, this problem became extremely acute. Industrial expansion, urban growth, and a new flood of immigration all coincided to produce congested areas in which thousands of people huddled in unbelievably inadequate housing deprived of some of the most elementary requirements of civilized life. Poverty, malnutrition, disease, and vice were widespread. The descriptions by Jacob Riis of slum conditions in New York equaled, if they did not surpass, the conditions depicted by Booth and Rowntree in England.

According to Justice Felix Frankfurter, "The domestic problems of our country after the Reconstruction period may be said to have revolved in the main around the responsibility of wealth to commonwealth." Health, housing, and social welfare were intimately connected with this larger question, which was present as well in England, Germany, and other industrialized countries. In fact, increases in wealth were even more spectacular in some cases than those of population. National wealth in the United States, for example, estimated at about $16,000,000,000 in 1860, rose to $65,000,000,000 in 1890, and to more than $300,000,000,000 by 1921. For the same dates, per capita wealth increased from $513 to $1035 to almost $3000. Similar trends might be cited for Great Britain and the European countries, but in all of them, this accumulation of wealth had important repercussions on the health of the people.

For one thing there was gross inequality in the distribution of wealth. At one end of the scale, the possession and control of vast wealth became concentrated in the hands of a small number of financial leaders. The tendency to business concentration, already evident in the late nineteenth century, moved through the stages of small and large corporations to the dominance of large combines, trusts, or cartels. At the other end of the scale was the stark poverty and social degradation that went hand in hand with economic and industrial development. Rapid industrialization required that a large part of the national income be devoted to capital equipment and accumulation. Furthermore, men engaged in industry and commerce for profit were little concerned about the consequences of their actions and inclined to regard the sacrifice of several generations of workers and their families to the claims of the industrial machine as a part of the natural order of things, or at most as a necessary evil.

Dislike of human suffering was not new. It had been an integral element in the movement for sanitary and factory reform. According to the tenets of economic liberalism, however, it was believed during most of the nineteenth century that increased production resulting from industrial advance would banish scarcity and thus eliminate poverty and decrease suffering as far as possible. The inescapable fact, at the turn of the century, of poverty, diseases, vice, and suffering as large-scale urban phenomena, and the increasing awareness that these were seemingly symptoms of a more deep-seated social malaise, made it increasingly impossible to rest content with the earlier belief. From the discontents and disorders that plagued England, America, Germany, and other similarly situated countries arose a stream of dissenting opinion manifesting itself concretely in various reform programs. While the origins and points of departure of this movement varied from country to country, in all of them there was a shift away from the free competitive order. To a greater or lesser degree, the necessity for state interference was accepted by the reformers. Adam Smith's idea of the "invisible hand" arranging the affairs of community life had never been fully accepted in Germany, and Bismarck's social insurance program showed how state action could be used to deal with social maladjustments. We have seen how, in England and the United States, the state had from time to time intervened for the health and welfare of the community, but it was only toward the end of the nineteenth century and the beginning of the present century that this approach was formulated as a theory and program of social action. The state was conceived by reformers to be an indispensable instrument for achieving desirable social goals. At the same time, this philosophy did not exclude voluntary action by independent citizens. Indeed, in many instances, public action in the form of regulation and legislation was obtained only after agitation by voluntary organizations. The point of view of this movement was characteristically expressed by Walter Lippman in 1914: "We can no longer treat life," he said, "as something that has trickled down to us. We have to deal with it deliberately, devise its social organization, alter its tools, formulate its method, educate and control it. In endless ways, we put intention where custom has reigned. We break up routines, make decisions, choose our ends, select means."

The orientation of this reform movement in the United States, and in varying degree in other countries, was empirical and pragmatic, with confidence in what might be accomplished by conscious social action. In the United States, it had no rigid system of ideas that had to be accepted in its entirety by those who participated. It was a broad movement concerned with problems of social welfare. This has been clearly expressed by Edward T. Devine, a pioneer of the movement. "Emerging social work in America in the nineties," he wrote, "was neither reactionary nor Utopian. Both liberal progressives and social-minded conservatives had part in it. Its embryonic philosophy was so formulated as not to exclude any who were willing to face the facts and to cooperate for the eradication of demonstrable evils, for the realization of demonstrable possibilities for a happier and better life, for the essentials of rational human existence for all." From such a point of view, one could undertake to deal with a diversity of problems: poverty and dependency, infant mortality, sweatshops, prostitution, tuberculosis prevention, and tenement house reform. It was clear, however, that ill health was the most constant of the attendants of poverty. In the homes of the poor, Devine said, "we find the dire consequences of death and disease, of unemployment and underemployment, of overwork and nervous strain, of dark and ill ventilated and overcrowded rooms, of undernourishment and exposure and poisoned food, of ignorance and maladjustment." It was on the basis of these ideas that socially minded citizens, physicians, clergymen, social workers, and government officials found a common ground for action, i.e., in the prevention of tuberculosis, to reduce health hazards in factories, to lower the infant mortality, to improve the health of school children, and the like.

THE WELFARE OF MOTHERS AND CHILDREN. An increasing concern with all phases of child life was a characteristic and prominent feature of the movement for social amelioration. This child welfare movement became noticeable in the industrialized countries of western Europe and in the United States about the turn of the century and was directed toward general hygiene for disease prevention, dietary improvement, and antepartum care.

The reasons for this concern are not hard to find. Political, economic, and humanitarian motivations all converged to reduce the large wastage of child life. Soon after 1870, a decrease in the number of births appeared in certain countries of western Europe, and somewhat later in England and the United States. Then it became evident in a number of countries that many young men examined for military service were physically unfit. Findings of this kind aroused concern in England at the time of the Boer War and in the United

States during the First World War. (Similar reactions developed in the United States over the large number of young men rejected by the armed forces as unfit for military service in the Second World War.) Clearly, here was a national resource that was being wasted. If a nation wanted to have enough healthy and fit young men to serve in its armed forces, conservation of its human resources was essential. It is certainly no accident that this trend coincided with a reappearance of mercantilist ideas and policies: efforts to acquire colonies, to secure markets and sources of raw materials, to define spheres of influence, and to increase population. Nor is it just coincidence that practical action to reduce child mortality on a scale commensurate with the need was first taken in France, where the birth rate was declining at an alarming rate and where an adequate number of fit young men was required if the conscript army was to be maintained.

Whatever its motivation, a community that placed a high value on child life could not long overlook the problem of infant mortality and its causes. Experts recognized that a large proportion of this mortality was preventable and that it was caused by malnourishment, parental ignorance, contaminated food, and other factors attributed entirely or in part to poverty. Some of these factors were removable, while the effects of others might be greatly lessened. As the problem had many ramifications, it would have to be attacked along a number of different lines: through the provision of clean milk; by instructing the mother in the proper feeding and care of the child; through legislation regulating the work of expectant mothers; and by providing facilities where babies of working mothers could be left.

The beginnings of child welfare at the turn of the century followed the same general lines in European and American urban communities. At first, stations were set up to provide clean milk; later these became well-child clinics where the health of infants and young children was supervised, and mothers were instructed in the care of the child at home. It was known that the diarrhea, from which so many babies younger than 2 years of age died, especially in the summer, was due largely to the unsafe, highly contaminated milk used to feed them. It was also known that the mortality among breast-fed babies was considerably lower than among those artificially fed. Consequently, the prime objective of all those concerned with infant health was to encourage breast feeding, or when this was not possible, to provide a safe and effective substitute.

Endeavors to improve child health along the lines initiated in the eighteenth century continued sporadically throughout the nineteenth century. John Bunnell Davis (1780–1824), an English physician, who in 1816 established a dispensary for children in London, showed a real understanding of the causes of infant mortality and of the measures needed to reduce it. Recognizing the need for instruction of mothers, he distributed pamphlets to them and organized a corps of visitors who went to the homes. In 1817, Davis outlined his views in a small book entitled *A Cursory Inquiry into some of the Principal Causes of Mortality among Children, with a View to Assist in Ameliorating the State of the Rising Generation in Health, Morals and Happiness.* Employing principles already developed and applied by Smellie, Armstrong, and Lettsom, Davis's work represents a transitional phase in the development of modern child hygiene and public health nursing.

Another important step along this road was taken in France, where since the eighteenth century problems of child health had been matters of concern to public officials and private individuals. In 1854, Morel, the mayor of Villiers-le-Duc, initiated a program to stem the wastage of infant life. By offering a bounty to every mother whose baby lived to the age of 1 year, he achieved a reduction of the village infant mortality from 300 to 200 per 1000 live births. This program lapsed after a while, but in 1893, 40 years later, Morel's son, who succeeded his father as mayor, revived the plan and set it up on a more thoroughgoing basis. This was a complete maternity and child welfare program. Every woman on reporting her pregnancy was at once visited by a physician, who later also examined the baby and attended it during illness. Babies were weighed every two weeks. An intensive campaign was launched to see that every mother nursed her baby for at least a year, and to provide a wetnurse if she could not do so. In addition, the community maintained a herd to supply clean milk to mothers and children. This program was so successful that for the decade 1893 to 1903 the infant mortality rate at Villiers-le-Duc was zero.

The goal achieved by the younger Morel had been envisaged as early as 1860 by Alfred Caron, a Paris physician, who developed the idea of a special branch of hygiene concerned with the health of well infants and children. He coined the name *puériculture* for this concept, which he explored at length in his book, *La puériculture ou la science d'élever hygièniquement et physologiquement les enfants* (*Puériculture or the Science of Raising Children in a Hygienic and Physiological Manner*). During subsequent decades, much work was done to investigate the physiology and pathology of the young child, chiefly in France and Germany. Somewhat later English and American physicians contributed to the growing specialty of pediatrics. The practice of weighing babies was first introduced in 1878 by Friedrich Ahlfeld of Leipzig. A major concern of the leading pediatricians of this period, among them Henoch, Heubner, Czerny, Finkelstein, Rotch, and Jacobi, was the problem of infant feeding.

There was as yet, however, little or no emphasis on community responsibility for the promotion of child health. First steps in this direction were taken by private organizations. In 1859, the New York Infirmary for Women and Children appointed a "sanitary visitor" whose duty was "to give simple, practical instruction to poor mothers on the management of infants and the preservation of the health of their families." The Civil War turned the attention of Americans to the problem of national survival, and it was not until the 1870s that further action was taken. A powerful impulse was furnished by the panic of 1873, whose black shadow falls across the succeeding years. When this period of hard times began, the New York Diet Kitchen set up food stations to feed the poor. In 1878, as conditions improved, the food station became a "milk station" for babies. About the same time, the New York City Health Department undertook to diminish infant mortality, especially in tenement houses. A simple leaflet on infant care was prepared and widely distributed in 1874. Two years later a summer corps of physicians was employed by the Health Department "to search out and treat cases of infant diarrhea."

As a result of the trends and developments described, facilities and programs for infant and child care began to appear in rapid succession during the 1890s and the subsequent decades. A milk distribution center is mentioned in Hamburg in 1899. In the same year, the American physician Henry Koplik (1858–1927) established a "milk station," which was actually a very simple consultation center for mothers and children, at the Good Samaritan Dispensary in New York. The following year a similar center was founded in Barcelona by Francisco Vidal Solares, a Cuban physician. None of these experiments had any other than local influence. However, demonstrations initiated in France along these lines exerted a wide effect in other countries. In 1890, François-Joseph Herrgott (1814–1907), professor at Nancy established an infant welfare center, a *consultation de nourrissons*. More important, however, was the work of Pierre Budin, professor of obstetrics at Paris. In 1892, he established a pioneer system of infant consultation centers, which served as a model for other countries. Budin worked unceasingly to promote child welfare clinics in France. In 1902, together with Roussel, Strauss, and Waldeck-Rousseau, he founded a league to combat infant mortality (*Ligue contre la mortalité infantile*). When he died in 1907, there were 497 clinics in France.

It was recognized that mothers, who could not feed their babies, naturally should be able to obtain clean cow's milk at a reasonable price. Early efforts to achieve this purpose have been mentioned, but the concept first took hold in France. Milk stations, known as *gouttes de lait*, were set up in Paris by two pediatricians. The first of these was established in 1890 by J. Comby, but the greater influence was exerted by Gaston Variot who created such milk stations in 1892. This example was soon followed in New York by the philanthropist Nathan Strauss, who was interested in health problems. In 1893, he began to establish a system of milk stations, which was widely copied and which he supported for 26 years until 1919. The milk was modified according to formula, pasteurized and dispensed in nursing bottles, and mothers were instructed on feeding their babies. In 1902, these stations distributed 250,000 bottles monthly.

The Strauss milk stations provided the impulse for governmental action along these lines. The pioneering was done at Rochester, New York, where in 1897 two milk stations were established under the direction of George W. Goler, a physician. Set up under health department auspices, experiments on child feeding were carried on in these stations, pasteurized milk was distributed at cost, and mothers were instructed in the proper care and feeding of infants. Two years later, the first station of this kind in England was opened by Drew Harris, medical officer of health for the borough of St. Helens. This was a six-room house provided with facilities for washing and sterilizing bottles and weighing babies. Cow's milk was modified by dilution with water and the addition of sugar and cream. A charge of two pence a day was made, and the infant received enough milk in nine bottles to last 24 hours. Two nipples were given for each child, and these had to be brought back periodically for examination.

In Liverpool, two milk stations were opened in 1901, and one each in Ashton-under-Lyme and Dunkenfeld. Similar facilities were created in Battersea in 1902 and Bradford in 1903. The movement soon extended to Scotland with the opening of milk stations at Leith in 1903 and at Glasgow and Dundee in 1904. Several of these establishments, notably those in York (1903) and Finsburg (1904), were created through voluntary efforts. An important advance was made at Battersea in 1905 when "infant consultations" of the kind advocated by Budin were incorporated into the activities of the milk station. This was also adopted at Glasgow in 1906. Health visitors were used to supplement the work of the station by instructing mothers at home.

Essentially, these activities were elements in a health education program. This was recognized in 1907 with the opening of a "school for nursing mothers" by Dr. Sykes, the medical officer of St. Paneras. A similar step was taken in the same year by C. O. Stallybrass, then a resident medical officer at the Liverpool Maternity Hospital. Influenced by Budin, he opened a clinic for infants discharged from that hospital.

German health workers also embarked upon activities of this type at this time. Tugendreich founded the first German infant consultation clinic at Berlin in 1905. By 1907, there were already 73 such establishments as well as 17 milk stations, and in 1910, there were 303 infant welfare establishments. At first these were created by voluntary organizations, as for instance the *Verein für Säuglingsfürsorge* (Society for Infant Welfare) at Düsseldorf. Later these functions were taken over by municipalities and other governmental units.

Teaching mothers to care for their babies, creation of clinics where this could be done properly, and the provision of clean milk were the three basic elements that entered into the development of well-child services. Toward the end of the first decade of the twentieth century, a number of private and governmental agencies in various countries had already demonstrated what might be accomplished along each of these lines in promoting child health. Recognition that the execution of these activities as a total program was a community responsibility to be borne by the agency officially concerned with the health of the community was first achieved in New York City.

The establishment in 1908 of a Division of Child Hygiene in the New York City Health Department is a landmark in the history of the child health movement. This unit was the first of its kind in the world and was to set a pattern for other health departments in the United States and abroad. S. Josephine Baker (1873–1945), a physician who had been a child health inspector in the Department, was put in charge. Early in the summer of 1908, she had shown how infant deaths could be greatly reduced through prevention. In a congested section of New York's Lower East Side the name and address of every newborn baby in the district was obtained from the registrar of records the day after its birth. On that day, a public health nurse visited the mother and taught her what to do to keep the baby well. When the results were tabulated after about two months, it was found that there were 1200 fewer deaths in the district than there had been in the preceding summer during the same period. The same purpose as in this demonstration, to give babies a healthy start in life, provided the basis for the work of the division.

One of its first achievements was to employ milk distribution as a way of coming into contact with mothers to teach them proper child care. Baby health stations were set up in 1910, at first with private funds provided by Mrs. J. Borden Harriman and later with public support, where the sale of bottled pasteurized milk, at a cost of a few cents less than that of loose grocery store milk, was combined with over-the-counter teaching in the care of infants. Attention was also directed to the condition of babies in foundling hospitals and to children of school age. Long before the idea of maternal deprivation was conceived, S. Josephine Baker pointed out that good mothering is as important as good hygienic conditions in the rearing of babies. Similarly, before the term "health education" was invented, the educational process was being employed as a fundamental tool in the campaign to save infant life. An instance is the development of the Little Mother's League. Recognizing that the "little mother," that is, the little girl in a poor family who is forced to take care of the next youngest child because her mother works, was a fertile source of infant mortality, Dr. Baker organized a flock of Little Mother's Leagues among school girls. These children were given practical instruction in child care and served as missionaries of the new gospel in tenements and slums.

The Division of Child Hygiene represented one avenue of attack on the preventable deaths of children. However, this was a battle waged simultaneously on many fronts. Of outstanding importance was the milk front. The need for clean milk had been recognized in the prebacteriological period, and, as a result of a campaign waged by Robert Hartley and Frank Leslie in New York City, conditions under which milk was produced were improved. Then came the era of bacteriology, and it was soon apparent that the problem was only partly solved. Milk is an ideal culture medium for bacteria, and the urban consumer, for a variety of reasons, generally obtained a product with a high degree of bacterial contamination.

William Taylor, of Penrith, England, had first incriminated milk as a transmitter of typhoid fever in 1857. However, it was not until 1881 that attention was first clearly called to the danger of the spread of epidemic disease by milk. That year, at the International Medical Congress in London, Ernest Hart cited 50 epidemics of typhoid fever, 15 epidemics of scarlet fever, and 4 epidemics of diphtheria attributed to this cause. In 1909, the U.S. Public Health Service issued its famous Bulletin 56, which listed 500 outbreaks of milk-borne disease between 1880 and 1907.

In 1901, W. H. Park of the New York City Bacteriological Laboratory showed that milk delivered to customers in the summer was generally highly contaminated with bacteria and might contain more than 5,000,000 organisms per cubic centimeter. Then, in 1902, together with L. Emmett Holt, the eminent pediatrician, he addressed himself to the problem of infantile diarrhea (cholera infantum) and its relation to the bacteriology of the milk consumed. The results were published in December, 1903, and clearly showed that during hot weather the kind of milk fed to infants influenced the amount of illness to which they were subject and their mortality. The effect of bacterial contamination was found to be marked when the milk was not heated before feeding. The next step was to endeavor to obtain a milk supply produced under clean and sanitary conditions. In 1902, the New York City Health Department assigned inspectors to visit dairy farms supplying the city; they were to investigate the conditions under which milk was produced and "to endeavor to educate farmers to the proper idea of sanitary milk production." Railway companies were advised of the necessity of having their milk cars properly refrigerated. Furthermore, the Department of Health began strictly to supervise the distribution and sale of milk within the city. These measures all contributed to improvement of the situation, but the protection of the consumer by any system of inspection and education alone left untouched the problem of the well-carrier who is the source of an outbreak. In August 1909, there was a sudden increase in the number of cases of typhoid fever in New York City. A certain milk supply proved to be the common element in several hundred cases, and ultimately, the source of infection was found to be a dairy man who was a chronic typhoid carrier. As a consequence of this and other outbreaks, the New York City Board of Health in 1910 adopted a requirement that all milk used for drinking purposes be properly pasteurized. Then in 1912, the Board of Health adopted a grading system and standards for all milk brought into the city for sale. Thereafter, clean milk became available for New York's babies, rich and poor. The degree to which infants benefited by measures for the improvement of milk is indicated by the virtual elimination of deaths from summer diarrhea. By 1923, scarcely a vestige remained of the great rise in infant mortality that generally came with the hot weather.

The beginnings of official action on behalf of child health in New York City have been described in some detail because they illustrate the elements and interrelationships that have entered into the development of this field of public health in the United States. What New York City had done on a local level was carried forward by the states and the Federal government. Louisiana in 1912 established a child hygiene unit in its state health department; other states followed in succeeding years. Federal recognition was accorded to the field of child health when President Taft on April 9, 1912, signed a bill creating a Children's Bureau, which was charged with investigating and reporting "upon all matters pertaining to the welfare of children and child life among all classes of our people." This broad mandate reflects the social context and the climate of ideas of which the Bureau was a product. The idea for such a Bureau came from Florence Kelley (1859–1932) and Lillian Wald (1867–1940), both members of that dedicated, militant group of men and women who at the end of the nineteenth century and during the first quarter of the present century undertook to curb some of the worst abuses of industrialization and prepared the way for the social legislation we take for granted today. Mrs. Kelley was the first Chief Inspector of Factories for Illinois and later General Secretary of the National Consumers League; Miss Wald founded public health nursing in America and established the Henry Street Settlement in New York. As early as 1900, Mrs. Kelley in a series of lectures on child labor proposed a National Commission to deal with such matters of immediate urgency as infant mortality, birth registration, orphanage, child labor, desertion, illegitimacy, and degeneracy. In 1903, Miss Wald suggested a Federal Children's Bureau, and the matter was brought to the attention of President Theodore Roosevelt, who promised his support. After several years of further study and of gathering support of community leaders, bills proposing a Children's Bureau were introduced into Congress in 1906. Six years of agitation, argument, and publicity elapsed before the measure was finally passed. Julia C. Lathrop, an associate of Jane Addams at Hull House, was appointed director of the Bureau. Its initial appropriation was only $26,640, and the Bureau wisely devoted much of its activity to a reconnaissance of the area assigned to it by Congress. Much of the data collected before the 1930s provided a solid basis of fact for later Federal action in the interest of maternal and child welfare.

That infancy could not be protected without the protection of maternity was one of the principles on which the Children's Bureau developed its program. This was not a new idea, having been expressed and put into practice more than two decades earlier. Adolph Pinard (1844–1934), a French obstetrician, in 1890 established the first "maternal dispensary" at the *Maternité Baudelocque* in Paris. It is worth noting that he also brought into prominence the term *Puériculture,* which had been coined by Caron 30 years earlier. Pinard was fully aware of the connection between maternal and child welfare, and he offered the proposition that a mother should be her child's paid nurse; in other words, when necessary, the mother should receive a pension, maternity benefits, or other allowances from the community to make sure that her child will receive proper care. According to René Sand, a similar institution was opened by Spencer, a London physician, in 1891. The attention of the medical profession was attracted to this subject, however, by the writings of John William Ballantyne (1861–1923), of the Simpson Memorial Maternity Hospital in Edinburgh. In a paper published in the *British Medical Journal* in 1901, he advocated the provision of prematernity beds. That year the hospital placed one bed at his disposal, and the number was increased over the next few years. In 1915, a prenatal center was established at the same institution, and nurses from the hospital began to make home visits to pregnant women. During this period, other maternity hospitals in Great Britain opened antepartum clinics. In 1942, 75.9 per cent of parturient women in England had received prenatal care.

During the same period, prenatal care also began to receive attention in the United States. The first organized program of health care during the prenatal period was provided in 1908 by the Pediatric Department of the New York Outdoor Medical Clinic. Visiting nurse service for pregnant women in their homes followed a year later in Boston, under the sponsorship of the Women's Municipal League. In 1912, such services were initiated in St. Louis. The Children's Bureau participated initially in the field of maternal health by studying maternal mortality, and by providing instruction for mothers. For the latter purpose, the Bureau, in 1913, published a pamphlet entitled *Prenatal Care,* which has been a best seller ever since. Since then, great strides have been taken in maternity care in the United States. In 1935, 63 per cent of all babies were born in places other than hospitals, and 13 per cent of all live births were not attended by physicians. By 1956, almost 95 per cent of all babies born in this country were delivered in hospitals, and 97 per cent of all registered births were attended by physicians. Furthermore, in recent years expectant mothers have averaged nine consultations for prenatal care with their physicians.

Public awareness of the value of maternity care coupled with advances in medical knowledge have been responsible over the past 30 years for the sharp declines in the mortality of mothers and infants, and the general improvement in their health. There are still areas and groups in the United States—

chiefly rural, low income, and of lower-than-average educational level—that do not fully enjoy these benefits, but even these have shown improvement in recent years. To a very considerable degree, this is a result of action by the Federal Government. During the First World War, health work for mothers and children, as a conservation measure, developed rapidly. England took a far-reaching step in 1918 with the passage of the Maternity and Child Welfare Act. Through the extension of grants-in-aid to private and public agencies, a strong stimulus was given to prenatal and child welfare work. Somewhat similar legislation was adopted in the United States in 1921 with the passage of the Maternity and Infancy Act, popularly known as the Sheppard-Towner Act. Since it was a direct outgrowth of the studies of infant and maternal mortality, it was the first measure to appropriate Federal funds for a health and social welfare purpose. For seven years, a successful program based on Federal-State cooperation was carried on, but in 1929, it failed to secure further appropriations from Congress. Six years later, however, it was reenacted on a much more ambitious scale as Title V of the Social Security Act. This section authorized grants to be made each year to the various states through the Children's Bureau to help them extend and improve their maternal and child health services, as well as services for handicapped children. During World War II, the Children's Bureau also administered through state agencies a vast emergency program of infant and maternity care (EMIC) for the wives of service men.

By holding unswervingly to a broad conception of child welfare as concerned with all the social aspects of child life, by insisting on the use of qualified personnel in all programs, and by encouraging communities on the local and state level to develop maternal and child welfare programs, the Children's Bureau has played a leading role in developing these aspects of community health in the United States. However, it is important to recognize in the development of maternal and child health work a pattern that has characterized community health action as a whole. Advances have come in waves determined by social, economic, and political conditions. The beginnings of the maternal and child health movement are deeply rooted in the abuses that characterized the advancing industrialization of the early years of this century. In the United States it has been a part of the larger movement for social reform that culminated politically in the Wilsonian New Freedom and socially in the endeavor to curb the exploitation of labor. While this wave receded in the normalcy of the 1920s, it provided a basis for the recrudescent wave of renovation that developed during the shattering depression of the 1930s into the Rooseveltian New Deal. The bitter experience of the depression provided a stimulus for renewed activity in the interest of the public health, merging in the 1940s with programs created to deal with the health needs of the war period.

THE HEALTH OF THE SCHOOL CHILD. Action in the interest of mothers and infants during this period is paralleled by the development of health services for school children. A few steps in this direction may be noted from the eighteenth century onward. In France, the principle of school medical inspections was approved by the Convention in 1793, but no action was actually taken until the nineteenth century. A law of 1833 and a Royal Ordinance of 1837 charged French school authorities with the duty of supervising the health of the children and of providing sanitary conditions in school buildings. For the most part, these laws were observed in the breach, and it was not until 1842 that the government issued a decree that all public schools in Paris had to be inspected by physicians. However, the present system of school medical inspection in Paris did not begin until 1879.

Germany was the second country to develop a system of health supervision of school children. A milestone in this development was the investigation by the oculist Hermann Cohn, in 1866, of the eyesight of 7568 children in the schools of Breslau. This painstaking study focused interest on the health of children in schools and led to further studies on the subject. During the next two decades in various countries, physicians began to visit schools, at first occasionally and then on a regular basis. They were concerned with the prevention of communicable diseases among the children and with the sanitary inspection of the school buildings. The first organized school medical services in Europe were instituted in Brussels (1874), throughout Sweden (1878), in Paris (1879), and in Lyons (1880). In England, action was first taken on a local level. The London School Board appointed James Kerr to such a post. It was not until 1907, however, with the passage of the Education (Administrative Provisions) Act, that action was taken on a national scale. As a result, a Medical Department was created at the Board of Education and to this Dr. Janet Campbell was appointed in 1908. George Newman had been appointed Chief Medical Officer to the Board in 1907. This department encouraged and stimulated local education authorities to arrange for the medical inspection of children in elementary schools as rapidly as possible.

School medical inspection in the United States began sporadically in the 1870s. Apparently, the first medical inspector of schools was the New York physician R. J. O'Sullivan, who was appointed by the Board of Education of New York in 1871. He vaccinated school children and carried out sanitary inspections of school buildings. Possibly owing to his criticism of existing conditions, his position was abolished in 1873. During the 1870s and 1880s physicians and interested laymen wrote on problems of school health and recommended medical inspection. Not until 1894, however, was organized medical inspection of schools finally established in the United States. This service was first started in Boston by Samuel H. Durgin, a physician who was chairman of the Board of Health. Medical inspection of school children was initiated here to control contagion. Faced with an epidemic of diphtheria, Durgin found it necessary to send physicians into the public schools to limit the spread of infection. For this purpose, he appointed 50 school physicians to examine children suspected of having the disease and to see that necessary sanitary precautions were taken. Philadelphia and Chicago instituted such systems in 1895, and New York followed suit two years later. In March 1897, 150 school medical inspectors were appointed, at a salary of $30.00 per month to visit public schools and examine children suspected of having communicable disease.

While these efforts marked an important advance, much of the early work in this field was sketchy. It was simply a crude method of screening out the worst cases of infectious diseases, and many minor ones could be brought to light by physicians who were conscientious and experienced. After a while, however, it was recognized that this was not enough. Aside from such conditions as diphtheria, measles, or scarlet fever, school children in large urban centers, especially in slum areas, suffered from skin diseases (pediculosis, scabies, ringworm, impetigo), eye conditions (trachoma), malnutrition, and physical defects. It was recognized that education of parent and child was necessary to combat these conditions. An effective method of dealing with the situation was first developed in New York City. In 1902, at the request of the Health Commissioner, Lillian Wald of the Henry Street Settlement loaned one of her best qualified nurses, Lina Rogers, to carry on experimental work in a particularly bad school. After a few months, she had evolved an educational approach that was effective in checking the minor infections. In consequence, Miss Rogers was appointed as the first full-time school nurse in the United States, and soon 12 more nurses were employed to work along the lines she had developed. This plan was eminently successful and contributed in large measure to the eventual disappearance of many of the conditions just listed.

In 1903, Vermont passed a law requiring annual eye examinations for all school children. Three years later, Massachusetts enacted a law that required that all children have an annual physical examination. The objectives of this measure were to discover and exclude communicable diseases, to detect physical defects, and to make it possible to have these corrected. With this law of 1906, Massachusetts introduced an important administrative precedent in the provision of school health services in the United States. Medical supervision of school children was made a responsibility of the Department of Education and not of the Health Department. This was done to ensure better care because numerous local health departments were poorly staffed, politically controlled, and therefore unable to provide competent service. This system was followed by some communities, but not by others, so that school health work as carried on in the United States today varies greatly from state to state and between localities in the same state. Partly for this reason, and as well for others still to be considered, school health work is nowhere quite what it should be.

Free clinics for school children were established in 1912 in New York City. This service remained a responsibility of the municipal health department. It comprised a general medical clinic, a skin clinic, an eye clinic, and a tonsil and adenoid clinic. Similar facilities have been established by other communities. Today, they may include dental clinics, mental hygiene clinics, as well as clinics for cardiac and other handicapped children.

With the passage of time, many changes have taken place in the provision of health services for school children. There has been a shift of emphasis from the initial limited objectives of school health to a broader concept of this field. From a concern with the control of contagion had come the introduction of public health nursing services in schools. The program was then expanded by the introduction of periodic medical examinations and follow-up procedures for the correction of discovered physical defects. Once interest in the health problems of children was aroused in the United States, developments occurred in a number of other directions.

The school lunch movement had its inception in New York in 1908 as an effort to supplement the diet of undernourished children. Robert Hunter, in his study of poverty in 1904, had estimated that in New York alone some sixty or seventy thousand children went hungry to school, and that poor classwork in many instances was due to malnutrition. This finding was further reinforced by John Spargo in his book *The Bitter Cry of the Children* (1906), in which he reported that thousands of slum children were undernourished. Philadelphia, Chicago, and other large centers followed the lead of New York in the supplementary feeding of poor children. For the most part, the movement was spread as a warm noon lunch for children who found it inconvenient to go home. The need for further work along these lines was indicated by Dr. Josephine Baker of the New York City Health Department who in 1917 estimated that 21 per cent of the children in the New York schools were undernourished. In 1918, Dr. Thomas Wood estimated that this was true of 15 to 25 per cent of the school children in the United States. The most important single factor in developing the school lunch program was the depression of the 1930s. Following the reorganization of the Federal Surplus Commodities Corporation in 1935, it undertook an active program of reducing agricultural surpluses. One phase of this work was the school lunch program. At the end of 1938, 45 states and the District of Columbia were participating in the program, and over a period of five years of operation about 130,000,000 meals had been served. There is no doubt that this program produced direct benefits in improving the health of children. At the same time, emphasis was also put on nutrition education, a subject that had been introduced into the public school curriculum in 1918 and has since become a regular part of both elementary and secondary education. This development was formalized in the National School Lunch Act of 1946, which provides grants-in-aid to states for state-administered school lunch programs. This Act has had a beneficial effect in stimulating the development of such programs throughout the United States.

Dental health services for children got off to a slow start in the United States. Only since the 1930s has there been a broad development of active programs. With the establishment in 1910 of the Forsyth Dental Infirmary in Boston, private philanthropy took the initiative in providing treatment for the children of indigent families. After the founding of the Infirmary, treatment services for school children, concerned largely with extractions, began to develop. Teaching children the need for brushing teeth was the earliest dental health activity in schools. The first dental hygienist was trained in 1913, in Bridgeport, Connecticut, to work with school children to teach them techniques of tooth brushing and to clean their teeth, thus saving the time of the dentist. Massachusetts recognized the services of dental hygienists two years later. In 1918, North Carolina organized the first dental unit in a state health department. The growth in public dental health programs since then is indicated by the organization in 1938 of the American Association of Public Health Dentists. Since 1948, the fluoridation of community water supplies promises to reduce considerably the burden of dental care in the population of school age.

It is manifestly impossible to develop in detail all the trends in school health work. One tendency, however, should be noted. Beginning in the 1920s and continuing into the 1930s, public health workers and educators began to question the conduct of school health work. It was felt that a hurried routine examination of a child without a parent present and with little attention to follow-up procedures was a sterile activity. To break out of this web of routine and to develop better means of providing health care, a number of studies were undertaken, beginning with that launched in 1923 by the American Child Health Association. Eventually, in July 1936, the Astoria Health District Study was initiated in New York City and carried on for four years to June 1940, under the direction of Dorothy B. Nyswander. Much of what has happened since then in the administration and practice of school health work is based on the Astoria demonstration and its results. Today, greater emphasis is placed on more adequate, though possibly less frequent, medical examinations by the family physician or the school physician. Teacher-nurse conferences on suspected health problems and special examinations by the school doctor are being used increasingly to see that children most urgently in need of care receive it. Nonetheless, full productivity in school health service in the United States is still a goal to be attained. One obstacle is the division of responsibility that exists in many communities between educational and health authorities in the administration of health services for school children. A second is the frequently unclear and truncated role of the school physician, who screens and diagnoses but does not treat, and his relation to the family doctor when a family has one. Thirdly, the child who needs dental care, or must have glasses, has to have a place to go and get what he needs. Finally, the family must work with teacher, doctor, and nurse to give the child the care he needs, and this, as we are only too well aware, is dependent in considerable degree on economic, social, and cultural factors. In short, as long as the "total" child is divided for care among several agencies and a variety of personnel, often inadequate in some respect, one cannot expect the full benefits of school health work.

While much remains to be done in the field of child health, a retrospective glance shows clearly how far we have come. The goal for the years ahead was set by the MidCentury White House Conference on Children and Youth of 1950. It took as its theme the total well-being of children or "how we can develop in children the mental, emotional and spiritual qualities essential to individual happiness and responsible citizenship and what physical, economic and social conditions are deemed necessary to this development." The Conference summed up what is known about the health of children and indicated the steps to be taken into the future.

Developments in the United States were paralleled by similar trends in Great Britain and Europe. In England, the Education Acts of 1918 and 1921 placed upon education authorities the duty of providing facilities for the treatment of defects and other conditions discovered in the course of medical inspections. Dental treatment also became compulsory. Examinations were to be carried out at least three times during the period of school attendance, generally when the child entered school, then between the ages of 8 and 12, and finally upon leaving the school. An act of 1944 extended these functions to students up to 18 years of age. The growth of the school medical services in England and Wales is indicated by the fact that from 1910 to 1935 the number of medical officers increased from 995 to 1412, school dentists, from 27 to 852, and school nurses, from 436 to 3429. The latter figure does not include 2215 district nurses employed in the school service on a part-time basis. The provision of treatment for conditions found in the course of medical examinations began with the treatment of minor ailments in school clinics. While in 1910 there were only 30 clinics for minor ailments, by 1935 the number rose to 2037. Special facilities were also developed for children with various physical and mental handicaps (deaf, deaf-mute, blind, mentally defective, and epileptic). Special attention was also given to the nutritional state of school children. At the time of the Boer War, a large number of volunteers for service were rejected on medical grounds. Evidence given before the Committee on Physical Deterioration in 1903 pointed to malnourishment among school children as an important causal factor. In 1904 the Provision of Meals Act was enacted permitting and empowering the educational authorities to make arrangement for the provision of meals for elementary school children. The initial limits set on these programs were removed in 1914. A further important advance was the introduction in 1934 of the milk in schools plan. Aided by public funds, school children were able to buy one third of a pint of milk a day at the nominal price of one half penny. In 1938, 160,000 elementary school children (8.9 per cent) received lunch in school, 110,000 were fed at public expense. In the same year, 2,500,000 children (55 per cent) received milk; 560,000 obtained the milk without payment. The Second World War led to a further expansion of these arrangements. The Education Act of 1944 and the Provision of Milk and Meals Regulations made it obligatory for all educational authorities to provide lunches for all children who wished to have them. Poor children received meals at no cost; others paid the actual cost, which was small. Since 1946, all children younger than 18 years can receive milk at public expense. In that year, 92.6 per cent of all pupils obtained milk in school. Since 1948, the various schemes mentioned have been transformed by the legislation, which originated in the seminal Beveridge Report of 1942. As a result of these developments, as well as of other social welfare measures, the physical and mental condition of British children underwent a remarkable improvement during the past 40 years. While measures for protection of children were by no means ideal, for example, many children died unnecessarily from diphtheria because immunization was not generally accepted until recently, children of the 1940s were better clothed, shod, and fed, on the whole, than they had been at the beginning of the twentieth century.

A NEW KIND OF NURSE APPEARS. In dealing with the health problems of mothers and children, it has been made clear that one of the basic tools is education. The desired goals can be attained by spreading knowledge, stimulating action, and in the last analysis by achieving changes in individual and group behavior. With the recognition and growth of this concept, organizations, techniques, and personnel were developed to reach the community as a whole, as well as particular groups and individuals in it. In working with individuals or with small groups, as in problems of maternal and child health, tuberculosis, venereal disease, or nutrition, it was essential to develop a health worker who could teach and work with people in a manner adapted to their particular needs. A number of health workers of this type have been developed in the past 50 years, among them the nutritionist and the dental hygienist. However, the first and most significant of these is the public health nurse, who today is an accepted member of the staff of any progressive public health agency.

Public health nursing as it exists at present is a recent development, but its roots extend far into the past. One of these derived from the didactic impulse of the Enlightenment, from the desire to improve the health status of the poor by providing them with information so that they might help themselves. The other was the charitable tradition of providing medical and nursing care to the sick poor. It was out of the interaction of these two trends within the social and health context of the late nineteenth and early twentieth centuries that public health nursing evolved in England, the United States, and to a lesser degree in other countries.

Efforts to provide home nursing on an organized basis for the sick poor were undertaken in several European and American communities during the earlier nineteenth century. It was in England, however, that district nursing first developed. Between 1854 and 1856, the Epidemiological Society of London promoted a plan to train suitable pauper women to go into the community and nurse the sick poor. It was felt that, if the nurse were of the same social class as the patient, she would be able to do her job more effectively. Furthermore, it would tend to increase the number of trained nurses available in the community. The plan failed, but in 1859 a scheme was initiated in Liverpool to provide nursing care to the poor. It owed its inception to William Rathbone, a Quaker, who recognized the need for such a service. He divided the community into 18 districts and assigned a nurse and a "lady visitor" to each one. These two women combined the functions of nursing, health education, and social work.

The success of this endeavor attracted attention in other communities, and the example set by Rathbone in Liverpool was followed by the organization of the Manchester and Salford Association in 1864, the Leicester Association in 1867, and the East London Nursing Society in 1868. Birmingham appointed its first district nurse in 1870 and Glasgow in 1875. The Metropolitan and National Nursing Association was founded in London in 1874 to train nurses for district work. Eventually, district nursing was placed on a national basis but remained associated with voluntary agencies.

At the same time, health visiting, another line of development that was to lead to public health nursing, was started in Manchester. In 1862, the Ladies Section of the Manchester and Salford Sanitary Association undertook to spread health information among the poor of the community. After discovering that the distribution of pamphlets brought only meager results, a woman of the working class was employed to make house to house visits among the poor and to teach them in matters of health and hygiene. This venture proved successful, and a number of other women were hired to develop the plan on a district basis. Other communities followed Manchester's example until by the turn of the century health visitors were to be found in many towns.

A tendency for nurses to become health visitors appeared early in the present century and was fostered particularly by the growth of the child health movement. In 1893, Florence Nightingale called attention to the need for "health nursing," and insisted that the district nurse should be a "health missioner" as well as a sick nurse. The following year she restated the importance of health teaching in the home, urging the training of health missioners for this purpose. Meanwhile, the Manchester Corporation in 1890 arranged with the Ladies Sanitary Association that 6 of 14 home visitors working for the latter be placed under the direction and supervision of the medical officer of health, their salaries to be paid by the municipality. Several years later a similar arrangement was arrived at between the Association and the Salford Corporation. By 1905, the work of the Association was being carried on in 23 districts each with its home visitor. In the same year a trained educated woman was appointed by the municipality to supervise the entire staff.

This pattern of collaboration between governmental and voluntary agencies was followed by other localities. Three visitors were employed on a full-time basis in 1892 by the country of Buckinghamshire, and five years later five "lady health missioners" were appointed by the Worcestershire County Council. Birmingham, Sheffield, and Chesterfield were among other communities that followed the example of Manchester. By 1905, some 50 communities had staffs consisting of voluntary visitors supplemented by employing women designed as sanitary inspectors or health visitors.

The function of these visitors was to promote the care and welfare of young children in the home. There was, however, little uniformity in the system. Some health visitors were drawn from the same social class as those among whom they worked; others were "ladies" with or without some special training; and a few were women doctors, trained nurses, or certified midwives. Experience showed higher education was a desirable qualification for this work, and steps were taken to improve the situation in this respect. Furthermore, since there was no statutory authority to appoint health visitors, it was common to hire them as sanitary inspectors. The first step to correct this situation was taken by the London County Council in 1908. It sponsored a bill that not only legalized the appointment of health visitors but also stipulated that the Local Government Board regulate their qualifications and duties. Regulations to this effect were issued in 1909. These set forth that a health visitor should have a medical degree, or be a fully trained nurse, or have the certificate of the Central Midwives Board, or in addition to having had some training in nursing must have a certificate from a society approved by the Local Government Board. Thus, the public health nurse in Great Britain came into existence legally.

There were no comparable requirements, however, for communities and health authorities outside London. As the years went by, the number of health visitors employed by local authorities continued to grow until in 1918 it reached the figure of 3038. Nevertheless, for many years there was no accepted course of study and training. The first important action to ensure proper training for health visitors was taken in 1908 when the Royal Sanitary Institute set up an examination for health visitors and school nurses. The following year the Board of Education prescribed the course of training and qualifications for health visitors. As a result, by the end of the second decade of the twentieth century, a number of training centers had been established. Some of the first in England and Wales were at King's College for Women, the Bedford College for Women, the Liverpool School of Hygiene, the Battersea Polytechnic, and the University College of South Wales. After the passage of the Maternity and Child Welfare Act of 1918, it became necessary for a health visitor to have the qualifications required by London, or others satisfactory to the Local Government Board. As a result, uniform training requirements were set forth in 1919, and in 1924 the Royal Sanitary Institute was made the central agency for conducting examinations and qualifying candidates for health visitor appointments. As of April 1, 1928, whole-time health visitors were required to have the certificate of the Royal Sanitary Institute. By the end of 1933, local authorities employed 2938 health visitors, and voluntary organizations employed 2546.

A tendency that characterized the growth of public health nursing in Great Britain and that can be observed as well for the United States, is the appearance initially of specialized nursing activities, e.g., district nursing, health visiting, and the like. In the course of the past 30 or 40 years others developed and were absorbed into the general stream of public health nursing. The school nurse, for example, appeared in England when medical inspection of school children was made compulsory in 1908, and the Board of Education urged the appointment of nurses. Thus at various times there appeared the tuberculosis nurse, the orthopedic nurse, the municipal midwife, and others. In recent years there has been an increasing trend to develop a generalized public health nurse, although some functions, such as midwifery, remain specialized. The role of the health visitor under the National Health Service is not fully clear, and it will undoubtedly change as public health develops in this new phase of community organization. Indicative is the fact that in September, 1953, the Ministers of Health and Education and the Secretary of State for Scotland appointed a group to advise on the proper field of work, the recruitment, and the training of health visitors in the National Health Service and in the school health service.

In the United States, as in England, public health nursing grew out of district nursing and home visiting. While these activities derived from Rathbone's work in Liverpool, it was not until 1877 that district nursing was introduced into America. The New York City Mission employed trained nurses to give care to the sick poor in their homes, and this endeavor was followed by the Society for Ethical Culture in the next year. The idea gradually spread to other communities. The first nursing associations organized directly for this purpose were in Buffalo in 1885, and in Boston and Philadelphia in 1886. Originally, those in Buffalo and Philadelphia were called District Nursing Societies, while that in Boston was named the Instructive District Nursing Association. Eventually, they all changed their names to Visiting Nurse Associations. The name of the Boston organization indicates that teaching was a recognized objective for the district nurse along with the care of the sick in their homes. In 1893, Lillian D. Wald and Mary Brewster opened the Henry Street District Nursing Service, an organization that has played an important role in the growth of public health nursing in the United States. These were all voluntary agencies depending for their support upon contributions and small service charges.

As the concept of public health expanded near the turn of the century and personal health services began to loom larger in the community health program, nurses began to be employed by health departments. Los Angeles was the first community to do so. In 1898, a nurse was employed by the health department to provide home nursing care to the sick poor. It was not until 1913, however, that the Los Angeles Health Department established a bureau of nursing. The use of trained nurses in health departments on any appreciable scale did not begin until 1902 when a Henry Street nurse was loaned to the New York City Health Department to work in a school. The successful outcome of this initial trial soon led to the employment of a group of nurses in the city schools. The following year (1903) the Department appointed three nurses at an annual salary of $900 each to visit patients with tuberculosis at home and to instruct them concerning sputum disposal and other elements of personal hygiene. In 1905, this service was increased to 14 nurses. Alabama in 1907 was the first state legally to approve the employment of public health nurses by local boards of health. Public health nursing developed rapidly and was accepted by school boards, local and state health departments, and eventually by the U.S. Public Health Service. The first public health nurse was appointed in the Service in 1913 for field work in trachoma. It was not until the early 1930s, after a survey to determine the needs of the Service in this area, that public health nursing was developed in this agency.

As in England, nurses were first appointed in American official and voluntary health agencies to deal with specific problems. The result was that most public health nursing programs originally developed on a specialized basis with nurses employed specifically as school nurses, tuberculosis nurses, maternal and child health nurses, communicable disease nurses, and so on. This trend was further strengthened by the activities of disease-centered voluntary agencies, by such legislation as the Sheppard-Towner Act, and by those interested in the health of school children. Evidence began to accumulate, however, that a generalized nursing program was more efficient and effective. Work with county health units sponsored by the Rockefeller Foundation, the U.S. Public Health Service, the Milbank Fund, and other agencies indicated the advantages of a generalized nursing program. Today, the generalized program is widely accepted, with the exception of such areas as industrial nursing.

An important agency in the advancement of this field has been the National Organization of Public Health Nursing, which was formed in 1912. It was concerned with improving the educational and service standards of the public health nurse, and with promoting public understanding of and respect for her work. By 1952, this group together with several other nursing organizations felt a need for coordination of activities, and so in that year they joined together to form the National League for Nursing.

In 1951, there were 25,461 public health nurses employed in the United States and its territories. Of these, 12,556 were engaged in local health work. Since then the number has increased somewhat, but there still exists a need for additional nurses to meet desirable standards.

Other countries have to a greater or lesser degree followed the same pattern as the United States and Great Britain. In Germany, nurses were developed in specific fields at first, for example, as baby nurses and midwives. From among these some were eventually drawn upon to work with health agencies. By 1922, there were enough public health nurses so that regulations for a certifying examination were set up. In 1950, the German Federal Republic had 3431 public health nurses (*Gesundheitsfürsorgerinnen*). Other countries have developed public health nursing even more recently. Denmark did not introduce public health nursing on a national basis until 1937.

VOLUNTARY ACTION FOR HEALTH. The promotion of health and the prevention of disease in a community are clearly responsibilities of government. Yet, it is also clear that in many instances voluntary action has preceded and indeed stimulated governmental action in the health field. Such action by private individuals or groups has frequently found its operational base in an organization developed specifically for the purpose of promoting an understanding of and action in the interest of solving certain community health problems. Voluntary action in public health is not a new phenomenon, and attention has been directed to it in earlier periods, especially in the eighteenth and nineteenth centuries. However, as a result of historical factors that have been operating for the past 50 or 60 years, a specific kind of organization, the voluntary health agency, has given concrete form to such endeavors.

In this sense, the voluntary health agency is a distinctly modern organization, which started out to furnish health services of a kind that had not previously been available. It was a pioneer in putting to use for the common welfare new facts or new conceptions about health and disease. While the voluntary health movement has had its fullest flowering in the United States, such voluntary organizations have not been confined to this country nor were they first developed here. Furthermore, it should occasion little surprise to find the voluntary health agencies reflecting the social and medical tendencies of the period in which they arose and came to maturity.

Historically, the voluntary health movement had two main sources of inspiration. On the one hand, the voluntary agencies arose and based their efforts on concepts of health and disease that had been developed and had gained acceptance at the end of the nineteenth century. Important in this respect was the concept of the etiological specificity of disease (bacteriology). Almost equally important was the trend to specialization in medicine, which was accelerated by the new discoveries. On the other hand, these health agencies developed out of the efforts to grapple with poverty and privation, which revealed the destructive role of ill health and disease in the lives of the poor, and the need for vigorous action to combat sickness and its consequences. Action was taken along various lines in the United States. Many of these organizations, such as the Henry Street Settlement and the Association for Improving the Condition of the Poor, both in New York, developed nursing or clinic services. The Charity Organization Society of New York established its Committee on Tuberculosis, which later became the New York Tuberculosis and Health Association. The social and economic environment within which this development occurred in America is that of industrialization, with its accompanying expansion of urban communities. It was the rapid economic growth which helped to create the problems that give rise to the voluntary health agencies and which made available resources and leisure that could be utilized to start new organizations of public significance.

By 1945, there were in the United States some 20,000 agencies enlisting the services of 300,000 members of boards and committees and a million or more volunteers, and raising from the public well more than $58,000,000 annually. These figures do not include such organizations as the American Red Cross, which occupies a quasi-official position, as well as the philanthropic foundations for health promotion, and organizations of physicians, dentists, nurses, and other professional groups concerned with health and disease. While professional associations have contributed greatly to the health and welfare of the community, their primary objectives are not those of the voluntary health agencies in the strict sense. The latter are concerned with furthering community health through education, demonstrating ways of improving health services, advancing related research or legislation, as well as guarding and representing the public interest in this field. Despite the great multiplicity and variety of such agencies, the voluntary health organizations tend generally to fall into four categories: (1) those concerned with specific diseases, such as tuberculosis, cancer, poliomyelitis, diabetes, and multiple sclerosis; (2) those concerned with disorders of certain organs of the body, such as the heart, defects of vision or hearing, dental defects, and diseases of the locomotor and skeletal systems;

(3) those concerned with the health and welfare of special groups in the community such as mothers and children, the aged, or the Negro; and (4) those that deal with health problems that affect the community as a whole, such as accident prevention, mental health, or planned parenthood.

Limitations of space preclude any detailed consideration of the history of even all the larger or national voluntary health organizations. Nevertheless, a brief survey of the origins and development of a few of these agencies will indicate the factors that have made them what they are today. The National Tuberculosis Association is the oldest agency of this type in the United States and its evolution epitomizes the whole voluntary health movement.

Only half a century ago, tuberculosis was not only the chief single cause of death in the United States, the Captain of the Men of Death, but it also produced an enormous amount of chronic illness and disability among the millions of its victims. At the same time, it was viewed by most physicians as a constitutional, hereditary disease related in some vague way to deleterious environmental conditions. Only a change of climate was regarded as holding out any hope for cure. Furthermore, there were practically no hospital facilities available to people with tuberculosis, and many looked upon these unfortunates as pariahs. To avoid being stigmatized, individuals and families with tuberculosis members made every effort to conceal the presence of the disease. These conditions undoubtedly helped to spread infections.

On March 24, 1882, Koch announced to the world his discovery of the tubercle bacillus as the etiologic agent of tuberculosis. The concept of tuberculosis as a disease entity, originally set up on purely clinical and pathological-anatomical grounds, was now confirmed by bacteriological discovery. Ten years elapsed, however, between the discovery of the tubercle bacillus and the commencement of the first organized campaign against the disease in the United States. Meanwhile, the implications for community action had been recognized in Great Britain, France, and several other European countries. Robert W. Philip (1857–1939), an Edinburgh physician, saw that "if the community as such was to benefit practically by the discovery, there appeared to be need of centralized effort in order to ascertain the extent of tuberculosis in a district, and to devise means for its limitation and prevention." The result was the opening in 1887 of the Victoria Dispensary for Consumption, the first tuberculosis dispensary in the world. Philip's program also included home visiting, health education, and an occupational farm colony for patients. This pioneer endeavor was followed in 1898 by the organization of the National Association for the Prevention of Consumption and other forms of tuberculosis for the purpose of preventing the ravages of the disease in Great Britain. Its objectives were to educate the public concerning the propagation and prevention of tuberculosis, to influence Parliament and other public bodies in matters relating to the prevention of the disease, and to establish branches of the Association to stimulate action on a local level.

Similar ideas were developed independently on the Continent. A French League Against Tuberculosis was founded early in 1891 by Armingaud of Bordeaux. In June of that year, the National League for the Campaign against Tuberculosis was organized in Denmark. In 1899, Albert Calmette (1863–1933), the great French student of tuberculosis, who introduced B.C.G. vaccine, conceived the idea of tuberculosis clinics for prevention, education, and ambulatory treatment. On February 1, 1901, he and his associates opened the *Dispensaire Émile Roux* at Lille. (A similar facility had been opened the preceding year at Liége by Ernest Malvoz.) By the end of 1905, there were no less than 62 of these establishments in France, of which 38 were in and around Paris. In November 1895, the German Central Committee for the Creation of Sanatoria for Patients with Pulmonary Disorders was organized to bring together all persons and agencies interested in combatting tuberculosis. At first concerned primarily with the development of sanatoria, it gradually shifted its interest to the larger field of tuberculosis control in the community and in 1906 changed its name to the German Central Committee for Combatting Tuberculosis. In 1903, Germany had 18 tuberculosis policlinics; by 1906 there were 68 dispensaries and policlinics.

The United States did not remain uninfluenced by these developments. As early as 1889, the implications of Koch's discovery for community action against tuberculosis had been drawn in a report prepared by Herman M. Biggs, J. Mitchell Prudden, and H. P. Loomis, consulting pathologists to the New York City Health Department. Emphasizing the preventability of tuberculosis, they recommended the surveillance of the disease by the department and education of the public concerning its changes. A leaflet on tuberculosis was printed and distributed, but owing to the cool reception given to the report by the medical profession, little more was done at this time. The matter was not dropped, however, and in 1894 the department began to require reporting of cases of tuberculosis by institutions, and in 1897 reporting by physicians. On September 30, 1893, the Michigan State Board of Health voted to require the reporting of tuberculosis to local health officers. Similar efforts were made by William Osier in Baltimore and Lawrence F. Flick in Philadelphia at this time.

Up to this point, however, the war against tuberculosis was a matter for the professional. The mobilization of the forces of the community for the control of a disease was first undertaken in the United States in the last decade of the nineteenth century. In form, this line of attack was directly related to earlier endeavors to procure sanitary reform and improved public health administration. What was new was the discovery of the potentialities of broad community organization as a means of controlling disease, a discovery that was to have far-reaching significance for the entire public health program. This novel and pregnant conception was introduced by the pioneers of the anti-tuberculosis movement, particularly the Philadelphia physician Lawrence F. Flick (1856–1934) and his associates, who organized the Pennsylvania Society for the Prevention of Tuberculosis in 1892. This was a pioneer association in several ways. Not only was it the first tuberculosis society in the United States, but it was also the first body to endeavor to marshal the forces of the community by combining lay and professional membership and to concentrate its activities against a single disease. In these respects it set a pattern that was to be widely followed up to the present. The objective of the Society—the prevention of tuberculosis—was to be achieved "(1) by promulgating the doctrine of the contagiousness of the disease; (2) by instructing the public in practical methods of avoidance and prevention; (3) by visiting the consumptive poor and supplying them with the necessary materials with which to protect themselves against the disease and instructing them in their use; (4) by furnishing the consumptive poor with hospital treatment; (5) by cooperating with boards of health in such measures as they may adopt for the prevention of disease; (6) by advocating the enactment of appropriate laws for the prevention of the disease; (7) by such other methods as the Society may from time to time adopt." In this respect as well, Flick and the Pennsylvania Society set a pattern for the voluntary health movement.

Flick's efforts were of more than just local consequence. Not only was he dauntless in propagating his ideas but like every true crusader he was also very persistent. The United States lagged behind Great Britain and Europe in its attack on tuberculosis, and Flick knew this. He had read with keen interest of Philip's work in Edinburgh in 1887, and corresponded with him concerning his methods. In 1902 he visited Europe where he met Calmette and other European leaders in anti-tuberculosis work. Most important of all, Flick corresponded with other Americans, among them the New York physician, S. Adolphus Knopf, urging the formation of a national organization. The example of the Pennsylvania Society had been followed elsewhere after the passage of a decade. In 1901 a second state tuberculosis society was organized in Ohio; and in 1902 the Committee for the Prevention of Tuberculosis of the Charity Organization Society of New York was organized. By 1904, 23 state and local associations had been formed. Finally, after a preliminary meeting at Baltimore in January, 1904, the idea of a nationwide organization was adopted and the National Association for the Study and Prevention of Tuberculosis was formed at Atlantic City in June of that year. (In 1918 the name was changed to the shorter National Tuberculosis Association.) Edward L. Trudeau (1848–1915), the physician who pioneered the sanatorium treatment of tuberculosis in America, was chosen as its first president. Among the other medical founders were William Osler, Hermann M. Biggs, Lawrence F. Flick, S. A. Knopf, William H. Welch,

George Sternberg, Henry B. Jacobs, and M. P. Ravenel. The six lay members of the board included Edward T. Devine, Homer Folks, and Samuel Gompers.

Financing was one of the first problems faced by the Association, and it was difficult to cope with initially. For 10 years, from 1907 to 1917, the Russell Sage Foundation assumed some responsibility. In 1907, Jacob Riis, the Danish-born journalist and social reformer, called attention to the idea of selling special stamps or seals as a means of raising money. This device had been hit upon by Einar Holboell, a postal clerk in Denmark, and was rapidly adopted in this country. From 1910 to 1919, the National Tuberculosis Association cooperated with the American Red Cross in the annual seal sale. Since that date, Christmas seals have been sold by the Association alone. In 1919 almost $4,000,000 was raised in this way, and in 1947 almost $19,000,000 were obtained through the sale of seals. From the beginning the National Tuberculosis Association decided to leave the bulk of the funds raised, 95 per cent, to the state and local affiliated groups, while retaining only 5 per cent for the national organization. Here too the Association set a pattern for others to follow. Extraordinarily successful in this respect has been the National Foundation for Infantile Paralysis with its March of Dimes. Two other agencies that have had a more modest success with such money-raising devices are the American Cancer Society with its Field Army and its label sale, and the National Society for Crippled Children with its Easter Seal sale.

The idea of organizing to control a specific disease or a group of disorders and of enlisting community support and action through a systematic and organized campaign of public health education soon spread to other fields. In 1905, Dr. Prince A. Morrow organized the Society for Social and Moral Prophylaxis to deal with the treatment and prevention of venereal diseases. Similar societies were formed in 11 states, and by 1910 these were united in the American Federation for Sex Hygiene, which in 1914 joined with the American Vigilance Association to form the American Social Hygiene Association. The National Committee for Mental Hygiene was organized in 1909, following the publication of *A Mind that Found Itself,* the autobiography of Clifford Beers. The American Society for the Control of Cancer was organized in 1913, the American Heart Association in 1922, the National Foundation for Infantile Paralysis in 1938, and the American Diabetes Association in 1940. One important voluntary agency that dissolved in 1935 was the American Child Health Association, which had grown out of the American Association for the Study and Prevention of Infant Mortality initially created in 1909.

By 1920, the multiplication of national health agencies raised questions in the minds of some community health leaders about the need for coordination, efficient use of funds, possible duplication of effort, and confusion of the public. To deal with these and related problems the National Health Council was formed in 1921. While it has many achievements to its credit, it has fallen short of the hopes originally placed in it. More recently it has been concerned with the development of community action for local health units, recruiting young people for health careers, and stimulating community programs for chronic illness. In 1941 the National Health Council sponsored, and the Rockefeller Foundation financed, a study of the extent and effectiveness of voluntary health work in the United States. The study involved field work and visits to more than 700 health agencies in 65 cities and 29 states. The final report of this study by S. M. Gunn and P. S. Platt devoted considerable attention to nationwide and statewide organizations and indicated their social values and functions as well as their defects. The authors deplored the lack of central direction and planning, pointing out that frequently individual health organizations have overlapped and duplicated one another's efforts. Furthermore, the various national organizations are dedicated to isolated combat with specific diseases or the diseases of specific organs, so that it has generally been a case of each specialized interest fending for itself. This state of affairs is reflected by the present separate, competitive money-raising appeals of the various voluntary health agencies. Gunn and Platt recommended the pooling of these appeals into a national health campaign so as to have a more equitable distribution of funds. They also proposed further coordination and consolidation of the agencies at the national level with wider coordination on state and local community levels. To accomplish this aim, the report urged the establishment of a health council in every community, to include representatives of all local health agencies. These proposals were made in the hope that they would ultimately lead to a unified community health program.

Since 1949 when Detroit, Michigan, organized its Torch Drive, approximately 900 communities have developed United Funds to finance the activities of voluntary health agencies, but there has been considerable opposition to this development.

One thing seems clear. The positive contributions of the voluntary health agencies are too considerable to be overlooked. Community health action in the United States could not have developed as it did in the absence of voluntary health agencies. Much that has been accomplished through research, demonstrations, professional education, and health teaching of the public can be placed to their credit. On the other hand is the fact that social, economic, and political conditions today are quite different from those that prevailed when the voluntary agencies appeared and developed. The role of the Federal Government has changed. It has become inordinately more active in the health field, and through categorical allotment of funds has made it possible for official health agencies to take over activities previously carried on by voluntary agencies. Then, due to higher rates of taxation, greater selectivity is being exercised in supporting voluntary health agencies. There has developed a "givers dilemma." Furthermore, as disease problems change, programs must inevitably be altered. Some agencies, for instance, tuberculosis associations, have tended to broaden their programs to include other health problems. The voluntary health movement is at present in a state of transition, nor is this undesirable.

TEACHING THE PEOPLE ABOUT HEALTH. In carrying on the new programs concerned with maternal and child health, school health, tuberculosis control, and related activities, official and voluntary health agencies inevitably found themselves engaged in a program of education. To promote health and prevent disease, it was necessary to combat ignorance. This emphasis, characteristic of the period that began toward the end of the nineteenth century, eventually led to a recognition of health education as a major function in the community health program.

Endeavors to impart health information and guidance have been described for earlier periods, and these continued along more or less similar lines into the nineteenth century. When health departments were established, they carried out such activities from time to time. The distribution of leaflets on infant care and diphtheria in 1874 and on tuberculosis in 1897 by the New York City Department of Health have been mentioned. In addition, however, there were other, even more significant influences that led to the development of health education as it exists in the United States today. On the one hand, there was a movement that led toward school health education. Through the 1880s and early 1890s a child study movement was inaugurated among educators, which endeavored to understand the needs of children. This became coupled with the teaching of physiology and hygiene when the latter was made mandatory around 1880 in consequence of a powerful propaganda movement sponsored by temperance interests. The basic purpose of this legislation was to require instruction on the effects of alcohol and narcotics, but most of these laws were so worded that this instruction became a part of a broader teaching program. Other activities that tended to further the evolution of health education have been the school lunch program, safety education and programs dealing with emotional, and mental health.

In large measure, however, the efforts of voluntary organizations, as they began to appear during and after the first decade of the present century, soon outstripped those of the official agencies. The trail blazer in public health education was the tuberculosis movement. John S. Fulton assembled the first tuberculosis exhibit in Baltimore in 1904. Owing to the nationwide attention it attracted, a similar exhibit was displayed the following year at the American Museum of Natural History in New York. In 1906, the recently organized National Association for the Study and Prevention of Tuberculosis built a traveling exhibit that was placed under the direction of Evart G. Routzahn. Soon another exhibit of this type was added. These exhibits were shown at fairs and in vacant stores in larger cities. They were created and manned by laymen, who were advised by some of the leading medical men of the period. Intended primarily to arouse public interest, the exhibits did this in a most direct and often crude manner. Tuberculous lungs, photographs of decrepit and unsanitary tenements, and other shocking facts were presented visually in the belief that they would prove the most compelling of arguments and that the public would become interested, impressed, and convinced. Other tools employed in the anti-tuberculosis campaign were newspaper publicity, leaflets and pamphlets, health talks, and lantern slides. Later the motion picture was added to this armamentarium. Throughout these endeavors, the major emphasis was on the presentation of facts by means of techniques developed in the fields of advertising and publicity.

During the second decade of the twentieth century, health departments intensified their educational activities and put them on an organized basis. Weekly bulletins began to be published in 1911 and 1912 by the Chicago and New York health departments. The former was intended for the lay public and was widely distributed in churches and schools. The New York City bulletin was intended primarily to further the education of the medical practitioner in the preventive aspects of his daily practice. Publication of this bulletin, which later became a monthly and finally a quarterly, was suspended only a few years ago (1955). In 1914, the New York City Health Department organized the first bureau for health education in an official health agency, and the same year witnessed the creation of a similar unit in the New York State Health Department. By 1929, 52 municipal and 35 state health departments were publishing bulletins on health subjects, generally on a monthly basis, and a few had full-time directors of health education.

The First World War greatly accelerated the evolution of health education and set the stage for its growth. War-time needs, especially the necessity to control venereal disease in the armed forces, led to increased emphasis on keeping fit as a patriotic duty. Neighborhood organizations and community councils made health a dominant concern. At the same time, continuing progress in the field of child health led to the first steps to differentiate health education as the most recent of the public health specialties. In 1918, the Child Health Organization of America was formed with L. Emmett Holt, the well-known pediatrician, and Sally Lucas Jean, a nurse, at its head. Rather than merely warning against disease, they stressed the potentialities of health promotion through education and nutrition. Since the organization operated chiefly through schools and was primarily interested in children, new notes of cheerfulness and humor were introduced. An attractively illustrated Child Health Alphabet was produced of which the first two lines were as follows:

A is for Apples, and also for Air
Children need both, and we have them to spare.

The health message was carried by such characters as the Health Fairy and Cho-Cho the Clown. While these efforts were undoubtedly superficial and overemphasized the "radiant" aspects of health, they were a useful corrective to the graphic gruesomeness of the earlier health education activities.

Probably more significant for its long-term consequences was the initial step taken at this time to recognize health education as a special field of endeavor in public health. The term "health education" was first proposed in 1919 at a conference called by the Child Health Organization, and the following year it offered its first fellowship in health education. In 1922, the Child Health Organization merged with the American Child Hygiene Association to form the American Child Health Association. That year, together with the United States Bureau of Education, it organized the Lake Mohonk Conference, which emphasized the proper training of teachers of health education. Furthermore, by 1922, the number of workers in public health agencies concerned with health education had become numerous enough to form a separate section in the American Public Health Association. Very few of these workers, however, gave their full time to health education activity, nor did they have any specialized training to equip them for this work. These pioneers were recruited from a number of health fields as well as related professions: medicine, nursing, teaching, publicity, and so on. The number of health education specialists grew slowly. In 1942, when the Subcommittee on Local Health Units of the American Public Health Association made its survey, only 13 states reported health educators as employed by state and local health departments. These 13 had a total of 44 workers. Recognizing the need for trained workers, the American Public Health Association in 1943 established qualifications for health educators in general. Educational standards for school health educators had been set by the Association in 1938. Also in 1943 schools of public health began to set up programs for the training of health educators. The results were very soon evident. A study made in 1947 revealed that 460 men and women were employed as health educators in official and voluntary health organizations. Of this group, 300 had completed graduate courses in recognized schools of public health. Graduate training in health education is presently offered at schools in the following universities: California, Columbia, Harvard, Michigan, Minnesota, North Carolina, Tulane, and Yale. The number of professional health educators was sufficiently numerous by 1951, so that the Society of Public Health Educators was formed as the group's professional organization. The need for trained health educators, however, is still great. As the health education specialist demonstrates the value of his skills in the community health program, the actual and potential demand for this relatively new member of the public health team likewise grows.

Coincident with this development, there have been changes in the objectives of health education. It has been recognized that it is not enough to impart information; what counts is what is done with this knowledge. Furthermore, it has been realized that the community is a unit and that in health education, as in other health work, a coordinated program is needed which will touch each segment of the community in accordance with its nature and its needs. Finally, it is recognized that when the members of a community have a chance to learn about their health problems and how to deal with them, the community health program is likely to be more solidly based. The idea of stimulating and encouraging citizens to work out their own health destinies was not new, but it had been obscured during the early decades of the century by an excessive emphasis on tools and techniques. Actually, the pattern had been set by the founders of the voluntary health organizations, and even earlier by the sanitary reformers. Adequate sewerage, water supply systems, and other community services were obtained because of the insistent demands of organized groups of citizens. Pioneer endeavors toward better community organization for health education were undertaken in a few cities, notably New York and Boston, in connection with district health centers. In 1938, however, a community-wide program was initiated in Hartford, Connecticut, which attracted national attention. This program, under the direction of Lucy Morgan, endeavored to enlist the entire community in a unified program of study and action. This was followed in 1941 by a report prepared by a committee of the American Public Health Association, titled *Community Organization for Health Education,* which has had a wide influence. Community organization is today an important element of the health education program in the United States.

Another trend of fundamental significance is the recognition that health education is concerned basically with human behavior and its alteration for the improvement and promotion of individual and community health, and that in consequence the health educator must turn to the social sciences for a better understanding of how to work with people individually or in groups. At the same time, health educators have become more critical of their activities and have begun to subject them to analysis and evaluation using methods and tools developed in the social sciences. This trend is only in its beginning, but there can be little doubt that as the social sciences contribute to a more precise knowledge of individual and group behavior the health educator will be able to carry out his important task in a more effective manner.

The last 30 odd years have also seen the introduction of important technical means of communication: radio and television, as well as the continued spread of urban culture over the United States, due in part to the effects of the inter-

nal combustion engine on transportation. Apparently the first health talk over
the radio was given by Dr. Charles A. Powers, President of the American Society for the Control of Cancer in November 1921. On December 6, 1921, the
U.S. Public Health Service began weekly health broadcasts, from the naval ob-
servatory station at Arlington, Virginia. The second official health agency to
give regular health programs was the New York State Health Department. On
March 24, 1922, a talk on "Keeping Well" was broadcast by the department
from the General Electric station in Schenectady, New York.

In the early 1920s, the New York Tuberculosis and Health Association extended its lecture program into the new field of radio, under the direction of
Dr. Iago Galdston. Other official and voluntary health agencies followed these
pioneers, and today the radio is an accepted tool for mass communication in
the health field. Television is still too new for its potentialities to have been fully
explored. Health agencies have utilized it for health education purposes, and
there can be little question that it is a powerful tool. It is for the future, however, to determine its true place in the armamentarium of the educator.

Health education in Europe has developed differently from that in the
United States in a number of important respects. First of all, with the possible exception of the Soviet Union, official health agencies have not engaged in
this function to the same extent. Secondly, voluntary health agencies are not so
well developed, and while health education is promoted by independent organizations, such as anti-tuberculosis groups, temperance societies, youth groups,
sickness insurance funds, and the like, the results have been sporadic and un-
coordinated. During the past two or three decades, efforts have been made in
a few countries to develop health education as a major activity in a coordinated
health program, but these have lagged far behind the United States.

Certain tools and channels of communication, on the other hand, were
more highly developed and more frequently employed than in the United
States. This is particularly true of the poster and the health museum. Poster
art reached a higher level in Europe and exerted an effect in the health field.
Similarly, the health museum was best exemplified by the German Hygiene
Museum established at Dresden in 1912. The influence of this institution has
been felt, directly or indirectly, all over the world. The first permanent health
museum in the United States, the Cleveland Health Museum, was established
under the direction of Dr. Bruno Gebhardt, formerly of the German Museum.
The Cleveland institution was incorporated in 1936 and opened its doors in
1940. A second health museum opened in Dallas, Texas, in October 1946. More
recently such institutions have been established at the Lankenau Hospital near
Philadelphia (1953), and at Hinsdale, Ill. (1957).

Health education in Germany first assumed an organized form in 1908 with the formation of the *Deutsche Verein für Volkshygiene* (German Society for Public Hygiene). This was followed in 1919 by the creation of the *Landesausschüsse für hygienische Volksbelehrung* (State Committees for Public Health Education); the following year (1920) they were united into a Reich Committee with headquarters first in Dresden, later in Berlin. Following the war and the de facto division of Germany, the Federal Republic on April 7, 1954, created a Federal Committee for Public Health Education. In 1957, it comprised 112 member organizations. While it receives government subvention, it remains a voluntary organization dedicated to the stimulation of activity on the part of individuals and groups in the interest of personal and community health. As yet the specialist health educator is unknown in Germany. While public health education is officially a function of the local health agency, practically, community health education is carried on almost exclusively by private voluntary organizations. Materials are prepared and made available by the Central Institute for Health Education, the German Health Museum, which was established in Köln after the war and the loss of the Dresden museum.

In France, health education is one of the recognized functions of the official health agency. Yet, in practice, a large part of this work is carried on by private organizations. Recognition was given to health education on an official level with the formation of the *Office National d'Hygiène Sociale* in 1924 at the suggestion of the Health Commission of the Rockefeller Foundation as an agency to combat tuberculosis. Eventually, it became an agency that endeavored to coordinate the efforts of private health and welfare organizations. While the *Office* was dissolved in 1935, its work provided the basis for the creation of the *Centre National d'Education Sanitaire, Démographique et Sociale* in the Ministry of Health, which is concerned with broad national programs of health education and prepares and distributes materials (printed materials, leaflets, posters, exhibit materials, films, and film projectors). This center has under its jurisdiction 25 interdepartmental centers that endeavor to implement such programs. The Social Security Agency, through its *Action Sanitaire et Sociale,* expends funds on various preventive programs that include a considerable educational element. Alongside the official organization there is the *Comité National d'Education Sanitaire Populaire,* a voluntary organization that endeavors to coordinate and to further all health education efforts. Furthermore, it played a large part in the formation in 1951 of the International Union for Health Education of the Public. On the local level, the status of health education in France is varied, differing from one *département* to another. In some localities where the official agency is interested in health education, there may be an active program. In numerous instances, voluntary agencies carry on educational activities. Sometimes official and voluntary agencies create a joint program. While there is an awareness of the concept of a full-time trained health educator, there are extremely few health workers of this type. There is as yet no uniform course of training for anyone desiring to enter upon such a career.

Organized health education in England has grown up around the Central Council for Health Education. Founded in 1927 as a result of the activity of the Society of Medical Officers of Health, the Council has no statutory powers, but it is officially recognized by the Minister of Health and the local authorities as the "responsible body for assisting local authorities in England and Wales in health education work." It does this by providing consultation and guidance, training courses for health workers, teaching aids and health education literature, as well as a variety of liaison activities with voluntary and public agencies. It publishes *The Health Education Journal,* a very useful periodical.

The Soviet Union has developed what is probably the most completely integrated system of health education. This is based, of course, on the prevailing system of socialized medicine. Actually, health education had been started before the Revolution of 1917. The Pirogoff Commission for the diffusion of health knowledge was established in 1893 and did much to introduce health education into schools. At the Hygiene Exhibition in Dresden in 1911, Russia had an exhibit illustrating mass health education. However, it was not until the Revolution that these efforts were expanded on a broad basis. Under Semashko, Commissar for Health, an organized program of health education was developed and steps were taken to put it into practice. Health education houses were established and these have become the main centers for the promotion of this work. They exist all over the Soviet Union and are staffed by people who have had special training in health education. A major center is the Moscow Central Research Institute for Health Education. This institution has three departments concerned with health education in schools, medical and prophylactic facilities, and in industrial establishments. In addition it concerns itself with research and evaluation, media and techniques, including press, radio, and visual aids. The Institute also publishes materials and prepares exhibits, photographs, and transparencies. Specialists in health education are trained there; these students take a three year course at public expense. Other health workers also study at the Institute. An interesting indication of this is the fact that in 1950 and 1952 some 2000 physicians in different medical specialties studied health education there.

Health education today is one of the most important expressions of the modern theory of community health action. Its value will undoubtedly increase even further as more is learned about human nature and its modifiability. There would seem to be no doubt that the late C.-E. A. Winslow struck to the heart of the matter when he said that the development of health education as a factor in preventive medicine is as important for us today as the germ theory of disease was for public health workers 40 years ago.

THE RISE OF SCIENTIFIC NUTRITION. The growing realization of the vital importance of the educational approach to health promotion and disease prevention has also been intimately linked to the acquisition of new knowledge in certain fields that had already been cultivated in earlier periods. Of these an increased understanding of the physiology and pathology of nutrition has been one of the most significant. The scientific foundations of this subject were created by Lavoisier in the eighteenth century. The great German chemist Justus von Liebig (1803–1873) created a unified concept of metabolic activity and exerted a far-reaching influence on nutrition and nutritional chemistry. Based on the work of the French physiologist François Magendie (1783–1855), he classified the nourishment of animals and men into three fundamental categories: protein, carbohydrate, and fat. He showed how the former was used to build up or repair the organism while the last two were used for fuel. Liebig's work was carried further by the German investigators Carl Voit (1831–1908), Max von Pettenkofer (1818–1901), and Max Rubner (1854–1932), and by the Americans Graham Lusk (1866–1932) and Wilbur O. Atwater (1864–1907). Their studies made it possible to analyze metabolic activities more precisely and to apply the results to clinical and theoretical problems. It was Rubner who in 1888 to 1890 finally produced incontrovertible experimental proof that the principle of the conservation of energy held for living systems. This was confirmed for man by Atwater and Benedict in 1903, and in the same year by Armsby on cattle. The researches of Voit, Rubner, and many others laid a firm basis for the study of intermediary metabolism, a subject that is being vigorously pursued at present. Related to this is the investigation of growth and its basis in metabolism.

Up to 1900, the study of nutrition was concerned almost exclusively with the caloric value—the amount of energy supplied by food. Studies of this type were carried out in 1886 by Atwater in collaboration with Carroll D. Wright (1840–1909), chief of the Massachusetts Bureau of Labor. As a result, he set the American standard requirement at 3500 calories per man per day. This standard has been revised since that date. Atwater also analyzed foods used in the American diet and determined the protein, fat, carbohydrate, and fuel value per pound of various foodstuffs. This compilation, published in 1896, is still a useful reference source for such data. At the same time, Atwater recognized that nutrition involved sociological and psychological aspects as well as laboratory experiments, and in 1888, he called on social scientists to help explain why the poor considered foods with the most delicate appearance and the highest price as most desirable.

Atwater felt that the consumer should obtain his dietary needs in the most economical manner consistent with good health. His ideas and work were followed with considerable interest by Edward Atkinson, an industrialist, who had similar ideas on the "pecuniary economy of food." In 1893, Atkinson advocated the establishment of food laboratories to be set up as part of the Agricultural Experiment Stations created several years before. Congressional reaction to this proposal was favorable, and the agricultural appropriation bill for the fiscal year ending June 30, 1895, contained $10,000 to enable the Secretary of Agriculture "to investigate and report upon the nutritive value of the various articles and commodities used for human food, with special suggestion of full, wholesome and edible rations less wasteful and more economical than those in common use." This amount was increased to $15,000 the next year. Under Atwater's supervision, the Office of Experiment Stations investigated the nutritive value and digestibility of various foods and surveyed the diets of various groups in the population.

It is proverbial that a little knowledge can be a dangerous thing and nowhere perhaps is this truth better illustrated than in the field of nutrition. With attention concentrated on the fuel values of food, and lacking knowledge of vitamins or of the role of minerals in nutrition, early workers often condemned foods that are today considered highly important. Atwater and Woods in 1897 deprecated the use of green vegetables, such as soup greens and sweet corn, since they contained only small amounts of protein and provided little energy. Similarly, canned tomatoes were found too costly as sources of protein and energy. It was felt that vegetables were necessary only to supply bulk and mineral salts and to render the diet palatable. Charles Longworthy, writing in 1907, felt that poor families could omit oranges from their diet without any material change in its nutritive value. Oranges simply added to the attractiveness of the diet, and green vegetables made food more appetizing.

At this very time, however, evidence was being collected, observations made, and inferences drawn that seemed to undermine all the accepted theories regarding the essential principles of diet and disease causation. It was slowly realized that disease could be due to the want of an essential substance, and that not only exogenous agents produced pathological conditions. To appreciate what this meant, one must remember that around the turn of the century, the world of medicine and public health was still adjusting itself to the revolutionary discoveries of Pasteur, Koch, and other microbiologists. Overwhelmingly, disease came to be considered as having its pathogenesis through exogenous agents: germs and toxins. Medical scientists investigating problems of disease turned naturally to microbial hypotheses. During the last two decades of the nineteenth century, however, there were already a few straws in the scientific wind, which in another climate of opinion might have led somewhat sooner to the recognition of disease caused by deficiency of nutrition elements. While the role of fresh fruit and vegetables, in particular, the juice of citrus fruits, in preventing scurvy had been recognized by the end of the eighteenth century, there was little further progress in this direction. Similarly, the use of cod liver oil in the treatment of rickets by German, French, and British physicians, introduced during the nineteenth century, did not lead to any greater understanding. These were purely empirical procedures and lacked any precise scientific foundation. For this purpose, chemistry had to advance further, and a new concept of disease causation was required. (A similar pattern of development has already been described in the case of Jennerian vaccination and the development of immunology.) By the end of the nineteenth century, a rational basis in biochemistry was available, and a new line of investigation could be opened up.

As early as 1881, N. I. Lunin (b. 1854), an assistant in Bunge's laboratory at the University of Basel, found that when young mice were fed on highly purified diets they survived only a very short time. The results were not better when he supplied all the necessary minerals in the form of the mineral ash of milk. However, mice fed on milk itself flourished. As a result, Lunin asked, "does milk contain, in addition to protein, fat, carbohydrates, other organic substances, which are also indispensable to the maintenance of life?" Unfortunately, this work was not carried further. Meanwhile, evidence was accumulating that some qualitative deficiency in the diet could produce disease. A naval surgeon, T. K. Takaki (1858–1920) in 1887 practically eradicated beriberi, the ancient scourge of the Far East, from the Japanese navy by adding fish, meat, and vegetables to the basic diet of rice. This was followed in 1889 by Bland-Sutton's demonstration at the London zoo that faulty diet was most probably the cause of rickets in lion cubs, and that it could be cured by feeding them crushed bone, milk, and cod-liver oil.

The first fundamental contribution on an experimental basis came, however, from the other side of the world. Several years earlier, in 1886, the Dutch had sent to the East Indies a commission headed by C. A. Pekelharing and Winkler to investigate the nature and cause of beriberi, which was highly prevalent. They were assisted by Christian Eijkman (1858–1930), a young Army doctor. It was natural enough at that time, the golden age of bacteriology, to think in terms of germs and infectivity. This hypothesis was pursued for some two years, and then a chance observation gave him the clue. He observed that chickens fed on polished rice developed symptoms reminiscent of beriberi, and that the birds promptly recovered when the food was changed. Either unpolished rice or the rice husks achieved a prompt cure. In the experiments based on these observations, Eijkman was assisted by G. Grijns (1865–1944), a physiologist, who in 1901 prepared extracts from the material removed when rice is polished and showed that it had a striking curative effect. Eijkman's great contribution, in his work with Grijns, was to show that a disease similar to beri-beri, characterized by polyneuritis, could be produced in birds by restricting them to a diet of polished rice, and that the condition was promptly relieved when whole rice was substituted. These findings were published in 1901 and were attributed by Eijkman to a neurotoxin. Grijns argued that the neuropathy of beriberi was caused by the lack of some essential substance present in the rice husk. Then, in 1905, Pekelharing, stimulated by Eijkman's work, began a series of experiments like those carried out by Lunin two decades earlier. The results supported Eijkman's observations but Pekelharing went even further and postulated the existence of accessory nutritional elements, now called vitamins. Essentially, the same concept was presented independently, in 1906, by Frederick Gowland Hopkins (1861–1947), the British biochemist. As a result of his work on the pathogenesis of rickets and scurvy, he postulated the existence of "minimal qualitative factors" other than the known basic nutritional elements (protein, carbohydrates, fat, minerals). Later, he termed these elements, "accessory nutritional factors." Finally, in 1912, Hopkins demonstrated in a series of convincing experiments that an animal diet must contain minute amounts of certain essential substances other than the hitherto accepted basic nutriments if the organism was to remain in good health. Meanwhile, in December 1911, Casimir Funk (b. 1884), a Polish-Jewish chemist, announced the isolation of a definite chemical substance possessing the antineuritic property. Believing that it belonged to the class of chemical compounds called amines, he added to this term the Latin word for life, *vita,* and invented the name "vitamine." This proposal has been generally adopted, and the final "e" was dropped when it became obvious that by no means all these substances were amines.

With the year 1912, the first chapter in the evolution of the modern concept of deficiency disease came to a close. It had been demonstrated that diets restricted to protein, carbohydrates, fat, and inorganic salts were inadequate for the maintenance of health and life and that a deficiency disease could be produced experimentally and cured by dietary supplementation; and a theory of vitamins had been proposed. The next chapter, which began after 1912, has been concerned with the elaboration and confirmation of this concept, and the application of the knowledge that has been acquired as a result. This work has proceeded along several lines. A variety of accessory dietary factors, vitamins, have been isolated and associated with specific diseases. As vitamins became known, efforts were made to determine their chemical nature and metabolic functions. Methods were developed to determine the vitamin content of foods and norms for optimal nutrition. Finally administrative and educational tools were developed to utilize this knowledge to improve individual and community health.

The first proof that there was more than one vitamin was supplied independently in 1913 by E. V. McCollum and A. Davis, and by T. B. Osborne and L. B. Mendel. Then, in 1916, McCollum showed that at least two factors were required for the normal growth of rats: a fat-soluble A factor found in butter and other fats, and a water-soluble B factor found in nonfatty foods and materials like rice polishings. These studies also set the precedent for labeling vitamins by letters of the alphabet. Shortly thereafter (1918 to 1922), McCollum in America and E. Mellanby in England demonstrated that the A factor contained two elements, one heat-stable and effective in curing rickets, the other heat-labile and capable of healing xerophthalmia. The former was named vitamin D, the latter remained vitamin A.

It now became possible to solve the riddle of rickets. During the late nineteenth and the early twentieth centuries, the disease was widespread in urban communities, especially in slum districts. By 1870, for example, it was believed that as many as one third of the poor children in such cities as London and Manchester suffered from obvious rickets. A survey stimulated by the Medical Congress of 1884 and published five years later showed that the distribution of rickets in Great Britain coincided with the density of the industrial population. In the Clyde district, for instance, almost every child examined was found to be affected. As late as 1921, McCollum, writing in the *Annals of the American Academy*, claimed that probably one half of the children in the cities of the United States had or had had rickets. For the greater part of the nineteenth century, doctors had no clear ideas on the causation of the disease. It was attributed to a wide variety of causes, but slowly two of these, faulty diet and poor living conditions, began to attract most attention. William Huntly, a medical missionary in India, on the basis of his observations in that country, concluded that while diet might play some part in rickets, lack of exercise in the open air and sunshine seemed to be the main factors responsible for the disease. The publication of these observations in 1889 led T. A. Palm to make a geographical survey of the distribution of rickets, and he found it prevalent where sunshine was scarce, and rare where sunshine was abundant. At the same time, it was known that cod liver oil cured rickets. This had been discovered empirically early in the nineteenth century, and in 1849, Trousseau the famous French clinician had shown that cod-liver oil was many times more antirachitic than butter. Bland-Sutton used it in his famous experiment on the lion cubs in 1889. Nonetheless, it had its ups and downs in medical favor for the simple reason that no one could explain how it worked, or what the connection was between cod-liver oil and living conditions, especially the presence or absence of sunshine.

The discovery of vitamin D and its antirachitic properties provided the link that tied together in a logical pattern the varied observations and experimental evidence concerning rickets. It was found that cod-liver oil was effective because it contained vitamin D. Furthermore, in 1919 Kurt Huldschinsky in

Germany had shown that rickets could be cured by exposing children to artificial sunlight. In 1924, H. Steenbock showed the development of rickets in
rats could be prevented by irradiating a ricket-producing diet, and A. F. Hess
demonstrated that naturally inactive fats like cottonseed or linseed oils could
be made antirachitic by exposure to the mercury-vapor lamp. The last pieces of
the jigsaw puzzle now fell into place. Sunshine acted on fats in the body to produce vitamin D. Thus, it became possible to take proper preventive measures
with the result that rickets is no longer the common cause of crippling among
children that it was only 30 years ago. Nevertheless, the disease has not been
eradicated. In 1945, there were about 400,000 children and young people in the
United States more or less seriously handicapped by orthopedic impairment.
Of these 4.4 per cent were due to rickets. In 1952, in England and Wales deaths
from rickets were still 3 per 100,000 inhabitants. Clearly, while men know that
rickets can be prevented, the disease still persists. This is due to the fact that
diet is determined not so much by knowledge alone as by social custom and by
what is available in a given place for a given income. Furthermore, housing or
other factors can also influence nutritional status. M'Gonigle and Kirby (1936),
in a famous study of rehoused slum dwellers at Stockton-on-Tees, England,
showed that they could actually be worse off in new housing because more of
the inadequate family income had to be spent for rent and less was left over for
food. As a result, the rehoused population was dying in greater numbers than
a comparable group of slum dwellers who continued to live in the slum area.

The role of economic and social factors in the causation of a disease due to
dietary deficiency probably was studied most intensively and thoroughly by Joseph Goldberger (1874–1929) and his associates in their investigations of pellagra. Beginning around 1907, there was an increase in the actual incidence
as well as in the recognition of the disease in the United States, especially in
the South. By the end of 1909, it was reported from 26 states. In 1916, pellagra
ranked second among the causes of death in South Carolina. Serious investigation of the disease was undertaken in 1909 in Illinois by competent research-
ers who attributed it to microbial infection. Goldberger was assigned by the
U.S. Public Health Service in 1914 to study the problem, and by the following
year he had demonstrated that the disease was due to some inadequacy in the
diet of pellagra sufferers. When the diet was improved by the addition of milk
and fresh meat, the disease disappeared, breaking out again when the faulty
diet was restored. But what was the exact element in the diet whose absence
caused pellagra? In 1917, Chittenden and Underhill at Yale showed that "black
tongue," a disease in dogs, could be produced by feeding them a diet that would
cause pellagra in man. Goldberger and his associate Wheeler then proved that
the two conditions were identical, and by 1920, he suggested that a vitamin factor—PP (pellagra preventive)—might be involved. Subsequently, Goldberger

demonstrated that the anti-beriberi substance, the B factor, was also a specific for pellagra, and in 1926, he reported that the B factor consisted of two components, the one effective against beriberi, the other against pellagra.

How pellagra could be prevented or cured was thus known in the second decade of our century, and yet in 1934, the disease caused 3602 deaths in the United States, with about 20 reported cases for each death. The reason lay not only in a lack of knowledge, but even more in the economic factors that affected the dietary of the cotton-raising South. Goldberger was fully aware of this component of the problem, and together with Edgar Syden-stricker carried out a series of classic studies in the social epidemiology of pellagra. Some were carried out in cotton mill villages, others among tenant farmers. An unmistakable inverse correlation between family income and pellagra incidence was demonstrated. As income increased, the pellagra rate declined. However, income was not the only factor involved. Sources of food supply and dietary habits played important roles as well. When families in mill villages were restricted to the mill store or commissary during the late winter or spring because of the absence of other sources of supply and given the restricted food pattern of the poorer class in the South, pellagra was almost inevitable. Goldberger could recommend the keeping of cows and chickens, and the planting of gardens, but he could not change the economics of the situation. As he wrote in 1927, referring to the rural population, "It is necessary to keep in mind two considerations of essential importance. The first is that the economic status of this population is bound up in the tenant system, which, in turn, is involved in single-crop agricultural production and the speculative character of agricultural finance as it is practiced in this area, the seasonal fluctuation in income of the tenant . . . and other factors of an economic nature."

As the newer knowledge of nutrition began to spread beyond medical and scientific circles, it could not remain without impact on the community. The United States Bureau of Chemistry (later became the Food and Drug Administration) believed the value of vitamins A and B to have been so effectively demonstrated that in 1917 it announced their significance to the public. The necessity to safeguard health while conserving food during the First World War led to the production of increased supplies of protective foods and a growing recognition of their value. Emphasis on scientific nutrition was pushed in the name of patriotism and the public took readily to the idea. Improved methods of producing and distributing perishable foods made protective foods more easily available in urban communities. The growth of cafeterias and chain restaurants also facilitated the distribution of perishable foods to consumers. Furthermore, the development of more effective advertising and merchandising methods for fruits, vegetables, milk, and other products led to an increased use of the health motive. Thus, by the third decade of this century, scientific nutrition had become in the United States not only an important branch of preventive medicine, but an important component of industry and commerce as well as a major instrument of social policy.

It is certainly not simply a coincidence that nutritionists were first employed by American health departments in 1917. Massachusetts and New York were the first states to do so, and they have maintained this service ever since. Nutrition education was not new. Attempts to influence the worker's choice of diet had been made in the 1870s and 1880s. A Free Training School for Women was formed in New York City in the early 1870s where volunteers gave weekly lectures on cookery. A decade later, Ellen Richards, a home economist, and Mrs. Mary Hinman Abel set up the New England Kitchen in Boston to help solve "one of the greatest problems of the age—how the poor might be economically and well fed." In line with this objective, the teaching of cookery and home economics was introduced into the curriculum of Eastern public schools in the 1880s. As the science of nutrition developed, it became necessary to have a health worker, the nutritionist, who specialized in guidance. In 1918, nutrition was introduced into the public school curriculum as a separate subject. At first nutritionists were merely specialized educators working essentially with the schools. Gradually, their activities expanded to include staff education, community education, and work with special groups as in tuberculosis clinics. Interest in improving the nutrition of children and of the mother during the child bearing period was furthered by the Maternity and Infancy (Sheppard-Towner) Act. Connecticut, Illinois, Michigan, and Mississippi initiated nutrition services largely as a result of funds made available at this time by the Federal government. Owing to their purpose, these activities were placed in the maternal and child health units of the respective state health departments. The passage of the Social Security Act of 1935 carried this development further. By the end of 1937, 15 states were employing a total of 27 nutritionists. At the same time, Agricultural Extension Service and other governmental agencies were also conducting nutrition services. The Depression and the Second World War made everyone more conscious than ever before of nutrition and its problems. One consequence was that by 1948, 50 out of 53 state and territorial health departments had funds for the employment of 70 nutritionists. During the same period, city health departments began to employ nutritionists. One of the first was Detroit, which in 1930 assigned a person to teach nutrition in prenatal and child health clinics. By the end of 1937, five staff nutritionists were providing this service.

Government action in relation to nutrition also took other forms. Much of this was stimulated by the world economic crisis of 1929–1936, when widespread malnutrition followed on the heels of mass unemployment, as well as by the special needs of the Second World War with its attendant food shortages, rationing, and the necessity for protecting workers in industry, as well as women and children.

The provision of food for school lunches and other programs by the Federal Surplus Commodities Corporation has already been mentioned. In May, 1939, the Food-Stamp Plan was inaugurated to supply families on relief and those with low incomes with food at public expense through local outlets. In 1940 and 1941, a total of $235,000,000 was available for the removal of agricultural surpluses to be distributed through the stamp plan, for free school lunches, and for relief agencies. These activities undoubtedly had a beneficial effect on the nutritional status and the food habits of a large segment of the American population. In Great Britain, the maintenance of the nutrition of the people generally, and especially of mothers and children, was a major preoccupation of the government during the war. The general policy was to see that all essential nutrients should be equally available to everyone to an extent necessary to maintain health. Certain foods, such as margarine and flour, were fortified by the addition of vitamins (A & D) and minerals (calcium). Enrichment of foods was also undertaken in the United States when War Food Order No. 1 went into effect on January 18, 1943. It required that white bread be enriched by the addition of niacin, riboflavin, thiamine, and iron. While this policy remained in effect only until the end of the war, various states continued it. Some 26 states as well as the territories of Hawaii and Puerto Rico now have such legislation.

The effects of such measures have been quite impressive. In Great Britain where supplementary goods were given to mothers and children, the number of stillbirths as well as infant and maternal deaths declined to a considerable degree. While the implications of these facts as well as of others derived from controlled studies are quite clear, the effects of dietary deficiency continue to occur even in the most prosperous areas of the world, such as the United States. Food is not just a necessity for the maintenance of life; it is also a commodity and is therefore inextricably linked with forms of economic organization. As a result, low-income groups in the United States suffer from deficiency diseases, sometimes only marginal in character. This situation is considerably worse in the so-called underdeveloped areas of the world. As de Castro has pointed out for Latin America, the food shortage is due largely to a semi-feudal agricultural regime, the colonial status of many of the countries involved where the land is exploited for export, inadequate communication facilities, an impoverished and ignorant population, and poor food habits. Nutrition education and research remain as necessary as ever, perhaps even more so, but it is evident that improvement of nutrition fundamentally involves economic, social, and political problems. It is to the solution of these problems that those who are concerned with community health will have to turn in the future.

THE HEALTH AND WELFARE OF THE WORKER. Effective concern with occupational health is of relatively recent origin in the United States. Fifty years ago the field of industrial medicine was still *terra incognita* to the American medical profession. Indifference to and ignorance of workers diseases often went hand in hand with scorn of the few doctors who endeavored to protect the health of the worker. The situation is well characterized in her autobiography by Alice Hamilton (1868–1970), whose name looms large in the beginnings of this field. When she attended the Fourth International Congress on Occupational Accidents and Diseases at Brussels in 1910, she found that "for an American it was not an occasion for national pride." Dr. Gilbert of the Belgian Labor Department was able to dispose of American activity with the curt statement, "It is well known that there is no industrial hygiene in the United States, *Ça n'existe pas.*"

That was not long ago; in fact it was the year in which the writer of this book was born. But what changes have taken place since 1910. Health problems arising out of exposure to noxious substances and dangerous working conditions have been recognized in numerous instances, and measures have been taken to prevent or to ameliorate the effects resulting from such exposure. Reforms have been brought about by the joint effort of organized labor, community leaders, legislators, and physicians. Furthermore, it has become increasingly evident that the health of the worker is of concern not only within the place of employment. What happens to the worker outside the plant may have an important bearing on his status as a producer and a wage earner. On the other hand, in-plant conditions affecting the worker's health may throw a burden on the community as a whole. Because of the complexity and the many ramifications of the problem of occupational health, it will probably be of increasing importance in the future. It represents an important challenge to the community and to all the groups in it concerned with the worker's health as a community asset.

The decade 1910 to 1920 saw the establishment of occupational health as a significant field of public health action. Emerging events during this period, however, were the product of cumulative developments extending back over several decades and influenced in some degree by European experience. Both in labor legislation as well as in the study of occupational disease, the United States had lagged behind England and the more progressive continental countries, especially Germany.

All the labor laws issued in England up to the early 1860s had been enacted to protect workers in textile plants and to a lesser degree those in mines. Beginning with the Act of 1864, however, industries other than textiles were included. Among these were the manufacture of matches, earthenware, percussion caps, and cartridges. This tendency was carried further by the Factory Act of 1867 and the Workshop Act of the same year, which brought under control a large number of hitherto unregulated industries. For the first time, certain groups of workers, such as boys younger than 12 years of age and women, were excluded from particular processes. This legislation was stimulated in large measure by the third and fourth reports of the Medical Officer to the Privy Council, based largely on E. H. Green-how's studies of dust diseases of the lungs. Further Acts dealing with the prevention of lead poisoning (1883), ventilation, sanitation, and safety in factories, workmen's compensation (1897), as well as other matters were enacted during the last three decades of the nineteenth century. The post of medical inspector was created in 1898, and Thomas M. Legge (1863–1932) received the first appointment. Thus, by the end of the nineteenth century, there had been created a code of factory law, comprising numerous acts and regulations and intended to provide for the health and safety of industrial workers. Admittedly, certain groups, for instance, those in home industries, were inadequately protected, but a firm basis for further action was present. The important consolidating Factory and Workshop Act was passed in 1901, thus bringing together all previous factory legislation and simplifying the procedure for establishing regulations in dangerous industries.

Increasing protection of the industrial worker by legislative enactment was the result of interacting political and economic trends. The Second Reform Bill of 1867 more than doubled the electorate, and in urban districts gave the vote to every male householder. It was not yet universal manhood suffrage, but it enfranchised the workers and projected the question of the unions' status into the forefront of politics. A trade union congress met in Manchester in 1868. Around 1873, the unions were given legal protection, and trade unionism became an accepted factor in English political and industrial life. The workers through the ballot and their organizations endeavored to improve their working conditions. At the same time, the old faith in laissez-faire was giving place to the belief that progress could be legislated. This ideological trend is most strikingly exemplified by the London Fabian Society, founded in 1884 for the purpose of "reconstructing society in accordance with the highest moral possibilities." Among the members were Sidney and Beatrice Webb, George Bernard Shaw, Graham Wallas, and others who were to be prominent in social reform. The Fabian doctrine of "the inevitability of gradualness" made it possible for many middle-class people to accept social change in the interest of labor. To use a favorite Fabian verb, they "permeated" the thought of labor leaders as well as of Conservative and Liberal politicians. Their influence, especially that of the Webbs is to be found in many quarters during this period, and we shall have occasion to deal with it later. Furthermore, as industry changed in scope and technology, new conditions were created with which the older factory legislation was unable to cope without expansion and amendment. Spectacular advances in organic chemistry, the application of electrical power to industrial production, and the increased use of new metals all tended to create problems of industrial disease that had not existed previously.

Further legislation was enacted and regulations issued during the first four decades of the present century. Laundries were brought under control in 1907. The following year the use of yellow phosphorus for the manufacture of matches was prohibited, previous acts relating to the employment of children in agriculture were amalgamated, and an eight hour law for miners was enacted to take effect in 1909. A Mines Accident Act and a Coal Mines Act were passed in 1910 and 1911, respectively. The former required the supply and maintenance of equipment and the training of personnel for rescue work, while the latter regulated the employment of women and young persons, required the provision of certain hygiene facilities, and wet drilling to reduce dust. The Police, Factories (Miscellaneous Provisions) Act of 1916 authorized the Secretary of State to compel employers to provide for the health and hygiene of workers by providing protective clothing, first aid arrangements, washing and dressing facilities, as well as accommodations for preparing and eating meals. During the same period, an increasing number of occupational diseases and accidents was made reportable. For the most part, these were industrial poisonings due to such materials as lead, arsenic, mercury, and aniline, but infections, such as anthrax, were also included. All previous acts and regulations were consolidated in the Factories Act, 1937, which not only strengthened provisions for safety and health, but also required the reporting of all industrial diseases, not just those specified in earlier legislation.

Paralleling legislative and regulatory activity were two other developments of equal importance. Effective handling of occupational health problems required an efficient system of factory inspection, as well as scientific investigation of illhealth among workers. The Factory and Workshop Act of 1878 created a centralized system of factory inspection with a chief inspector in London. Alexander Redgrave was the first to hold this position. In 1883 and 1884, he had a staff of 5 superintending inspectors, 30 inspectors, and 10 juniors distributed throughout the country. The first woman inspector was appointed in 1893, followed five years later by the appointment of Legge as the first medical inspector. Arthur Whitelegge, the first medical man to occupy the post of chief inspector, had been appointed in 1896. An electrical inspector as well as an inspector for dangerous trades were brought into the system in 1902 and 1903, respectively. By 1910, the authorized factory inspectorate consisted of 200 persons, in 1939, of 320, and in 1944, of 440 persons.

Legislation and regulation must be based on knowledge, and important studies were carried on by government physicians, factory inspectors, and others concerned with occupational health. The reports of Greenhow and other phy-

TABLE 7
The Year of Appointment of the First Medical Inspectors

Country	Year	Appointee
Belgium	1895	D. Gilbert
England	1898	T. M. Legge
Netherlands	1903	E. Wintgens, W. E. R. Kranenborg
Baden	1906	F. Holtzmann
Bavaria	1909	F. Koelsch
Italy	1912	G. Loriga
Austria	1919	Jenny Adler-Herzmark
Prussia	1921	L. Teleky, H. Gerbis
Saxony	1921	A. Thiele
France	1942	H. Desville

sicians in the 1860s were followed by many other governmental investigations. Among the noteworthy British publications from 1890 on are the classic *Hygiene, Diseases and Mortality of Occupations* (1892) by J. T. Arlidge, the monumental collaborative work, *Dangerous Trades* (1902), edited by Thomas Oliver, which is still useful today, the important study on *Lead Poisoning and Lead Absorption* by Legge and K. W. Goadby in 1912, and the splendid book on *The Health of the Industrial Worker* (1921) by E. L. Collis and M. Greenwood.

Throughout this period, other countries proceeded in the same direction as Great Britain in dealing with the health and welfare of the worker. Sometimes this was done in the same way as in Britain, sometimes in other ways, depending on the state of industrial development as well as on the political and social organization of the country. For example, physicians were appointed as factory inspectors with specifically medical duties at the end of the nineteenth century in some countries, but not until well into the present century in others. Table 7 shows the first medical inspectors in a number of European countries with the year of appointment.

Action in the German Empire was based upon the Industrial Code (*Gewerbeordnung*) of the North German Confederation (1869), which was extended to the entire Reich in 1873. Part VII of the Code, which dealt with workers, was amended in 1878, and particularly in 1891 by a law for the protection of workers (*Arbeiterschutzgesetz*). Further changes were made in 1897, 1900, 1908, 1918, and 1920. In 1914, a law was passed dealing with the special problem of home workers. The right to issue protective regulations for individual trades was vested in the Federal Council (*Bundesrat*) under the Empire, and after 1918 in the National Minister of Labor (*Reichsarbeits-minister*). The first of these regulations issued in 1893 dealt with the manufacture of lead paint, mirrors, and cigars. In 1903 a law was enacted to govern the dangerous manufacture of phosphorus matches. Later regulations were issued to cover lead and zinc smelters, quarries, and various chemicals. At the beginning of the Second World War, there were 33 such regulations in force. Where the national authority did not issue regulations, governments of individual states or localities had the right to do so.

When factory inspection was extended throughout the whole of Germany in 1878, inspectors were given the rights of local police. Until 1937, however, they did not have the power to inflict penalties under the national law. Some states did grant factory inspectors the right to issue police orders (Hamburg, 1898; Prussia, 1909). Factory inspectors were required to submit annual reports to the Federal Council and the *Reichstag*, which were published. In 1909, Prussia had 285 inspectors; by 1912 the number increased to 328. In 1940, Prussia had 449 inspectors, as well as eight medical inspectors. Developments in other German states were similar to those in Prussia.

Beginning in the 1880s, the Imperial Health Office (*Kaiserliche Gesundheit-samt, after 1918 Reichsgesund-heitsamt*) undertook to carry out studies in the field of industrial health when requested to do so by governmental authorities. This continued to be the practice up to World War II. Between 1889 and 1938, among several hundred public health investigations, there were 46 on industrial health. They dealt with lead and mercury poisoning, anthrax, ankylostomiasis, and the inhalation of Thomas slag. Numerous important contributions were also made by clinicians and research workers in the universities.

Throughout western Europe, occupational health and welfare have been the concern of Ministries of Labor. This has been true of Germany, the Scandinavian countries (Norway, Sweden, Denmark, Finland), France, and Belgium. On the other hand, following the November Revolution in 1917, the Soviet Union made industrial health one of the responsibilities of the Commissariat of Health. Other patterns have been developing in Latin America, Asia, and Africa, as countries there become industrialized. Generally, there tends to be a sharing of administrative responsibility, with the Ministry of Labor maintaining a system of factory inspection, and the Health Ministry carrying out the health and sanitary supervision of working places.

The process of evolution in the United States has differed from these patterns owing to the division of political and administrative responsibilities between the Federal government and the states. Concern for the health of the worker in the United States came later than in Great Britain and the more industrialized European nations. However, a number of events, all occurring in 1910, gave evidence that interest in this area was growing in America as well. In that eventful year, the first National Conference on Industrial Diseases was held in Chicago; the United States Bureau of Mines was created; the first clinic for occupational diseases was established by W. Gilman Thompson at Cornell University Medical College in New York; Alice Hamilton began her pioneering work with the publication of a report on lead poisoning; John B. Andrews published his studies on phosphorus poisoning in the American match industry; and the United States Bureau of Labor issued a list of industrial poisons. These events, however, were all part of a movement whose roots lay in the latter decades of the nineteenth century and were nourished in a broad sense by the quest for social justice that characterized the first decades of the present century. One of these roots was the governmental machinery that had been created, first by the states and then by the Federal government, to deal with the interests of labor. Following the Civil War, labor unions and their leaders demanded government units devoted to the problems of the wage earner. The first agency of this kind was the Massachusetts Bureau of the Statistics of Labor, formed in 1869, the year in which the State Health Department was constituted. Fourteen states created similar bureaus before the Federal government in 1885 set up a Bureau of Labor in the Department of the Interior. Soon thereafter, the Knights of Labor, the leading labor union of the period, demanded a department of labor. This was created in 1888, but in 1903 it was merged with the Department of Commerce to become the Department of Commerce and Labor. The present U.S. Department of Labor was established in 1913 to "foster, promote and develop the welfare of the wage-earners, to improve their working conditions and to advance their opportunities for profitable employment." The early American state labor bureaus were agencies for investigating labor conditions and making recommendations to the legislatures. The worker's health was one of the problems that early attracted the attention of these bureaus. Between 1889 and 1895, for example, New Jersey published a series of reports on the effects of occupation upon longevity. The subject of the effect of occupation upon health was touched on in studies published by New Jersey (1883), Wisconsin (1887 and 1888), and Montana (1893).

At the same time, such agencies provided a useful basis for an attack on the conditions under which women and children were employed. Long hours and appalling sanitary conditions in factories characterized the employment of women and children. From 1870 to 1900, increasing numbers of children were caught in the tentacles of the spreading factory system. Some measure of social legislation for children and women had been secured in the older industrial states during the nineteenth century, but by 1890 these laws were largely ignored. By 1900, the number of children younger than 16 years of age engaged in gainful occupation was at least 1,700,000, and some students of the problem felt the figure was even greater. The worst conditions prevailed in manufacturing and especially in sweated industries. The spectacle of thousands of children caught in a ruthless economic system, which blasted their physical and mental energies before they had barely emerged from infancy, roused a number of socially minded citizens and government officials to determined action. The situation in Illinois is illustrative. Carroll D. Wright, chief of the Massachusetts labor bureau from 1873 to 1885, had been appointed head of the Federal bureau when it was created. Several years later he initiated an inquiry into the slums of great cities, and, in 1892, appointed Florence Kelly to cover the Chicago area. The outstanding fact that emerged was the ubiquity of tenement sweatshops, employing men, women, and children, the latter down to 3 years of age. To make these facts known to the general public, Mrs. Kelly proposed that the Illinois Bureau of Labor look into the matter, and eventually a legislative committee, set up to consider remedial legislation, recommended the first factory law in Illinois. For the first time in the United States, a proposal was made to limit the employment of women in factories to an eight hour day. The employment of children younger than 14 years in factories was prohibited; steps were proposed to control tenement sweatshops; and a Factory Inspection Department was created. Mrs. Kelly became the first Chief Inspector of Factories for Illinois in July 1893. With a staff of 12 and an appropriation of $14,000, she proceeded vigorously and tenaciously to enforce the new law and to eliminate child labor, sweatshops, and the other abuses of industrial life. In 1895, the state supreme court declared unconstitutional the eight-hour day for women, and in 1897 under a new governor Mrs. Kelly was removed from office. Transferring her activities to the national level, she became the head of the National Consumer's League, which was to become a most potent influence in protecting employed women and children. Working through labor unions, women's clubs, and other organizations, the movement for child labor legislation grew and gathered momentum. An important step was taken in 1904 with the formation of the National Child Labor Committee. Between 1905 and 1907, some of the first results of these efforts began to appear, when about two thirds of the states either initiated protective legislation or strengthened existing laws. Then, in 1907, Congress appropriated $150,000 for a study of the conditions of women and children engaged in industry, which resulted in an exhaustive report published in 19 volumes and which aroused public horror at its findings. The Pittsburgh Survey, also initiated in 1907 and financed by the Russell Sage Foundation, brought similarly shocking revelations to the attention of the public. It was these activities, as well as those previously described, that led to the creation in 1912 of the Children's Bureau. State laws relating to child labor adopted during this period generally prohibited certain employments as dangerous to health and morals, fixed a minimum age limit, limited the number of hours, and in some cases set up an educational requirement. An important judicial event was the act of the United States Supreme Court in 1908 in upholding the Oregon law of 1903 prohibiting the hiring of women in industry for more than 10 hours a day. Employing the novel method of "sociological" jurisprudence, Louis D. Brandeis convinced the Court that excessive hours had a direct bearing on the health of women and the stability of the family. Consequently, the state had a right to protect the health, safety, morals, and well-being of its citizens.

It was obvious to a small number of socially conscious physicians that there were problems of occupational disease that were not receiving adequate attention, and throughout the first decade of the present century, with slowly growing momentum, attention began to turn to this subject. There is no doubt that Americans were influenced by contemporary developments in England and on the Continent. In 1896, a striking editorial on industrial hygiene appeared in the *Transactions* of the American Public Health Association. The editorial discussed the report of a parliamentary committee in Great Britain which dealt with 134 factories involving such procedures or products as bronzing, use of inflammable paint, dry cleaning, India rubber, aerated waters, and steam locomotives. In 1902, George M. Kober (1850–1931), professor of state medicine at Georgetown Medical College, upon request of Commissioner of Labor Wright, recommended his former student C. F. W. Doehring to investigate the manufacture of white lead, paint, linseed oil, varnishes, tallow fertilizers, and a number of other products. The results of this study, the first of its kind in the United States, were published in January 1903. The first state to recognize that occupational health was a responsibility of the health department was Massachusetts. In 1905, the State Board of Health submitted a brief report on the conditions affecting the health and safety of employees in factories and other establishments. Health inspectors were appointed, and they checked factories, workshops, tenements, and similar structures. Their reports, like those of the New York inspectors appointed in 1907, emphasized the importance of public control over shop hygiene. (It must be noted, however, that the New York inspectors were employed by the State Labor Department.) W. L. Hanson, a physician, was in charge of industrial hygiene and in 1907 issued a more exhaustive report with particular emphasis on the health hazards of the dusty trades. This was also the era of the "muckrake," and by 1907 the popular magazines were beginning to devote space to the industrial health movement. That year *Munsey's Magazine* published an article by William Hard entitled "Where Poison Haunts Man's Daily Work."

By the end of the decade, the movement to improve health conditions in industry was in full swing. In 1908, Kober, who had been appointed to President Roosevelt's Homes Commission, made a comprehensive report on health hazards in a number of industries, with suggestions for legal and other measures to cope with the situation. The same year and the following year, the Bureau of Labor published Frederick L. Hoffman's study of *Mortality from Consumption in Dusty Trades,* which was to have an important impact on American labor legislation as well as on the campaign to control tuberculosis. Within the next few years, laws requiring the removal of dust by exhaust fans or other methods became one of the common provisions of factory codes. The year 1908 also saw the publication of *Diseases of Occupation* by Thomas Oliver (1853–1942), an English pioneer of industrial hygiene. This volume was widely read in the United States, by members of labor and health departments as well as by interested physicians. Another significant event in 1908 was the appointment by Illinois of the first state Commission on Occupational Diseases, although it did not begin its activities until 1910. Meanwhile, nationwide discussion of health problems was aroused by the publication in 1909 of the *Report on National Vitality, Its Wastes and Conservation* by Irving Fisher, the Yale economist. He urged the Federal and state governments as well as the municipalities to undertake vigorous action so as to protect the people from disease, and thus conserve a basic national resource.

Leadership in the campaign against occupational disease was assumed in 1910 by the American Association for Labor Legislation when it organized the First National Conference on Industrial Diseases. Two years later, a second conference was held in Atlantic City under the joint sponsorship of the Association and the American Medical Association. Representatives of a wide variety of professional and economic groups interested in occupational disease were present, and the conference proceedings indicate clearly that a firm foundation had been created for a vigorous advance over the next decades.

Between these two conferences, a number of notable advances were made. The memorable study by John B. Andrews of phosphorus poisoning in the match industry—"phossy jaw"—was published in 1910 and led to the enactment of the Esch law in 1912. This law imposed such a high tax on white phosphorus matches that it became unprofitable to manufacture them. (Andrews had founded the American Association for Labor Legislation in 1906 and served as its secretary with zeal and devotion. It passed out of existence in 1942.) In 1910, the Illinois Commission on Occupational Diseases began its labors and by 1911 made a final report that is a valuable pioneer work in this field. The most elaborate study in it is that by Alice Hamilton on industrial lead poisoning. Her interest in industrial diseases had been aroused after she became a resident in 1897 of Hull House, the pioneer settlement house founded in 1889 by Jane Addams. Here she learned to know at first hand the pressing social problems of our society and also that something could be done about them. Dr. Hamilton's work with the Illinois Commission led to her pioneering studies of lead poisoning among pottery workers and painters (1912 and 1913). For the next 30 odd years her energies were devoted to the discovery and prevention of occupational disease, particularly industrial poisoning.

Concurrently attention was directed to other kinds of health hazards. In 1909, a Senate *Report on Condition of Woman and Child Wage Earners in the*

United States emphasized the conditions in the glass, textile, clothing, and other industries which produced illnesses among women and children. In these instances, morbidity was due not to poisons but to speed, noise, excessively long hours, poor ventilation, and similar conditions. The following year, in September, the Joint Board of Sanitary Control of the Cloak, Suit and Skirt Industry of Greater New York began the study and control of health conditions in clothing factories and shops. This was the first instance in American industrial history in which an employer's association and a union undertook to establish and enforce healthful working conditions. The situation in the needle trades was brought dramatically to public attention in New York by the disastrous Triangle Waist Factory fire in 1911, which caused the death of 145 workers, mostly young women. Public opinion was aroused and a Factory Investigating Commission was appointed to study safety and health conditions. The Commission was led by Alfred E. Smith, later Governor of New York, and Robert F. Wagner, who became U.S. Senator; both men later became outstanding advocates of social legislation. Between 1912 and 1915, the commission succeeded in remaking the labor laws of New York. It may be noted also that studies in 1914 among garment workers in New York City by J. W. Schereschewsky, a Public Health Service physician, brought to light an excessive prevalence of tuberculosis, and this led in part to the establishment of the Union Health Center of the International Ladies Garment Workers Union, a pioneer facility that has continued to serve union members uninterruptedly up to the present.

Simultaneously, the movement to protect and conserve the worker's health was taking organizational form in a number of different places. The National Safety Council was organized in 1911 and later created a Section on Health Service. As early as 1910, the U.S. Public Health Service had begun to take cognizance of dangers to health in the working environment, and in 1914 a Division of Industrial Hygiene and Sanitation, headed by J. W. Schereschewsky, was set up. The same year a Section on Industrial Hygiene was organized by the American Public Health Association.

Serious attention to the health of employees is of considerable benefit to industry and was recognized early by a few far-sighted employers. By the second decade of the twentieth century, there were several hundred physicians throughout the country who had contractual arrangements with industrial concerns to provide care for employees accidentally injured in the course of their work. Some also gave medical examinations to employees. For example, in 1909, the physician H. E. Mock introduced the practice of medical examinations for employees in the Sears, Roebuck Company of Chicago. On April 14, 1914, a group of physicians, who were directors of industrial medical departments, formed the Conference Board of Physicians in Industry. This organization became the adviser on medical problems in industry to the National

Industrial Conference Board. Then, in 1916, the American Association of Industrial Physicians and Surgeons was organized.

Organized health service in industry developed chiefly after 1910 as a consequence of the workmen's compensation movement. Interest in workmen's compensation in this country may be dated from the publication in 1893 of John Graham Brook's report on Compulsory Insurance in Germany. The Federal government was the first to compensate its employees for accidents (1908), but the law was notoriously inadequate. Montana followed in 1909 with compensation for accidents to miners. What may be called the first modern American compensation law was enacted in 1910 by New York. While the law was promptly declared invalid by the state supreme court, it stimulated the spread of compensation legislation. In 1911, 10 states enacted such laws, and 11 more did so in 1912 and 1913. Then, in 1917, the United States Supreme Court upheld the constitutionality of such laws, so that legislation enacted after this date tended to be compulsory. By the end of 1932, only four states were left without compensation laws covering accidents. At first, these laws covered only industrial accidents and not occupational diseases. In 1911, six states (California, Connecticut, Illinois, Michigan, New York, and Wisconsin) had enacted legislation requiring the reporting of occupational diseases to the state health department. However, it was not until after 1917 that the courts began to interpret compensation laws to cover occupational diseases. By 1948, compensation for occupational diseases existed in 33 states, the District of Columbia, and four territories. At the present time, occupational disease is not covered in seven states. Workmen's compensation laws exerted a beneficial influence on the occupational health situation in the United States by throwing a large portion of the financial costs of injury and disease upon employers. Since employers must carry insurance to cover such costs, and the premiums are determined by the experience of the plant and the quality of its safety and health facilities, insurance companies have contributed to improvements in accident prevention and the control of industrial disease. At the same time, one cannot overlook the limitations of workmen's compensation and the lack of uniformity in the laws, as well as the limits of establishing specified categories of disease.

While the Massachusetts state health department had begun to concern itself with occupational health as early as 1905, official health agencies in other states followed this lead very slowly. As in so many other health areas, the passage of the Social Security Act in 1935 and the needs created by the Second World War stimulated interest and activity in this field. Through grants-in-aid to the states, industrial hygiene units have been created in state health departments. In 1940, more than a fourth of the state health agencies did not carry on any occupational health activities. By 1950, 51 state and territorial health departments were participating in some way in activities concerned with occupational health. Furthermore, in 1953, nine cities and counties were reported as having programs in this area.

Progress in dealing with problems of occupational health has been due in part as well to professional and educational advances. The *Journal of Industrial Hygiene* was established in May 1919, and for many years remained the only American periodical in the field. Not until 1930 did the second journal devoted to occupational health, *Industrial Medicine,* begin to appear. Several professional organizations have had a significant part in advancing the occupational health program. In 1926, the American College of Surgeons organized its Committee on Industrial Medicine and Traumatic Surgery, which has done excellent work in setting minimum standards for medical services in industry, in surveying the medical departments of industrial plants, and accrediting those that measure up to specified standards. Just 10 years later, in 1937, the American Medical Association formed its Council on Industrial Health to coordinate efforts in this field and to carry on educational work. The first courses on the subject were presented by Kober in 1890 at Georgetown University and C.-E. A. Winslow at the Massachusetts Institute of Technology in 1905. Since then, the subject has been taught in medical schools and schools of public health.

The growth of interest and facilities in relation to occupational health has also led to the appearance of another specialist, the industrial nurse. Actually, industrial nursing is a branch of public health nursing. In England, the first nurse was employed in a factory in 1878. In the United States, this service had its beginnings in the 1890s. As the area of occupational health has expanded, the number of nurses has slowly increased. A count made by the United States Public Health Service in 1940 listed a total of 3271 industrial nurses. The National Organization for Public Health Nursing recognized the importance of this development by forming a section on industrial nursing in 1930 and by adding an industrial nurse consultant in April 1941. A similar consultant was added to its staff of nurses by the U.S Public Health Service in the same year. The American Association of Industrial Nurses was organized a year later in 1942. For many years, the Metropolitan Life Insurance Company of New York maintained a nursing service for its industrial policy holders. This service began in 1909 and was discontinued in 1950. Beginning in 1928, Employers Mutual of Wisconsin, a compensation insurance company, developed a nursing service for the purpose of visiting industry. In 1943, this service comprised a staff of 16 nurses.

It is obvious that the field of occupational health is large and complex and is likely to become even more so as industry changes and develops in the wake of scientific and technological advance. It is equally obvious, also, that important advances have been made over the past 40 years and that a firm foundation now exists on which to build further. While an immense amount of research has been done much knowledge still remains unapplied. Furthermore, we can now see that the health of the worker in the plant cannot be compartmentalized. Conditions of life in the home as well as conditions of work in the factory have important effects on the worker's health, and we cannot effectively prevent ill health unless this is fully recognized. It is being increasingly recognized that industrial medical care must be coordinated with the general medical care received by workers and their families. This is one of the major health problems that we face in the United States as more and more people are employed in commerce and industry. The ultimate solution will no doubt be shaped by the way in which the organization of medical care will develop, particularly under the influence of prepayment.

BETTER MEDICAL CARE FOR THE PEOPLE. Twenty-five years ago, prepaid medical care hardly existed in the United States; in fact, the principle of health insurance was still being hotly debated. In 1932, the Committee on the Costs of Medical Care published its *Final Report,* thus providing the point of departure for the emergence of present developments in health insurance in this country. While the problem of the organization and distribution of medical services has appeared in an acute form only recently on the American scene, the need for adequate methods of providing medical care appeared in England and on the Continent as early as the seventeenth and eighteenth centuries.

The problem of the laboring poor, concretely symbolized in the figure of the pauper, occupied a strategic position in the social logic of the eighteenth century. It was in relation to the question of poverty that several social pioneers began to explore the problem of provision against the needs of sickness, inclusive of medical care. For the most part, medical care for the sick poor was provided by local, often parochial, authorities. In England, the Elizabethan Poor Law had laid upon the parish authorities the responsibility for providing assistance to the poor, and in time, this came to include medical care. The parish officers, however, had neither training nor desire to deal with such problems. This gave rise to the common practice of contracting with private persons to perform public tasks. Following this general pattern, parish officers often contracted with a local practitioner for medical treatment of their poor. These contracts varied from parish to parish. Sometimes, the medical practitioner agreed to attend all the poor who were living in the parish, or only those for whom the parish was legally responsible, and to supply medicine as well. Occasionally, a separate agreement was made with an apothecary. Other contracts exempted such items as smallpox inoculation or epidemic diseases. Some parishes paid per head, others on a fee for service basis. This practice was popular because it was regarded as offering an opportunity for reducing taxes. A system of this kind was bound to lead to abuses. Nevertheless, one must recognize that medical care of a sort was provided and that the pattern of administration developed for this purpose had an influence in shaping later schemes for the provision of medical care.

At the same time, a few far-sighted individuals concerned with the laboring poor suggested ways and means whereby the poor might be enabled to pay for their own care and to receive it in an effective manner. One of these was Daniel Defoe, hack journalist and novelist. In 1697, there appeared his *Essay Upon Projects,* in which he pours out suggestion after suggestion for the common good. Among these is "The Proposal for a Pension Office," which Defoe offers "as an attempt for the relief of the poor." With strong faith in business methods, he proposed the application to the poor of the insurance principle. As part of this scheme, Defoe included the provision of medical care. More imaginative, unmeasurably broader in scope, and based on considerably greater insight into the socioeconomic aspects of health was the plan proposed in 1714 by John Bellers, a Quaker cloth merchant of London. In his *Essay Towards the Improvement of Physick,* he set forth a plan for a national health service. Neither problems nor plans, however, were an English monopoly, for in 1754, Claude Humbert Piarron de Chamousset, a wealthy Parisian philanthropist, published his *Plan d'une maison d'association,* outlining a scheme for medical care and hospitalization insurance. Specifically, he proposed an organization that in return for a monthly payment would, in case of illness, provide its members with medical care at home or in a hospital. Chamousset envisaged group enrollment at reduced rates and suggested that apprentices, workmen, or servants might collectively be enrolled by their employers. Such groups would be represented on the board of administration. As a measure of prudence, Chamousset suggested certain limitations on admission of members and provision of service to them. For pregnant women, the only qualification would be membership for at least nine months. Persons with venereal diseases or incurable conditions would be excluded. Physicians and surgeons would be selected with all possible care and appointed on a salaried basis. Patients who preferred a medical attendant not associated with the organization could have his services but would have to pay the fee themselves. A well-managed, well-stocked pharmacy would provide the necessary medicaments. Careful records would be kept on all patients, and the doctors would prescribe diets and drugs in writing.

The projects of Defoe, Bellers, and Chamousset never materialized, but several plans for the relief of the unemployed, which also provided medical care, did come into operation at Bristol, Hamburg, and Munich. At Hamburg, the program was financed by taxation and by voluntary contributions. Physicians, surgeons, and midwives provided care on a district basis upon request by the overseer of the poor. In 1790, a similar system was started in Munich by Benjamin Thompson, Count Rumford. Equally significant at this time are the efforts made by employed laborers and artisans to protect themselves against the exigencies of illness. The most characteristic expression of this endeavor was the urban trade club, or Friendly Society. Medieval guilds had their schemes for mutual help, and on the Continent they continued to fill this function until the nineteenth century, especially in Germany. In England, and also in France, the societies of which we speak did not come into existence until the end of the seventeenth century. Friendly societies, for example, were founded in 1687, 1703, and 1708 by Huguenot workmen in Spitalfields. Throughout the eighteenth century, there was a steady growth of friendly societies of many types in England. Their basic purpose was to provide help in case of sickness, unemployment, death, or other misfortune.

Defoe in his project had proposed that compulsion be employed for certain population groups that neglected or refused to join a scheme such as he suggested. It is also worth noting that compulsory schemes to provide for disabled seamen were actually set up by Colbert in France in 1693, and by the English government in 1696 at the Greenwich Hospital. (Noteworthy too is the circumstance that a century later, in 1798, the United States also set up a scheme of compulsory insurance for sick and disabled seamen, out of which the Public Health Service eventually developed.) Of interest in this connection is an act passed by the Parliament in 1757 "for the relief of coal-heavers working upon the river Thames." To create a fund out of which benefits were to be paid in case of sickness, disability, old age, and death, employers were required to withhold from the wages paid to their employees an amount equivalent to 2 shillings in the pound. However, the scheme was abused by the employers and in 1770 was abolished by an act of Parliament.

About this time, voluntary insurance schemes began to make their appearance in increasing numbers. For example, at Gnosall, Staffordshire, the parish records included the minutes of a friendly society, formed at least as early as 1766. Regarded as tending to decrease parish taxes for the poor, this society enjoyed the blessing of the parish authorities, so that occasionally the overseers of the poor even paid the subscriptions of members who were in difficulties. A similar society is recorded at Wimbledon, Surrey, from 1776 to 1787. Various mutual aid organizations providing medical care for their members also developed in France. In the French glass industry, benefits to the workers in some cases included medical attention, monetary assistance during sickness, and old age pensions. The gravediggers guild of Paris provided hospitalization for its sick members. An association of domestic workers organized at Paris provided medical attention for its members when sick.

Proposals to further the development and extension of such organizations were put forth in increasing number during the late eighteenth century. These proposals reflect both the growth of the friendly societies as well as the development of insurance on sounder actuarial lines. Bills embodying plans for enabling the laboring poor to provide for themselves in sickness and old age were approved by the Commons in 1773 and 1789 but were rejected by the House of Lords. The first Act of Parliament relating to friendly societies was not passed until 1793. This act, sponsored by George Rose, a friend and colleague of William Pitt, was intended to facilitate the establishment of friendly societies among wage earners. It permitted individuals to combine and to raise funds for mutual assistance, provided the rules of the organization created for this purpose were approved by a justice of the peace. Rose's Act stimulated the growth of friendly societies, and by 1801, their number was estimated at more than 7000 in England and Wales, with a membership between 600,000 and 700,000. Their growth continued slowly during the nineteenth century, and by 1872, there were almost 2,000,000 members in Great Britain. Over the next two years, however, there was an astonishingly rapid increase, membership in England and Wales alone amounting to 4,000,000 people. When wives, children, and other dependents are considered, about 8,000,000 persons received some protection. There were about 32,000 societies with assets of about £11,000,000. Between 1793 and the major consolidating Act of 1875, 19 Acts relating to friendly societies were passed by Parliament. The Act of 1875 consolidated the existing position of the societies and put them under government supervision with regard to their financial soundness.

While the friendly societies served a considerable segment of the working class, there were many workers who for one reason or another could not belong to them. This was particularly the case with those who came under the jurisdiction of the Poor Law. Beginning with the Poor Law Amendment Act of 1834, the medical relief of the sick poor was taken over by the Poor Law authorities. After a few ineffectual attempts to reduce the provision of medical relief, steps were taken to provide medical care through Poor Law doctors who received fixed salaries plus an additional payment per case. Care was also given through Poor Law infirmaries and dispensaries. Critics of the system insisted, however, that the provision of medical care should be separated from poor relief. It was pointed out that medical care was beyond the means of half the English population. Realization of this situation led to the proposal of various solutions. One was to have "a set of public officers distributed through the country having no private practice, but attending entirely to the sick poor and matters of public health." This awareness of the importance of the people's health was not primarily a humanitarian viewpoint, but one that was based on very practical considerations. It was recognized to an increasing degree that a sick labor force was a health menace. Thus, while economic liberalism was still the dominant social philosophy, the establishment of a system of free medical advice to all wage earners in England and Wales was seriously considered by the Poor Law Board in 1870. At the same time, there persisted right into the twentieth century the belief that giving medical care to the poor led inevitably to pauperism and that it should be provided only under the stringent deterrent conditions of the Poor Law. Nevertheless, changing economic conditions during the last quarter of the nineteenth century imposed the necessity of reconsidering the whole problem of medical care for the poor.

Two highly significant attempts to solve the problem of providing medical care for a large population were made in Europe during the second half of the nineteenth century. These endeavors were to change the pattern of medical care over a large part of the world in the present century. One was the path taken by Russia. This was a solution suitable to an agricultural country where the overwhelming majority of the indigent sick were peasants. As part of the program of reform, following the liberation of the serfs in 1861, Russia in 1864 established a system of public medical service in the rural districts. This was the so-called *Zemstvo* system. The administration of welfare and health was placed in the hands of the local government of the district or provincial *Zemstvo* or council. These authorities appointed physicians, whose salaries were paid out of tax funds; they built hospitals and endeavored to provide auxiliary medical personnel (the *feldsher*) when physicians could not be obtained. These developments coincided with certain political and economic trends. During this period, the Industrial Revolution slowly began to affect Russia, and the liberated serfs began to move into the factories. Simultaneously, political liberals began to urge constitutional and social changes and to look to the people for support. The first attempts were made at this time to alleviate the condition of factory workers. For example, a law of 1866 required factory owners to provide a bed for every hundred workers. This was the system that existed, alongside the private practice of medicine, at the time of the 1917 Revolution, and it provided the basis for the present Soviet medical organization. This is a complete system of medical and public health services supported through taxation and available to all the people. With modifications, this method of providing medical care has been adopted by a number of European and Asian countries.

The other path toward the provision of medical care for low-income groups was taken by Germany when Otto von Bismarck inaugurated a system of social insurance (1883 to 1889). This system was comprehensive, including insurance against industrial accidents, sickness, invalidity, and old age, and it had its roots in German experience. Following the Napoleonic wars in 1818, the Duchy of Nassau had developed a complete system of public medical services in which physicians were civil servants. The system operated until 1861 when the duchy became a part of Prussia. Then some of the guild funds continued to operate. Among the oldest of these funds were those of the miners (*Knappschaftskassen*), which remained in existence until the latter part of the nineteenth century. When Bismarck introduced social insurance legislation in 1883, it was based in part upon the existing miners' benefit funds. Finally, as in England and other European countries, wage earners were organized in mutual benefit societies that provided sickness benefits, including medical care. From 1869 on, communities in Bavaria, Baden, and Württemberg were authorized to establish public sickness insurance funds, membership in which could be made compulsory for all unmarried wage earners not living with their parents. In short, the idea of prepaid medical care, partly on a voluntary and partly on a compulsory basis, was accepted in Germany long before Bismarck extended it to the entire nation. Bismarck wanted a unified, centralized system of insurance to embrace all economically underprivileged persons in industry and agriculture. The final product was a compromise, which was supported by contributions from employers, employees, and the state. While the result did not satisfy everybody, a beginning had been made, and Germany's example has since been followed by other countries. The German system was satisfactory enough to be retained in essence under the Weimar Republic, the Third Reich, and at present in the German Federal Republic. Noteworthy also is the circumstance that when Alsace-Lorraine returned to France after 1918, its people insisted on retaining the German social insurance system. Eventually, in 1928, France established a similar plan for the entire country.

Other countries that followed the German plan were Austria (1888), Hungary (1891), Luxemburg (1901), Norway (1909), Switzerland (1911), and Great Britain (1911). One of the most interesting developments in this area has occurred in the latter country during the past 50 years. The 1880s saw mounting unemployment and pauperism, and it became increasingly evident that Poor Law administration could not be separated from questions of economic fluctuations and seasonal employment. The workers and their representatives called for less reliance on the invisible hand and more positive action by government. Simultaneously, it was becoming abundantly clear that there was great confusion with respect to poor relief between various local authorities and the boards of guardians originally responsible for this function. Furthermore, there was a feeling in some circles that the principle of deterrence, which underlay the Poor Law of 1834, was being abandoned. As a result, a Royal Commission was appointed in 1905 to examine the problem of the Poor Law in all its aspects. When the *Report of the Poor Law Commission* was issued in 1909, it recommended the official abandonment of the concept of deterrence. Despite a large measure of agreement on the basic issues, the Commissioners nevertheless issued a Majority and Minority Report, each showing a profoundly different approach.

The Minority Report, largely the work of Beatrice Webb, proposed a unified state medical service, to combine the Poor Law medical services with those provided by public health authorities, the whole to be administered by a national health department as part of a social security system. In effect, this was the plan that 40 years later became the National Health Service. The Majority Report proposed a less radical and more piecemeal approach. Among the measures proposed were labor exchanges, unemployment insurance, and health insurance. The first two proposals were actually the work of two civil servants at the Board of Trade: William Beveridge and Hubert Llewellyn Smith. In 1909, the former published his important study, *Unemployment: A Problem of Industry*, which was the first step on the road toward the Beveridge Report of 1942. Unemployment insurance was sponsored by Winston Churchill, then President of the Board of Trade, and in 1911, the proposal was incorporated into the health insurance measure sponsored by Lloyd George, then Chancellor of the Exchequer. The Act of 1911 was entitled "An Act to provide for Insurance against Loss of Health and for the Prevention and Care of Sickness, and for Insurance against Unemployment and for purposes incidental thereto." It was modelled on the Bismarckian legislation for Germany. Finally, in 1919, another recommendation of the Poor Law Commission became a reality with the establishment in 1919 of the Ministry of Health "for the purpose of promoting the health of the people throughout England and Wales." The Ministry took over the health functions of the Local Government Board, the health insurance organization, the health and medical inspection duties of the Ministry of Education, as well as all other matters relating to health, such as sanitation, epidemics, and housing.

While these measures provided a basis for a coordinated health service, no further action was taken in the ensuing years. Personal health services developed by public health authorities, especially for mothers and children, hospital services, and the general practitioner services available to insured persons continued to develop side by side without any real planning or coordination. Between 1920 and 1939, a number of notable studies and reports on health policy and the provisions of health services were made. All indicated a need for change and improvement, yet for 20 years little direct action commensurate with the need was taken. The coming of the Second World War thrust upon Britain the need for national planning, and not least in health. There was considerable evidence of the existence of a vast amount of avoidable ill health, in part a legacy of the great depression. The emergency of the war burst through the barriers of inertia, hesitation, and party politics and carried through reforms long overdue. The Beveridge Committee was appointed in June, 1941, and in November, 1942, Sir William Beveridge presented his report, *Social Insurance and Allied Services*. In it he pointed out that the parts of a national social policy are so intimately related that social security cannot be fully developed unless health is cared for along comprehensive lines. This is the content of the famous Assumption B. The goal was to have a National Health Service that would provide "full preventive and curative treatment of a kind to every citizen without exceptions, without remuneration limit and without an economic barrier at any point to delay recourse to it." In February, 1943, the coalition government formally announced its approval of the policy of a National Health Service. Three more years were required to develop the necessary legislation; finally on November 6, 1946, the National Health Service Act received the Royal Assent and became the law of the land. The actual operation of the National Health Service began on July 5, 1948, and it is today an established part of British life. It was launched as a great experiment, and as an embodiment of an ideal of social justice and welfare. The effect of the Service on the health of the British people will not be easy to determine precisely over a short period. Details, practice, and shortcomings still have to be worked out. Nevertheless, the fact remains that a modern industrialized community has undertaken to organize existing health resources in democratic fashion for the benefit of all the people, a historic milestone in the evolution of community health action.

In the United States, some recognition of special and limited problems in the provision of medical care can be traced to the colonial period. Care was provided for the sick poor through municipal physicians and midwives. Mention has already been made of the provision of medical care for sick and disabled seamen through a sickness insurance system in 1798. Some awareness of a rural health problem can be traced at least to the Civil War period when the report of the first Commissioner of Agriculture to President Lincoln devoted a section to the health problems of farm families.

It was not, however, until the present century that the problem of medical care began to intrude itself into public consciousness. The environment within this process occurred is that of industrialization. American society during the nineteenth century shifted from a locally subsisting agricultural economy, with handicraft production, to an urban mechanized industrial economy, with wide income variation, in which men no longer made their living but worked for wages. These changes in working and living conditions created significant health problems in both urban and rural communities and have decisively influenced the provision of medical care.

Simultaneously, the advance of medical science led to the use of new diagnostic and curative procedures and instruments. Urbanization also contributed to the centralization of medical care in the hospital. These developments facilitated access to medical care, but at the same time, the cost of medical care increased and complicated the problem of its distribution. The fact is that the cost of medical care increased more rapidly than purchasing power, and it was realized by some that to serve the new industrialized American society, medicine required new forms of organization.

The first extensive movement for a comprehensive system of compulsory sickness insurance in the United States was launched in 1912 by the American Association for Labor Legislation. This step was taken one year after the passage of the National Health Insurance Act in England and was no doubt influenced by that fact. More immediately, however, it appeared as a natural and logical sequence to the successful campaign for workmen's compensation during the preceding five years. The problem of illness and protection against its economic consequences seemed to be most pressing, and, under the slogan, "Health Insurance—the next step in social progress," the Association proceeded to act.

The idea of medical care insurance was known in the United States before this time. Fraternal orders and trade unions with their sickness benefit schemes helped to establish the basic idea. Lodges and similar organizations among immigrant groups worked in the same direction. Also, as early as 1890, group hospital care plans were developed. Between 1890 and 1920, hospital care and insurance was represented by company and single-hospital plans. These early plans were few in number, however, their financial structure was weak due to small membership (in this respect similar to the early Friendly Society), and there was no uniformity of rates. These early plans were for workers in mining, lumbering, or railroading in areas in which medical care was not easily provided.

Furthermore, even before the first movement for sickness insurance, proposals had been made for far-reaching reform of the provision of medical care. Most interesting are those of Gustav A. Kleene (1868–1946), professor of economics at Trinity College in Hartford, Connecticut. In 1904, Kleene published a discussion of medical relief to the indigent in which he advocated free medical care for all. In 1907, he went on to propose measures by government for unemployment and old age insurance, but such ideas were somewhat ahead of their time in the United States.

The first American movement for compulsory health insurance developed in the atmosphere of the Wilsonian New Freedom and shared its decline. The period of 10 years from 1910 to 1920 has a character of its own both in health and in general social policy. The rising energy of reform since the turn of the century reached its peak during this decade, and its application to a wide variety of community health problems—maternal and child health, tuberculosis, malnutrition, industrial diseases—has already been described. Among the leaders who conceived and sustained the movement were economists, lawyers, physicians, social workers, and political scientists, as well as others concerned with social problems. John B. Andrews, I. M. Rubinow, Jane Addams, and Edward T. Devine were actively involved. In 1912, the American Association for Labor Legislation formed a Committee on Social Insurance, which over the next few years carried the major burden of the campaign for compulsory medical care insurance. Three medical men on the Committee, Alexander Lambert, I. M. Rubinow, and S. S. Goldwater, were also members of a Social Insurance Committee established by the American Medical Association in 1915. The Association for Labor Legislation devoted the major part of its seventh annual meeting in December 1913, to health insurance; an American Conference on Social Insurance was held the same year; and the subject was brought before the 1914 National Conference of Charities and Corrections. By the end of 1915, the Committee on Social Insurance had drafted a model bill to be introduced into state legislatures the following year. Eleven state commissions on health insurance were appointed between 1915 and 1920. Bills were introduced in 16 state legislatures. Discussions were promoted; local committees were developed. Striking success was achieved in making American students of social problems "health insurance conscious." Beyond this rather limited group, the movement won little support. After a brief but brilliant period of activity, vehement opposition from diverse groups brought about collapse of the movement.

The reasons for the failure are illuminating. Basically, it was due to the fact that the proponents of health insurance had neglected to consider and to deal with the economic, ideological, and other interests of the groups that would be involved in this social innovation. It was assumed that the intrinsic merits of the idea of health insurance would be enough to enable it to triumph over opposition. However, various important groups were aroused, and they combined to form a united front to fight health insurance. In general, popular prejudice against intellectuals and "do-gooders" was played up and proved quite detrimental. At the same time, the climate of opinion created by the First World War and postwar period was also adverse to any rational consideration of the problem. Our enemy, Germany, had developed sickness insurance and consequently it was un-American to favor it.

Most important among the opposed groups were the following interests. Employers were generally antagonistic on the ground that their costs would be increased. Commercial life insurance companies were perhaps the most active opponents, largely because they feared the loss of a large and lucrative business. Symbolic is the resignation of Frederick L. Hoffman, statistician for the Prudential Insurance Company of America, from the Committee on Social Insurance in 1916 when it endorsed compulsory medical care insurance. There were in force some 44 million industrial insurance policies amounting to about six billion dollars. It was feared that the funeral benefit proposed in health insurance would practically eliminate that business. Fraternal societies writing insurance were opposed largely for the same reason. "By including the funeral benefit," said I. M. Rubinow, "the health insurance movement signed its own death warrant."

Certain labor leaders, especially Samuel Gompers, president of the American Federation of Labor, opposed compulsory social insurance schemes operated by government on the ground that this would lead to control of the union movement. Workers were suspicious because deductions would be made from the pay envelope. It should be noted, however, that at least 11 state federations were favorable to health insurance, especially in New York.

The medical profession was for a brief time interested in securing provisions in pending bills that would safeguard its interests. In 1915, the American Medical Association created a committee to compile information on this subject and "to do everything in their power to secure such constructions of the proposed laws as will work the most harmonious adjustment of the new sociologic relations between physicians and laymen which will necessarily result therefrom. . . ." There were some in the profession who favored insurance. Most of these were teachers in medical schools, public health officials, and salaried physicians in other employment. A majority of the profession, however, were alarmed at the prospect of a system of compulsory health insurance. Vindictively antagonistic to all forms of contract practice, this opposition was in large measure transferred to health insurance on the ground that it would lead to a reduction of income, bring about restrictions on freedom of practice, and create extra clerical work. Dentists, pharmacists, and practitioners of healing cults supported the physicians. By 1920, the American Medical Association established its basic policy of opposition to compulsory health insurance, which still remains unchanged.

This attitude of the organized medical profession is noteworthy, because it differed so much from the reaction of the German physicians in 1883 and the English profession in 1911. The German physicians were not consulted and in large measure the medical profession was indifferent to the problem. In England, there was some opposition from the British Medical Association, but it was largely concerned with administrative and financial arrangements so as to eliminate evils that had existed under earlier contractual arrangements with friendly societies. In the United States, however, the opposition of organized medicine to compulsory health insurance has radiated to many other forms of government action in the interest of health. The Sheppard-Towner Act, for example, was disapproved officially by the House of Delegates at the annual meeting of the American Medical Association in 1922.

During the period of the 1920s, there was little action for medical insurance. Nevertheless, the idea never completely disappeared. Mounting concern over the cost and organization of medical care led in 1925 to the Washington Conference on the Economic Factors Affecting the Organization of Medicine. Another Conference was held in 1926. These meetings led to the establishment in 1927 of the Committee on the Costs of Medical Care, with Dr. Ray Lyman Wilbur, Secretary of the Interior, as chairman, and C.-E. A. Winslow, an outstanding public health leader as vice-chairman. The Committee was financed by six foundations and had at its disposal a large and able research staff headed by I. S. Falk. It was a thoroughly representative committee, comprising 49 members of whom 18 were medical practitioners, 6 were public health workers, 10 represented medical schools and other institutions concerned with medicine, 6 were social scientists, and 9 represented the public at large. The Committee planned and carried out a five-year program of research and study and published its findings and recommendations in 28 major volumes, as well as in a number of subsidiary reports. *Medical Care for the American People,* the final report of the Committee appeared in November 1932, when the country was almost at the lowest point in this period of black depression.

When the Committee drew up its recommendations, it split into a majority and a minority. An important and penetrating individual statement was made by Walton A. Hamilton, professor of law at Yale University. The majority favored medical and hospital care insurance on a voluntary basis, until adequate experience could be accumulated to serve as a sound basis for a comprehensive system based on compulsory tax deductions. The majority also approved group medical practice organized around health centers. It favored government grants-in-aid to provide hospitals, doctors, and nurses in poor and thinly populated areas. The cost of medical care for the indigent, the tubercular, and the mentally ill should be borne by the state. While the minority agreed in many respects with the majority, it had little to offer that was constructive. It reaffirmed the opposition of the medical and dental organizations to prepaid medical care even on a voluntary basis and objected particularly to the proposal for group practice. The minority opposed insurance plans unless sponsored and controlled by organized medicine. *The Journal of the American Medical Association* went even further and indicted the majority report as "inciting to revolution."

Nevertheless, the recommendations of the Committee on the Costs of Medical Care indicated the issues that were to be fought over and acted on in the next 25 years. Concurrently, other forces were at work, which added impetus to the movement for better organization and financing of medical care. President Roosevelt in a special message to Congress on June 8, 1934, announced that he was seeking a "sound means" to provide more security for the common man. Late in June, he appointed the Committee on Economic Security consisting of the Secretaries of Labor, Agriculture, and the Treasury, as well as the Attorney General and the Federal Emergency Relief Administrator. Health insurance was considered by the Committee, but nothing was done about it. The original social security bill did provide that the Social Security Board study the problem of health insurance and report its findings and recommendations to Congress. However, this simple proposal aroused so much opposition that the Ways and Means Committee struck the clause out of the bill. There is no reference to health insurance in the Social Security Act, but it is a duty of the Administration to study the most effective means of providing economic security through social insurance and to make recommendations for this purpose. Studies on health insurance have been carried out and in general the Social Security Act strengthened action in the field of medical care.

As a result of the developments described as well as of several other factors to be mentioned, public interest in health insurance revived. The deepening of the Depression threw into stark and bold relief the connection between economics and medical care. Labor shifted from opposition to advocacy of health insurance in 1935. This movement was given further impetus by several studies carried out during the latter part of the 1930s. Of the extent of illness and disability, one study has given us fairly comprehensive, although far from precise data. This was the National Health Survey, which was sponsored by the U.S. Public Health Service and carried out from October 1935, to the end of March 1936. The study covered more than 700,000 urban households in 18 states and 37,000 rural households in 3 states, comprising a total of 3 million persons. The National Health Survey showed that the frequency of illness was disproportionately higher among the poor and the jobless than among the well-to-do and the employed. Disabling illness occurred 57 per cent more frequently among families on relief than among families with an annual income of $3000 or more. Chronic illnesses were 87 per cent higher for relief families. Non-relief families with an income of less than $1000 had twice as much illness disability as families with an annual income of more than $1000. Other surveys, notably one carried out by the Cost of Living Division of the Department of Labor on the family expenditures of 14,469 wage earning and clerical families in 42 large cities, substantiated further the fact that the amount and quality of medical care received was closely correlated with the family's income. The receipt of hospital care by the low-income groups paralleled their experience with medical care.

Out of a realization of the disparity existing between the receipt and the cost of medical care and because of the inability of low-income groups to pay for such care, there developed various efforts to achieve a more equitable distribution of medical care and its costs. These efforts have proceeded along two basic lines: to secure reorganization of medical care through government action, and to achieve this goal by developing private prepaid medical care programs.

Many attempts have been made since 1935 to secure the enactment of a national health insurance law, or to stimulate the passage of state legislation, and many different bills have been proposed. Up to the present, all these efforts have failed. Nonetheless, these bills have stimulated the spread of voluntary health and hospitalization insurance and thereby fostered the movement for better distribution of medical care. Most significant in this connection was the bill introduced by Senator Robert F. Wagner in the Seventy-Sixth Congress in 1939, which was stimulated by the findings of the National Health Survey and the National Health Conference held in Washington, D.C., in July, 1938. The Wagner-Murray-Dingell Bill, introduced in the Senate in November 1945, marks the peak of the recent movement to establish a compulsory national health insurance system. Opponents of this bill, although successful in the fight against it, were thoroughly aroused by the growing strength of the movement for government action. The consequence was the appearance in 1947 of the first counter-proposal to compulsory medical care insurance in the bill sponsored by Senator Robert A. Taft and others to assist states in providing medical care for the indigent.

The National Health Assembly, a conference of professional and community leaders, was held in Washington in May 1948. Contributory insurance was recommended as the basic method of financing care for the large majority of the American people, but opinions varied on how to put this principle into practice. In 1949, the Truman administration, on the recommendation of Oscar R. Ewing, the Federal Security Administrator, urged the enactment of compulsory medical care insurance, while the opposition in Congress proposed a voluntary approach by providing Federal grants to assist voluntary prepayment plans in extending their services to those wishing to use them. Two years later (1951) President Truman created a Commission on the Health Needs of the Nation, which made an extensive study of the problem and made a number of recommendations. The advent of the Eisenhower Administration in 1952 has been followed by a diminution of Congressional interest in the problem of national health insurance.

Although the legislative results have been extremely meager, there have been definite gains since 1935. These have occurred chiefly because of the growth of voluntary prepayment programs for hospitalization and medical care. The growth of plans to cover hospital costs has been phenomenal, especially since 1937. There was one Blue Cross Hospital service plan with an enrollment of 2000 in 1933. As of January 1, 1953, some 59 per cent of the civilian population of the United States had hospitalization insurance of some kind. There were 41.8 million persons under Blue Cross, 48.7 million under commercial insurance company plans, and an estimated 6.7 million under other types of plans. Even though much has been achieved in this field, 41 per cent of the population, or 64 million persons, were without prepaid hospital protection. For the most part, this group is in the lower income levels and to a large extent is situated in the Southern states and in the Mountain and Pacific regions of the country.

While the issue of national compulsory health insurance was still enveloped in controversy, experiments in prepaid medical care were being made in various parts of the United States. By 1935, the doctrinal winds had shifted sufficiently so that the House of Delegates of the American Medical Association offered "its encouragement to local medical organizations to establish plans for the provision of adequate medical service for all of the people, adjusted to present economic conditions, by voluntary budgeting to meet the costs of illness. . . ." One year earlier, however, the Michigan State Medical Society had already worked out a plan for voluntary health insurance. Active antagonism to group practice continued. The matter came to a head in the case of the Group Health Association in Washington, D.C., which had been established in 1937 at the urging of Federal Home Loan Bank employees. Various acts of hostility against this organization led to the criminal conviction under the Sherman Anti-Trust Act of the American Medical Association and the District of Columbia Medical Society, and the affirmation of this conviction by the United States Supreme Court in 1943. In the same year, the House of Delegates created a Council of Medical Service and Public Relations, which soon set about interesting state medical societies in making some type of health insurance plan available to the public. To coordinate these plans, Associated Medical Care Plans was created in 1945 and incorporated as a trade association. This organization adopted the Blue Shield as its symbol just as Blue Cross designated hospital insurance plans. From about 750,000 members in 1942 the Blue Shield plans grew to almost 20 million in 1950.

Another significant development during the past few decades has been the development of prepaid group practice plans offering comprehensive services to their members. Most important in this area are the Health Insurance Plan of Greater New York established in 1947, and the Permanente Foundation in California. Something over 3 million people are served by such plans at present. During the Second World War, another element was introduced into the medical care picture. Unable to obtain increased wages, labor unions in negotiating contracts began to bargain for so-called fringe benefits. Among these, demands for health and welfare funds have been prominent. At the same time and partly as a result, unions have expanded their efforts to create medical care centers. Perhaps one of the most widely known programs organized by a union is that of the United Mine Workers.

None of the voluntary plans have so far provided a completely adequate answer to the problem of providing medical care of good quality to people when they need it. The comprehensive group practice plans have probably come closest to this goal. Yet there are many people who need medical care and cannot be reached by any of the existing plans. This is true of the low-income group that needs medical care most. Furthermore, the absence of coordination among these varied organizations also hinders the realization of the full potentialities of modern medical care for the people of the community. The relationship of prepaid medical care plans to the official health agencies and to other voluntary health agencies also remains to be clarified. The significance of organized medical care for the health of the community was recognized by the public health profession with the formation of the Medical Care Section by the American Public Health Association in 1948.

Nevertheless, the fact remains that the evolution of prepaid medical and hospital care in the United States has been a considerable improvement over previously existing conditions and has provided some degree of protection against the heaviest costs of illness. Concern with the problem of medical care also contributed to the enactment of the important Hospital Survey and Construction (Hill-Burton) Act of 1946, which has brought about a substantial increase in hospital and health center facilities where they are needed. While recognizing the achievements discussed, it seems clear that further progress toward better health for the American people will demand more efficient organization of health resources and services. All available evidence points to the imperative need for action on local community, state, and Federal levels to achieve the close coordination among individuals and groups who work for health, which alone can provide the basis for obtaining the full potentialities of modern medicine and public health.

THE RESPONSIBILITY OF GOVERNMENT FOR THE ADVANCEMENT OF HEALTH. It was inevitable that the transformation of the United States from a rural, agricultural nation into one predominantly urban and industrial should have a profound effect upon its civil institutions. The resulting expansion of governmental functions was already evident during the latter part of the nineteenth century, but the full impact of public undertaking in relation to health was not felt until well into the twentieth century. The decade between 1910 and 1920 marked the first great period in the formulation of American social policy and of legislation in relation to health. The keynote for the period was struck by Hermann Biggs in 1911.

"Disease is largely a removable evil," he wrote, "it continues to afflict humanity, not only because of incomplete knowledge of its causes and lack of individual and public hygiene, but also because it is extensively fostered by harsh economic and industrial conditions and by wretched housing in congested communities. These conditions and consequently the diseases which spring from them can be removed by better social organization. No duty of society, acting through its governmental agencies, is paramount to this obligation to attack the removable causes of disease. . . . The reduction of the death rate is the principal statistical expression and index of human and social progress. It means the saving and lengthening of the lives of thousands of citizens, the extension of the vigorous working period well into the old age, and the prevention of inefficiency, misery, and suffering. These advances can be made by organized social effort."

Numerous studies demonstrated the toll levied by sickness upon society. The valuable report on *National Vitality* prepared in 1909 by Irving Fisher has been mentioned. Further evidence was provided by the sickness surveys carried out by the Metropolitan Life Insurance Company from 1915 to 1917, and the reports of various state commissions on social and health insurance that were appointed between 1915 and 1920. To meet the exigencies of industrial expansion and the challenge of economic insecurity, legislation was passed for the protection of women and children, workmen's compensation schemes were inaugurated, interest was aroused in the organization and the provision of medical care, and government tended more and more to assume responsibility for stimulating action by the states and localities.

These developments must be seen, however, not alone as events peculiar to the United States, but in the perspective of a worldwide historical evolution that has brought into being the modern state with its concern for individual, family, and community needs for organized social security and service. There is probably no more fascinating process in recent history than that through which the laissez-faire "night-watchman" state of the nineteenth century has been transformed into the present day "welfare" state. The process was, of course, gradual and was in effect a result of the Industrial Revolution. As early as 1815, Robert Owen pleaded for state action to curb extreme forms of exploitation, and by the 1880s Herbert Spencer was already fighting a losing, rearguard action in defence of sound laissez-faire principles.

The same broad developments occurred in all the leading industrial countries, though with numerous variations and, above all, differences in tempo due to varying historical antecedents and economic conditions. Today, the principle of state intervention and control in health matters is admitted; the only difference is in the greater or lesser efficiency of the intervention and in the greater or lesser frankness with which the role of the state is admitted. Its emergence has resulted from the interaction of important economic and social trends. For one thing, during this period, the typical trend of economic organization has been the continuous and progressive replacement of smaller units by larger ones. However, the further this process advanced the more untenable has become the conception of non-interference by the state. No one has solicited state intervention more widely in the United States than the small business man seeking protection against the large producer and competitor. The state has also had to intervene to protect the worker, hence, the development of factory legislation, social insurance, wage fixing, and the like. Analogous means, such as price fixing and quality controls, are used to protect the consumer. These developments have necessarily led to the widespread acceptance of a strong, unified, central authority, entrusted with large powers to promote social well-being. This acceptance is a product as well of a new climate of opinion that emerged toward the end of the nineteenth century, first in the highly advanced countries of industrialism, England and Germany, and somewhat later in other countries like the United States. By the first decade of the present century, it was no longer possible seriously to consider poverty as the "natural" punishment of the poor for their shortcomings, and poverty came to be diagnosed as a social disease. It was equally clear that the consequences of poverty for health must be dealt with if the national economy was to be maintained in a healthy state.

In part, this was due to the gradual, but progressive, growth of trade unionism. As the trade union substituted group solidarity for unlimited competition among the workers, demands began to be made for state action to provide better living as well as working conditions. Two factors hastened this process: one was unemployment, the other was war. Waves of unemployment around the turn of the century, after the First World War, and during the great depression of the 1930s drove home the fact that unemployment was a problem of society, affecting equally the just and the unjust, the competent and the incompetent, and that its causes were beyond the ability of any one individual to alter. War has been the other motive force behind this change. The need for national efficiency and the planned utilization of resources, animate as well as inanimate, led to the assumption of responsibility by central governments. Under the influence of those stimuli, national governments have developed a concern with health services, nutrition, and social security in general.

To handle the expanding interests of government in these areas, national administrative systems have had to be created. Generally, each system is centered in a national ministry or department. In England, for example, the Ministry of Health Act was passed in 1919, abolishing the Local Government Board and creating the Ministry of Health. For the most part, various health functions of other departments were brought into the new ministry, whose scope went beyond the concept of health in a narrow sense. Among its responsibilities were housing, the poor law administration, the health insurance scheme, and local government, as well as the initiation and direction of research and measures concerned with health of all the people. Thus, by the slow but inexorable logic of events, just over 70 years after the creation of the General Board of Health (1848), England had a National Department of Health, with a Minister of Health responsible to Parliament and, in the words of John Simon, with a mandate "in the widest sense to care for the physical necessities of human life."

The creation of a national health agency was not achieved until 1953 in the United States. The Public Health Service developed rapidly after 1912 under the stimulus of the needs of an increasingly industrialized complex society. Despite the increasing scope of its operations, it remained as a unit within the Treasury Department. In 1938, as a part of his executive reorganization program, President Roosevelt proposed to set up two new cabinet departments, Social Welfare and Public Works. While the plan was not accepted, a Federal Security Agency was created in 1939 to bring together most of the health, welfare, and educational services of the Federal government. In 1946, the Agency was expanded by the transfer to it of the Children's Bureau and the Food and Drug Administration. Then in 1953, President Eisenhower proposed that the Federal Security Agency be made a cabinet department. On April 11, 1953, Congress established the Department of Health, Education, and Welfare. Seventy years after the National Board of Health went out of existence, the United States again had a national health agency.

The modern conception that the national government is responsible for the health of the people is but a natural extension of the previous view where the local community provided for such needs. As the center of gravity has moved from the small political unit to the large one, this has had its effect on the provision of health services. By and large, the trend today is for the national health agency to wield the greatest influence in endeavoring to remove those notorious obstacles to human improvement, the five giants of Lord Beveridge: want, disease, ignorance, squalor, and idleness. Most recently, in fact, this trend has moved beyond the national community to the world community with the creation of the World Health Organization. While the duty of health promotion and protection is today lodged basically in the executive organ of the national community, localities as well as groups and individuals in them must still take an important part in the preservation of individual and collective health. The relations of the national health service to local health services and personnel show the widest variations throughout the world. Nevertheless, the increasing complexity of social life, especially in the economically more advanced countries has revealed new and delicate problems that have not been solved as yet. Physicians and other professional groups that had traditionally enjoyed a large measure of autonomy in the laissez-faire state now find that their professional work involves them in more intimate contacts and intricate relationships with public authorities. This problem involves also the relation between action by public authorities and voluntary associations. Lord Beveridge followed up his epoch-making report on *Social Insurance and Allied Services* with a less well known, but no less important, examination of *Voluntary Action* (1948). The original Beveridge Report laid down the principle that "social security must be achieved by cooperation between the state and the individual." In the later study, he elaborated this principle, urging that the state encourage, protect, and even support out of public funds, every kind of voluntary action for social advance and social service. This is one of the basic problems today in countries such as the United States. What is the best functional division in the provision of health services? Which services are best provided by government, which are best provided by independent voluntary action, and which by state-aided voluntary action? Obviously such developments will be influenced by historical traditions, local psychology, vested interests, and national assessment of needs, but there is also need for a comprehensive theory of public health administration to develop principles upon which such distinction can be made.

In countries in which a national government exercises direct authority over a locality, a health program that has been formulated can readily be put into effect. In other countries, like the United States, the national health authority deals with international and interstate quarantine, carries out and stimulates extensive programs of research, and stimulates state and local health departments through grants-in-aid. Here suasion and indirect influence are employed. While a national or central health organization provides direction and guidance to the local health authorities, or gives specialized technical services that cannot be procured at a local level, the ultimate success of any public health program depends on the degree to which it is brought close to the people whom it is intended to serve, and the understanding of it which they have acquired. The Preamble to the Constitution of the World Health Organization has affirmed this principle in the statement: "Informed opinion and active cooperation on the part of the public are of the utmost importance in the improvement of the health of the people." Implied in this is a reciprocity of rights and duties shared by the individual and the community. In brief, it is necessary that every member of a community become an active participant in the work needed to improve individual and collective health. Health education is the fundamental tool for this purpose.

To bring public health work close to the people, the concept of district health administration and the idea of the health center were developed during the second and third decades of this century and applied in a variety of ways in different countries. In the United States, as methods of controlling tuberculosis and infant mortality became more effective, those concerned with these problems began to explore ways and means of applying these methods in an organized manner to the largest possible numbers of people. Gradually, the health district concept was developed. Efforts to relate services to a delimited population or to the population in a definite area began to take practical form between 1910 and 1915. For such a plan to function with high efficiency, it was soon realized that a focal point of administration, a health center, was needed.

Significant activities in this direction were initiated by health and welfare workers in a number of American communities in the decade before the First World War. In 1910, William Charles White in Pittsburgh and Wilbur C. Philips in Wilkes-Barre adapted the department store idea to the health field by housing several clinics under the same roof. The autonomy of each clinic was maintained. The importance of health planning for a given region or area was recognized by the New York City Health Department in 1914 and led to the establishment of Health District No. 1 in the Lower East Side in 1915. A year later the first district health unit was opened in Boston. Also, 1916 was the year in which the National Social Unit Organization was formed, under the leadership of Wilbur C. Philips, with headquarters in New York City. The purpose of this group was "to promote the type of democratic community organization through which the citizenship as a whole can participate directly in the control of community affairs, while at the same time making constant use of the highest technical skill available." After some deliberation, the Mohawk-Brighton district of Cincinnati was selected for the purpose of carrying out a "social unit" community experiment on a large scale and a sum of money was appropriated by the national organization for this purpose. This demonstration was developed around a center. All segments of the district were represented: workers, teachers, social workers, and so forth. The work of this unit included antepartum care, well-child care, nursing service, tuberculosis control, and medical care, the last to a limited degree. On the whole, this was one of the most seminal experiments in social organization for health undertaken in the United States. Indeed, the objectives set up by this plan are in many instances only now being explored.

In New York City, the initial health district started in 1915 proved so satisfactory that in 1916 Commissioner of Health Haven Emerson extended it to the borough of Queens where four districts were created. At the same time, a Division of Health Districts was established. Initially, community organization, health education, child health, and control of preventable diseases were emphasized. Later other activities, for example, school medical inspection, food handler's examinations, supervision of midwives, inspections for industrial hygiene, as well as many others were added. Unfortunately, at this time, there was a change in the city government, and the new administration slipped smoothly back into the established rut of the *status quo ante*. Among other achievements, it halted the plans to extend health district administration to other parts of the city, and it was not until more than 12 years later that district health centers began to be established in New York City. Nevertheless, experience had been gained for such a program, and the advantages to be derived from decentralized public health administration demonstrated.

During the First World War and the period after the war, health demonstrations and health centers financed by voluntary agencies, foundations, or other social welfare organizations were established in many parts of the United States. Following the war, the American Red Cross as part of its peacetime program undertook the establishment of health centers by local chapters. During the latter part of 1919, the Red Cross made a preliminary survey of 76 health centers in the United States. Analyses of the existing and proposed centers studied shows that at the time of the report, published in March, 1920, 33 were administered entirely by public authorities, 27 were under private control, and 16 were under combined public and private control. The Red Cross was concerned in 19 instances. There was considerable variation in the work and aims of the existing health centers. In 40 communities having health centers in operation, 37 contained clinics of some type, 34 carried on visiting nursing, 29 did child welfare work, and 27 did anti-tuberculosis work. Twenty-two had venereal disease clinics, 14 had dental clinics, and 11 had eye, ear, nose, and throat clinics. Only 10 had laboratories and 9 had milk stations.

While health center types and the scope of district administration associated with them varied considerably, the succeeding decades witnessed a great deal of development and experimentation. In 1930, a subcommittee on health centers collected information for the White House Conference on Child Health and Protection. It obtained data for 1511 major and minor health centers throughout the country. Eighty per cent had been established since 1910. Of the total number, 725 were operated by private agencies, 729 by county or municipal health departments, and a small number by the Red Cross, hospitals, tuberculosis associations, case-work agencies, and the like. In nearly half these centers, the principal support came from public funds, while supplementary aid came through community chests, or from private or voluntary funds.

The concept of the health center as a neighborhood or district service developed as a direct consequence of the problems created by the increasing expansion of the scope of community health action and the impact on health departments. The district health center, coordinating hitherto separated clinics and services was inaugurated to replace centralized control of each particular service. In the United States, the health center is generally a part of an official health agency, while most medical care concerned with diagnosis and therapy remains outside the sphere of activity of health centers. Far-sighted leaders in the health field realized that the health center principle might be employed to improve the provision of medical care. The "social unit" experiment in Cincinnati touched on this problem, but the most imaginative approach was made by Hermann Biggs in 1920 when he endeavored to deal with health service for rural areas in New York State. As Commissioner of Health, he proposed the establishment of local health centers to include one or more of the following elements: hospital, clinics (for tuberculosis, venereal diseases, prenatal and child welfare, mental diseases, dental defects, as well as for medical care), laboratories, district health administration, and public health nursing. The centers could be established in any community with the approval of the State Health Commissioner. In addition to coordinating public health services, these centers were intended "to encourage and provide facilities for an annual medical examination to detect physical defects and disease;" and "to provide for the residents of rural districts, for industrial workers and all others in need of such

service, scientific medical and surgical treatment, hospital and dispensary facilities and nursing care at a cost within their means or, if necessary, free." State
aid in the form of 50 per cent cash grants for buildings, a cash allowance for
the treatment of free patients, together with certain allowances toward maintenance, were to be furnished to all communities fulfilling the requirements of
the State Health Department. While a large number of community organizations supported these proposals, the Sage-Machold bill, which embodied this
health center program, was defeated in the New York State Legislature. The
whole idea was far ahead of public opinion, and especially of opinion in the
New York medical profession.

Biggs realized quite early that the next step in the development of community health services required a coalescence of preventive and curative medicine. Since 1920, this seminal concept has evolved in several directions. Among
these, the idea of prepaid group practice, as exemplified in the Health Insurance Plan of Greater New York and the Kaiser-Permanente Foundation,
has been demonstrated as practicable. Another approach was promoted by the
late Dr. Joseph W. Mountin (1891–1952), based on his belief that hospitals and
health departments must eventually combine or coordinate their facilities and
resources to provide a more nearly complete health service for the communities they serve. As part of such a plan, he proposed to correlate the health center with the general hospital in the community.

Meanwhile, significant health district programs were created and developed
in a number of American communities, notably in Baltimore and New York. In
1932, plans initially started by William H. Welch eventuated in the establishment of the Eastern Health District as a cooperative endeavor of the Baltimore
City Health Department, the Johns Hopkins School of Hygiene and Public
Health, as well as several voluntary agencies. This district has made possible
the intensive study of public health problems and has provided a field for the
testing of new administrative procedures and for the training of personnel. A
second district was organized in 1935.

In New York, a program of district health administration was developed
after 1929, and a group of health centers were opened beginning in 1930. Actually, this program grew out of two demonstrations inaugurated in the 1920s.
The East Harlem Health Center was initiated in 1921 by the New York County
Chapter of the Red Cross with the cooperation of 21 public and voluntary agencies. Eventually this center became one of the district health units. While East
Harlem was the first general health center, the Bellevue-Yorkville Health Demonstration, organized in 1924 and opened to the public in 1926, led eventually
to the adoption by New York City of the principle of district health administration. Financed by the Milbank Memorial Fund and the Health Department,

the Demonstration was carried on for 10 years in cooperation with more than 80 official and voluntary health and welfare agencies.

The development in the United States of health services on a district basis and organized around a central facility has been followed by the establishment of similar services in various countries. One of the features of the National Health Service Act, 1946, which captured the imagination of many people was the provision for health centers to house the clinics of local authorities as well as offices of physicians and dentists. It was hoped that this would make possible teamwork and facilitate the coordination of all health services in a given neighborhood. Actually the idea was not new in England. Under the Ministry of Health Act of 1919, a consultative council on medical and allied services had been appointed. Known as the Dawson Committee, the council submitted a report in 1920 in which it recommended the creation of a system of health centers, in two categories: to provide preventive and curative care in a given district through general practitioners, nurses, midwives, dentists, and so on; and to provide specialist and consultant services. It is noteworthy that both Hermann Biggs and Lord Dawson offered similar proposals for the organization of health services. Despite similar recommendations in later studies, progress in the development of health centers has been slower than in the United States.

Centers first began to appear in the 1930s. Bristol constructed one in 1935 and by 1946 had five health centers. By that time there were health centers as well in Gloucestershire, Glasgow, Finsbury, Darwen, Fulham, Swindon, Tottenham, and Slough. The last-named center was organized in some degree on the lines of the Peckham experiment, one of the most unusual developments in the organization of medical care. The Pioneer Health Center at Peckham, London, was developed by two physicians, Innes H. Pearse and G. Scott Williamson, to provide a facility for families where "health is supervised by medical examination and vitality is raised by the opportunities of personal expression offered to each individual." A pilot center had been created in 1926, and on the basis of this experience a second center was established in 1935. After the war, the Center was taken over by the London County Council as an element in its system of health facilities. For a time after the Second World War, the building situation in Great Britain rendered impossible the development of health centers as originally envisaged in the National Health Service Act. With increasing recovery, however, attention began to turn again to this facet of the health services. London took the lead with the construction of the Woodbery Down center to serve a population of 20,000 people. Since then, other localities have also established centers.

Health centers have been and are being set up in many parts of the world. Such facilities have been created in a number of South American countries in recent years. The Soviet system of medical care outside of hospitals is based on a network of policlinics, which are essentially health centers of the type envisaged by the Dawson committee. The South African National Health Services Commission of 1944 recommended the unification of preventive and curative services, and its report led to the institution of a health center service. The pioneer unit is the Pholela Health Center in South-West Natal. It was later associated with the Institute of Family and Community Health, an institution created by the South African Health Department in 1945. A program for rural health centers has been projected for Egypt in the past decade, and a number of pilot centers have been established, notably at Qalyub in the Delta. A noteworthy aspect of the Egyptian program is that this development is part of a much broader program of national planning intended to raise the standard of living through improvement of agriculture, education, and housing, as well as health. This program is illustrative as well of certain recent trends, namely, the efforts of underdeveloped countries to improve the health of their people, and the increasing prominence that international health problems have come to occupy in the thinking of health workers.

"NO MAN IS AN ILAND . . ." A major fact about the international scene today is the revolt of Asia and Africa against political, economic, and racial inequity, as exemplified by European rule over "backward" peoples. While demands are raised for political independence and equality, there is also a realization that these are no longer enough. The lesson has been thoroughly learned and digested that these achievements are hollow unless backed up by the application of scientific and technical knowledge to produce modern industry, achieve a high standard of living, and develop widespread education. It has also been recognized that these goals require a healthy population, and yet it is these very countries that have the worst health conditions. Poverty and disease are linked in a vicious cycle, which must be broken if such countries are to occupy their rightful places in the modern world. The essence of the problem is summed up in Table 8.

At this point, it is appropriate to comment briefly on a related problem, namely, population development. It has become fashionable in some quarters in recent years to take a dim view of the possibility of improving the lot of the underdeveloped countries. The dimness of the prospect results from the heavy overcast of neo-Malthusianism. Decline of mortality due to improved hygienic conditions coupled with a high and rising birth rate are seen as leading to a continually accelerating increase of population. In turn, such a development is regarded as leading to an ever increasing gap between the available food and the demand for it by avid population masses. The only hope to escape catastrophe is said to lie in the adoption of drastic measures to curb expansion of

TABLE 8

The Importance of Economic and Social Factors on the Health of the People

	Developed Areas	Intermediate Areas	Underdeveloped Areas
Proportion of world population	One-fifth	Less than one-sixth	Two-thirds
Annual per capita income, in U.S. dollars	461	154	41
Food supply, calories per day	3040	2760	2150
Physicians per 100,000 population	106	78	17
Life expectancy at birth, in years	63	52	30

population. Although the regulation of population growth may be desirable on various grounds, this argument is basically fallacious. It is not true that miserable living standards, poverty, malnutrition, and disease necessarily go hand in hand with dense or rapidly increasing populations. The facts are that some of the highest population densities are to be found in advanced countries such as Belgium, Great Britain, Holland, France, and Italy, that underdeveloped areas may have much lower population densities, that these areas share certain characteristics—they are industrially underdeveloped and many of them have been exploited to their detriment by other countries, and finally that there is a direct correlation between living conditions, health status, and industrialization. Economic growth tends to reduce death rates and to improve the health and productive efficiency of a population. To be sure, industrialization also creates health problems, but the means for dealing with them are known in many cases. Economic development is, therefore, the crucial element if living standards are to be raised and health conditions improved.

Poverty and disease are linked through inadequate nutrition, housing, clothing, and insanitary living conditions. Furthermore, these in turn are based on low income and lack of education. The importance of economic, social, and political factors in determining the health status of a people renders imperative the creation of a comprehensive program. In many parts of the world, health aims cannot be attained without improvement of agriculture, development of industry, creation of competent administrative services, and improvement in the educational status of the population. In short, the underdeveloped areas of the world confront the twentieth century on a global scale with the same kind of problem that the sanitary reformers faced on a national scale about a hundred years ago. Just as Chadwick, Southwood Smith, and the other sanitary reformers recognized that no community can continue to exist indefinitely half sick and half well, so today men realize that the international community must assist its underprivileged members to solve their health problems within a broad framework of social and economic assistance.

As with many other important concepts, this one is not entirely new. International health cooperation has grown out of a broadening realization that in a world that for more than a hundred years has been contracting because of technological evolution and increasingly complex international economic and political interdependence, the presence of disease in one area constituted a continuing danger for many others. Even as recently as 50 years ago, the health officer of every port in the world knew that he was sitting on an epidemiological volcano. His first news of plague in China might be the appearance in the harbor of a ship with the yellow jack at her mast head. Coordination of quarantine procedures was an urgent problem, and the Pan American Sanitary Bureau, the oldest of the international health organizations, was created in 1902 to deal with this problem in the American hemisphere. Five years later, in 1907, an agreement was signed at Rome establishing the Office Internationale d'Hygiène Publique (International Office of Public Health), the first worldwide international health organization. Its chief function was to gather and distribute epidemiological information, especially with regard to plague, cholera, smallpox, typhus fever, and yellow fever. This was the culmination of the various sanitary conferences that had been held during the nineteenth century.

The next important step in the development of international health work was taken in 1923 with the creation of the Health Organization of the League of Nations. One of the most important functions of the Health Organization was its Epidemiological Intelligence Service. At the same time, it was becoming apparent that there were other health problems beside quarantine and the control of communicable disease that called for international action. One of the valuable contributions of the Health Organization was also the least spectacular. It carried out important studies in a variety of fields, such as rural hygiene, housing, the health of the school child, health centers, health insurance, and physical education, and in general it endeavored to develop the concept of health promotion. Furthermore, as a result of technical studies, it was possible to obtain international agreement on such important matters as the serological diagnosis of syphilis and the standardization of biological products employed therapeutically.

However, more significant than any of these in the long run was the fact that the Health Organization was the first attempt to create an effective mechanism for a continuing global attack on problems of disease. A disastrous spread of malaria had been one of the consequences of the First World War, and the Health Organization through its Malaria Commission tackled the problem. As a result of extended field study and repeated conferences, the Commission succeeded in developing a sound program that could be accepted by health workers in Europe, Asia, and the Americas as a basis for action. Similar constructive approaches were taken in relation to tuberculosis, syphilis, rabies, leprosy, cancer, and sleeping sickness. In addition to these activities, direct service was given to individual nations. The Greek Government in 1928 asked for aid in reorganizing its public health system, and expert personnel as well as funds were provided for this purpose. A similar service was rendered to Bolivia, where improvement of sanitary conditions was the major objective. Direct technical aid was also given to China in 1929 to develop a health program, to Poland and Rumania for the control of typhus fever after the First World War, and to other countries.

Some of these activities were carried on in cooperation with the Rockefeller Foundation and other organizations. As early as 1913, the Foundation established an International Health Commission (now the International Health Division), as a result of the work of the Rockefeller Sanitary Commission created in 1909 for the eradication of hookworm in the United States. Its basic policy was based on the principle that community health is a function of government and that long-term, effective results can be achieved only as countries are helped to help themselves by developing national and local health agencies, including personnel and resources on which to build in the future. This goal has been approached by (1) carrying on and supporting basic research, (2) educating and training public health personnel either through the provision of financial aid or the creation of training centers, and (3) by setting up demonstrations or providing personnel and funds on a temporary basis to establish sound community health services. In essence these are the principles on which international health work, and in particular programs of technical assistance have developed since the Second World War. Among the more notable achievements of the Rockefeller Foundation in this field have been the development of an effective yellow fever vaccine, the successful campaign to repel *Anopheles gambiae,* which had invaded Brazil from Africa in 1938, and its widespread educational program for health workers.

The Health Organization of the League, as well as the work of the International Office of Public Health and the Rockefeller Foundation, accustomed the nations to the idea of international cooperation in many areas of health and provided a large fund of useful experience. What was created up to the outbreak of the Second World War was not abandoned, but it provided the foundation on which international public health activities have been developed in the decade from 1946 to 1956. The World Health Organization was created in 1946 and took over the duties and powers of the Health Organization of the League, the International Office, and the United Nations Relief and Rehabilitation Administration (UNRRA). It came into official existence in 1948 when its constitution was ratified by the necessary 26 nations. The principle of mutual aid in dealing with social and health problems was contemplated by the Charter of the United Nations, and the World Health Organization (WHO) has approached the tasks of international health on a very broad basis, recognizing that health is "one of the fundamental rights of every human being without distinction of race, religion, political belief, economic or social condition." On this basis, WHO has become the worldwide coordinating official agency in the field of international health. Its work is supplemented by and correlated with the activities of several other organization, notably the United Nations Children's Fund, the Food and Agriculture Organization, the International Labor Organization, and the United Nations Educational Scientific and Cultural Organization.

Still more recently, international health work, and particularly technical assistance, has become intimately associated with foreign policy. In 1942, the American Republics agreed to take such steps as were necessary to solve problems of community health in the Americas through bilateral and other agreements. The United States accepted the responsibility for leadership and established the organization known today as the Institute of Inter-American Affairs. Through this agency, programs for technical assistance in the health field were developed. These emphasized chiefly the development of local health services through health centers, sanitation of the environment (water supply, sewage disposal, insect control), public health education, and training and employment of professional public health personnel. In brief, the stress has been on community health action under trained direction. This program has continued actively to the present.

On January 20, 1949, in his Inaugural Address, President Truman proposed the addition of an additional element to American foreign policy. As "Point Four," he urged that the United States "embark on a bold new program for making the benefits of our scientific advances and industrial progress available for the improvement and growth of underdeveloped areas. . ." Since then, this proposal has been developed into a widespread program. As a result in 1953, the Federal government set up an overall agency, the Foreign Operations Administration, to be responsible for all international technical assistance activities of the United States. In 1955, bilateral health programs were being carried on in 38 countries.

What the outcome of all this will be cannot yet be fully appreciated. The field of international cooperation for the advancement of health is still comparatively new. Nonetheless, the basic objectives and approaches are quite clear. As the WHO program for 1950 stated: "Public health officers have for long affirmed that economic development and public health are inseparable and complementary and that the social, cultural and economic development of a community, and its state of health, are interdependent." If properly carried out, technical assistance to the underprivileged areas of the world is a way of providing help so that their people can improve standards of living in their own way. Consequently, plans for the development of health programs must be fully integrated into this larger program. The task of improving the environment and the health services of the underdeveloped countries of the world will continue to be a challenge to all health workers in the coming years and will undoubtedly continue to be an important part of the expanding frontier of public health.

"THAT UNTRAVELL'D WORLD, WHOSE MARGIN FADES . . ." The past 50 years have witnessed an unprecedented overall trend toward the improvement of community health. Yet, this advance has not been uniform either within communities or between various parts of the world. A large group of countries generally underdeveloped in an economic and technological sense, and often new as independent nations, still have problems of preventable disease like those with which the countries of western Europe and the United States had to cope 75 to 50 years ago. Their problems are still the control of infectious diseases, the provision of un-contaminated water supplies and proper sewerage, and the elevation of the general standard of living to a minimum acceptable level. However, in economically more fortunate countries, such as the United States, Great Britain, and a number of others in western Europe, the actual problems of community health are very different. To be sure, much unfinished business remains in environmental sanitation, control of communicable diseases, health education, and nutrition. Nevertheless, a whole set of newer problems has appeared, and it is with these that the community health program of the next fifty years will have to be concerned.

These problems are in large measure a consequence of the success achieved by community action for health and welfare over the past half century. The diseases of infancy, youth, and early adulthood have been reduced to such an extent that people are no longer dying of them in great numbers. As a result of the increased life expectancy at birth, people live into the older years and the community must concern itself increasingly with the health problems of a maturing population. In 1900, only 13,000,000 persons, or 18 per cent of the population of the United States, were in the age group over 45 years. Fifty years later, this group comprised 43,000,000 persons, or 30 per cent of the population. In consequence, among the actual problems that confront us today are the control of the much less remediable chronic or degenerative diseases—cancer, cardiovascular-renal conditions, diabetes mellitus, arthritis, musculoskeletal diseases, and mental changes associated with aging.

At the same time, as the problems of communicable disease have declined in urgency, the community health program has broadened to include, wherever feasible, other elements and situations that may adversely affect the physical and mental well-being of people in the community. The widening horizons of public health have in recent years come to include such problems as accident prevention and mental health, as well as renewed emphasis on the control of the physical environment. With our expanding and changing industrial technology have come environmental alterations of increasing complexity. The once dominant problems of bacterially contaminated air, water, and food have now been replaced in considerable degree by chemical pollution, and the possible relation of this condition to the induction of cancer. Recent years have also brought an increasing amount of discussion of the social and economic changes accompanying our expanding industrialism. On the one hand, there is the continuing flight from the farm to the city, on the other, a countervailing flight from city to suburbia. In either case, the consequences for community health must be kept in mind and investigated. It is in these and related areas that the expanding frontiers of public health are to be sought. What does this mean then for the immediate future of community health action?

Recent years have brought an increasing awareness of the problem of atmospheric pollution, similar to the established concern with water pollution. As yet, it is impossible to give a complete answer to the question of the effect of air pollution on individual and community health. Nevertheless, much has been learned in recent years from epidemic outbreaks of illness and death caused by polluted fog (smog), as well as from the study of atmospheric carcinogens and their relation to lung cancer. Smog epidemics occurred in and around Liège, Belgium, during 1930, at Donora, Pennsylvania, in 1948, at Poza Rica, Mexico, in 1950, and at various times in London, England. These have been shown to be due to meteorologie conditions and a high concentration of toxic aerial contaminants. An even more difficult problem is the long-term effect of atmospheric contaminants. Pertinent data are gradually accumulating on carcinogenic agents in the atmosphere. Stocks and Campbell in England, studying the problem of lung cancer, have reported that concentrations of smoke, sulfur dioxide, benzpyrene, and other polycyclic hydrocarbons rise with increasing urbanization. In Liverpool it was found that the concentration of benzpyrene in the air was 8 to 11 times greater than in rural areas. Elsewhere, it has also been found that the concentration of benzpyrene in smog-filled air was about four times greater than in ordinary air. In short, the atmosphere of the modern industrial community is a carcinogenic sea, polluted and made murky by many sorts of individual waste. In such an environment it is hardly possible to avoid daily contact with cancer-producing agents. Such contamination may have contributed to the increase in cancer as a cause of death during the past 50 years. However, inherent difficulties have so far prevented a full epidemiological and technical solution of the problem. The causes of atmospheric pollution are many and complex, adequate standards and measuring instruments are still being developed, and a large number of interests, governmental, business, and industrial, are involved. Legislative control is still in the earliest stages. California enacted the most extensive legislation in 1947. A few cities, notably Pittsburgh, have been active in seeking to reduce air pollution. It is obvious, however, that this is an area for research and action.

In the same category is the new and important field of radiological health. The disposal of radioactive wastes, protection against damaging radiation, the creation of healthful conditions for workers engaged in the production of power from nuclear energy, or in research involving nuclear processes, as well as activities still to come indicate that this will be of increasing importance for community health in the immediate future.

Then there is the problem of housing. The health aspects of the home are manifold and are still quite unexplored. Recent work in social and preventive medicine has laid renewed emphasis on the importance of the family in the promotion of health and the prevention and treatment of sickness. A Committee on the Hygiene of Housing was established in 1937 by the American Public Health Association, and over the past 20 years this group has studied the components of healthful housing in terms of physical, physiological, and psychological needs. Much research is still needed on the effects of unsatisfactory housing on health. Nevertheless, there is a good deal of evidence to show that overcrowded, deteriorated housing is closely associated with physical and mental ill health. The problem of housing, like that of medical care, is fundamentally economic. The provision of decent housing for slum dwellers has been undertaken in many industrial countries by a system of government subsidy for low-rent housing.

The Federal government first provided public housing in 1918 when the United States Shipping Board and the United States Housing Corporation (in the Department of Labor) built 16,000 units for war workers. After the First World War, this housing was sold to private owners, but with the emergency of the depression more public housing came into existence. The Emergency Relief and Construction Act of 1932, a product of the Hoover Administration, authorized Federal loans to certain corporations for the construction of houses. The following year the National Industrial Recovery Act provided for slum clearance and low-cost housing. During this period, the Public Works Administration built about 50 projects, amounting to well over 20,000 units in 30 cities. Then, in 1937, the National Housing Act was passed to encourage the creation by local communities of independent agencies, chartered by the states and empowered to receive Federal grants to build and manage housing. The major purpose of the Act was slum clearance. Between 1939 and 1942, about 170,000 dwelling units were built under this program in more than 260 communities.

During the Second World War, the Federal government financed the building for civilians of 805,000 units of housing, of which 195,000 were of permanent construction. Much of this was built and managed for the Federal government by local authorities. Finally, several lines of policy development were brought together in the Housing Act of 1949, which authorized loans and subsidies as well as Federal credit for the development of vacant land. By November 30, 1953, about 110,000 units had been completed, more were under construction, and sites had been approved for 263,875 units in 1761 projects.

This has not been a startling achievement, but it must be seen in the light of a number of interacting factors. The period following the Second World War has been one of increasing conservatism in social policy. Some communities readily accepted all the housing they could get, while in others bitter controversy retarded or prevented such action. Opponents of public housing introduced such questions as the maintenance of racial segregation, especially after the Supreme Court in 1948 acted against racially restrictive covenants. Other trends also began to make themselves felt. The 1950 census showed that for the first time since industrialization began in America, more people owned homes than rented them. The trend is also connected with the trek to suburbia, which will be considered shortly. This is part of a wave of prosperity that developed since the war and changed the views of many people.

Despite the creation of low-cost housing, slums remain and the problem of housing is one with which health workers most concern themselves. However, it must be made clear that housing is a complex problem that involves governmental action on various levels as well as participation of agencies concerned not only with health, but also fire protection, traffic engineering, schools, recreation, and others. Nevertheless, the modern health department should have a thorough knowledge of the housing of the community.

One of the outstanding features of modern American life is the extensive movement of peoples from one place to another by some form of transportation. The most important element in this development has been the internal combustion engine. By permitting people to move to the fringe of the urban community, or even beyond, a sizable portion of the American population today lives in suburban communities. At the time of the 1950 census, approximately 20,900,000 people lived in such areas. These communities are of concern to the modern health worker because frequently, if they are new, they are apt to suffer from inadequate provision of water, sewerage, recreation, street lights, and other public services. Furthermore, both old and new suburban communities are often governed by antiquated political and administrative jurisdictions unable to develop and finance community services regarded as necessary.

Closely related to both housing and the internal combustion engine, in the form of the motor vehicle, is the problem of accidents. At present in the United States, about 11 people are killed every hour, and 1210 are injured. Accidents involving motor vehicles tend to attract and monopolize public attention. Actually, accidents in the home outnumber those involving automobiles. On the other hand, occupational injuries and deaths are declining. As an important community health problem, public health agencies have begun to study accidents and their prevention. Epidemiology, statistical analysis, health education, safety engineering, mental hygiene, and many other fields of health action are being brought to bear on this problem.

The question of mental health has been found to be intimately involved not only with accident prevention, but also with many other community health problems. When the "mental hygiene" movement was launched following the publication of Clifford Beers's courageous autobiography, it was practically concerned with improving the institutional care of the mentally ill. To do this, appalling conditions in psychiatric asylums were uncovered, community pressure was brought to bear on legislative and administrative bodies, and conspicuous improvements were achieved. Credit for this goes to the National Committee for Mental Hygiene, created in 1909, and the various state and local groups affiliated with it. The intervening years have seen an increasing expansion in the number and variety of activities and facilities loosely ranged under the overarching rubric "mental hygiene." From the care of the mentally ill, interest and attention have shifted to the possible prevention and control of mental disease. It has been only recently, however, that governmental action has been taken. The passage in 1946 of the National Mental Health Act provided a great stimulus to mental health programs and activities in the states, by providing grants-in-aid for research, training of personnel, and the establishment and development of community mental health programs. The great interest shown in the community mental health program is an increasingly prominent trend, and health workers have to be trained to work successfully in such an endeavor. There is also a great need for research in this area. Until now, the problem of the criteria to be used in defining mental health and disease has remained in the background. No definite answer has yet been found, and it remains for the future to see how it can be solved.

To deal with these matters as well as with those discussed in preceding chapters, trained personnel are needed. It is presently recognized that we have a deficit in this respect, and the Federal government as well as other agencies are now endeavoring to recruit new workers for the field of public health. Today, it is possible to do so because there are 10 schools of public health in the United States accredited to grant degrees in this field. Actually, this is a recent development that has occurred over the past 40 odd years. Until 1910, there were no facilities for the training of public health workers in the United States. In that year the University of Michigan awarded the first specific public health degree. The first school, however, was organized in 1912 by William T. Sedgwick at the Massachusetts Institute of Technology. In 1913, Sedgwick joined forces with Milton J. Rosenau, professor of preventive medicine at the Harvard Medical School, and George C. Whipple, statistician and sanitary engineer, also of Harvard, to form a school of public health. In 1918, the Johns Hopkins School of Hygiene was opened with William H. Welch as its first director. It had been envisioned by him as an institution for the training of public health personnel, and also as contributing to the training of physicians going into medical practice. While it did not entirely realize his goals, this school set the pattern for the training of American public health workers up to the present. Within the last decade, however, as the problems of community health have begun to change, the schools have also begun to reorient themselves to the future. The professionalization of public health has been enhanced as well by several recent developments. In 1945, a system of accreditation of schools of public health was set up under the aegis of the American Public Health Association. Four years later, a specialty board, the American Board of Preventive Medicine and Public Health, was established so that medical men in the field of public health could stand among their fellow physicians on an equivalent basis of specialization.

We are now in a position to look back and to see clearly the road that has been traversed in dealing with the health problems of the community. The manner in which these have been handled has always been connected with the way of life of the community and the scientific and technical knowledge available to it. Today, the community is in a better position than ever before to control its environment and so to preserve health and avert disease. More and more, man can consciously plan and organize his campaign for better health because available knowledge and resources make it possible for him in many instances to act with a clear understanding of what he is doing. This does not imply that there are no more problems. Indeed, the worker in the field of community health might well agree with Tennyson:

Yet all experience is an arch wherethro'
Gleams that untravell'd world, whose margin fades
Forever and forever when I move.

Many health problems have been solved in theory, and this knowledge awaits application in practice. This is true of much preventable ill health in all countries and particularly in underdeveloped lands. In all countries there are problems of community health that require social and political action guided by available knowledge. This is true of such matters as the provision of public health services or the organization of medical care. Furthermore, the horizon of health workers today can no longer be limited to the local or even the national community but must extend to the international community. Today, we are all members one of another; and so each in our own community, we must strive toward a goal of freedom from disease, want, and fear. We must strive to enhance and hand on the noble legacy that has come down to us. And may the outcome be a happy one!

Access to Primary Sources in the History of Public Health

A vast number of books have been scanned and made available online since 1993, when a bibliography of primary sources in public health was published in the expanded edition of George Rosen's *A History of Public Health*. In particular, several leading medical history collections have collaborated to create the online Medical Heritage Library (www.medical heritage.org). The home page of the Medical Heritage Library provides the means to search for rare books and other historical books in the catalogs of the

U.S. National Library of Medicine
Countway Library of Medicine at Harvard University
Library of the New York Academy of Medicine
Library of the College of Physicians of Philadelphia
Cushing/Whitney Medical Library at Yale University
Welch Medical Library at Johns Hopkins University
Wellcome Library (London, UK)

as well as in smaller historical and archival collections at other institutions in the United States and Canada.

As of 2014, virtually all printed material published in 1923 or earlier is in the public domain, which means it can be freely copied (including by digital scanning) and made available online. All public domain material scanned as part of the Medical Heritage Library is being mounted by the Internet Archive (www.archive.org). The Internet Archive provides page images in a number of formats, as well as in several formats that are accessible nonvisually, using text-to-speech screen readers.

There are other sources of full-text scanned historical books available online, most notably Google Books (books.google.com). Google Books and others sources may provide access to some items that are not part of the Medical Heritage Library. Those associated with institutions whose libraries have contracts with Google Books, UPCC, or J-STOR (for periodicals) may also have access to digital editions of material that is copyright protected.

This edition of George Rosen's *A History of Public Health* forgoes a selected list of primary sources. Instead the editors urge interested readers to search for primary sources in the Medical Heritage Library and other online sources.

Classified Bibliography of Secondary Sources

This bibliography lists the major English-language book-length works on aspects of the history of public health originally cited by George Rosen in 1958. In addition, it incorporates a large sample of significant books in English on public health history published between 1958 and 2014. As interest in the history of public health has grown significantly over the past two decades, the majority of the works cited were published since 1993.

This bibliography is organized according to the following classification:

I.   General
II. Specific diseases
   a. AIDS; Other Sexually Transmitted Diseases
   b. Anthrax
   c. Beriberi
   d. Bilharzia; Schistosomiasis
   e. Cancer
   f. Cholera
   g. Diphtheria
   h. Hookworm
   i. Influenza
   j. Leprosy
   k. Malaria
   l. Measles
   m. Pellagra
   n. Plague
   o. Polio
   p. Rabies
   q. Rheumatic Fever
   r. SARS
   s. Scurvy
   t. Sickle-Cell Anemia
   u. Smallpox
   v. Trypanosomiasis
   w. Tuberculosis
   x. Typhoid Fever
   y. Typhus
   z. Yellow Fever
III. Historical periods before 1801
   a. Ancient; before 500 CE
   b. European Middle Ages; Other Parts of the World: 500 to 1450
   c. European Renaissance; Early Modern Europe; Other Parts of the World: 1450 to 1800
IV. Geographical divisions
   a. United States
   b. Canada
   c. Minorities, Immigration, Race, and Health in North America

Each item is cited only once, under the most pertinent subject heading, with cross-references provided to other relevant subjects. Since the overwhelming majority of entries deal with the nineteenth, twentieth, and twenty-first centuries, these eras are excluded from the chronological listing (III). Similarly, since most of the books deal with the United States or Great Britain and Ireland, there are no cross-references to or from the subject headings "United States" or "Ireland and Great Britain." All items that deal with the period since 1800—or with specific diseases or areas of public health concern in the United States, Great Britain or Ireland—are listed only under the specific disease or area of concern. Likewise, materials about pre-modern Europe are cited under relevant diseases and areas of concern, and in the appropriate chronological category, but not under "Europe" in the geographical listings.

This bibliography was derived from the LocatorPlus database maintained by the U.S. National Library of Medicine (NLM). LocatorPlus will remain the best source for citations to books published in 2014 and later. The NLM's companion database, PUBMED, should be utilized for citations to journal articles and other sources. When searching either of these databases for secondary historical material, the word "history" should be included as a MESH subject heading.

I. GENERAL

1. Ackerknecht, Erwin. *A History and Geography of the Most Important Diseases.* New York: Hafner, 1965.
2. Alchon, Suzanne. *A Pest in the Land: New World Epidemics in a Global Perspective.* Albuquerque: University of New Mexico Press, 2003.
3. Bashford, Alison, and Claire Hooker, eds. *Contagion: Historical and Cultural Studies.* New York: Routledge, 2001.
4. Berridge, Virginia, Martin Gorsky, and Alex Mold. *Public Health in History.* Maidenhead, Berkshire, UK: Open University Press, 2011.
5. Bollet, Alfred J. *Plagues and Poxes: The Impact of Human History on Epidemic Disease.* New York: Demos, 2004.
6. Brandt, Allan, and Paul Rozin. *Morality and Health.* New York: Routledge, 1997.
7. Cohen, Mark Nathan. *Health and the Rise of Civilization.* New Haven, CT: Yale University Press, 1989.
8. Crosby, Alfred W., Jr. *Ecological Imperialism: The Biological Expansion of Europe, 900–1900.* New York: Cambridge University Press, 1986.
9. Goodall, Edward Wilberforce. *A Short History of the Epidemic Infectious Diseases.* London: Bale & Danielsson, 1934.
10. Greenblatt, Charles, and Mark Spigelman. *Emerging Pathogens: The Archaeology, Ecology, and Evolution of Infectious Disease.* New York: Oxford University Press, 2003.
11. Harrison, Mark. *Contagion: How Commerce Has Spread Disease.* New Haven, CT: Yale University Press, 2012.
12. Hays, J. N. *The Burdens of Disease: Epidemics and Human Response in Western History.* New Brunswick, NJ: Rutgers University Press, 2009.
13. Herring, D. Ann, and Alan C. Swedlund. *Plagues and Epidemics: Infected Spaces Past and Present.* Oxford: Berg, 2010.
14. Kiple, Kenneth. *Plagues, Pox, and Pestilence.* London: Weidenfeld & Nicolson, 1997.
15. Kohn, George C. *Encyclopedia of Plague and Pestilence: From Ancient Times to the Present.* Rev. ed. New York: Facts on File, 2001.
16. McGuire, Robert, and Philip R.P. Coelho. *Parasites, Pathogens, and Progress: Diseases and Economic Development.* Cambridge MA: MIT Press, 2011.
17. McKeown, Thomas. *The Origins of Human Disease.* New York: Basil Blackwell, 1988.
18. McKeown, Thomas. *The Role of Medicine: Dream, Mirage, or Nemesis?* Princeton, NJ: Princeton University Press, 1979.
19. McNeill, William H. *Plagues and Peoples.* Garden City, NY: Anchor Press, 1976.
20. Newman, George. *The Rise of Preventive Medicine.* London: Oxford University Press, 1932.

21. Ogawa, Teizo, ed. *Public Health*. Tokyo: Saikon, 1981.

22. Oldstone, Michael B. A. *Viruses, Plagues, and History: Past, Present, and Future*. Rev. and updated ed. New York: Oxford University Press, 2010.

23. Packard, Randall M., Peter J. Brown, Ruth Berkelman, and Howard Frumkin, eds. 2004. *Emerging Illnesses and Society: Negotiating the Public Health Agenda*. Baltimore: Johns Hopkins University Press, 2004.

24. Porter, Dorothy. *Health, Civilization, and the State: A History of Public Health from Ancient to Modern Times*. New York: Routledge, 1999.

25. Riley, James C. *Rising Life Expectancy: A Global History*. New York: Cambridge University Press, 2001.

26. Rodríguez-Ocaña, Esteban. *The Politics of the Healthy Life: An International Perspective*. Sheffield, UK: European Association for the History of Medicine and Health Publications, 2002.

27. Rothstein, William G. *Public Health and the Risk Factor: A History of an Uneven Medical Revolution*. Rochester, NY: University of Rochester Press, 2003.

28. Rosen, George. *From Medical Police to Social Medicine: Essays on the History of Health Care*. New York: Science History Publications, 1974.

29. Sigerist, Henry E. *Civilization and Disease*. Ithaca, NY: Cornell University Press, 1941.

30. Sigerist, Henry E. *Landmarks in the History of Hygiene*. New York: Oxford University Press, 1956.

31. Spink, Wesley. *Infectious Diseases: Prevention and Treatment in the Nineteenth and Twentieth Centuries*. Minneapolis: University of Minnesota Press, 1978.

32. Sprinkle, Robert Hunt. *Profession of Conscience: The Making and Meaning of Life Science Liberalism*. Princeton, NJ: Princeton University Press, 1994.

33. Steckel, Richard H., and Roderick Floud. *Health and Welfare during Industrialization*. Chicago: University of Chicago Press, 1997.

34. Szreter, Simon. *Health and Wealth: Studies in History and Policy*. Rochester, NY: University of Rochester Press, 2005.

35. Tulchinsky, Thodore H., and Elena A. Varavikova. *The New Public Health: An Introduction for the 21st Century*. San Diego, CA: Academic Press, 2000.

36. Waitzkin, Howard. *Medicine and Public Health at the End of Empire*. Boulder, CO: Paradigm Publishers, 2011.

37. Watts, Sheldon. *Epidemics and History: Disease, Power, and Imperialism*. New Haven, CT: Yale University Press, 2007.

38. Webster, Charles, ed. *Caring for Health: History and Diversity*. Philadelphia: Open University, 2001.

39. Winslow, Charles-Edward Amory. *The Conquest of Epidemic Disease: A Chapter in the History of Ideas*. Princeton, NJ: Princeton University Press, 1943.

40. Winslow, Charles-Edward Amory. *The Evolution and Significance of the Modern Public Health Campaign*. New Haven, CT: Yale University Press, 1923.

II. SPECIFIC DISEASES

AIDS; Other Sexually Transmitted Diseases (see also 224, 284, 294, 295, 343, 353, 470, 493, 564, and 690)

41. Aisenberg, Andrew R. *Contagion: Disease, Government, and the "Social Question" in Nineteenth-Century France*. Stanford, CA: Stanford University Press, 1999.

42. Baldwin, Peter. *Disease and Democracy: The Industrialized World Faces AIDS*. New York: Milbank Memorial Fund, 2005.

43. Bayer, Ronald. *Private Acts, Social Consequences: AIDS and the Politics of Public Health*. New York: Free Press, 1989.

44. Behrman, Greg. *The Invisible People: How the U.S. Has Slept through the Global AIDS Pandemic, the Greatest Humanitarian Catastrophe of Our Time*. New York: Free Press, 2004.

45. Berridge, Virginia. *AIDS in the UK: The Making of Policy*. New York: Oxford University Press, 1996.

46. Berridge, Virginia, and Philip Strong, eds. *AIDS and Contemporary History*. New York: Cambridge University Press, 1993.

47. Brandt, Allan M. *No Magic Bullet: A Social History of Venereal Disease in the United States since 1880*. Expanded ed. New York: Oxford University Press, 1987.

48. Brier, Jennifer. *Infectious Ideas: U.S. Political Responses to the AIDS Crisis*. Chapel Hill: University of North Carolina Press, 2009.

49. Cassel, Jay. *The Secret Plague: Venereal Disease in Canada, 1838–1939*. Toronto: University of Toronto Press, 1987.

50. Cochrane, Michelle. *When AIDS Began: San Francisco and the Making of an Epidemic*. New York: Routledge, 2004.

51. Fee, Elizabeth, and Daniel M. Fox, eds. *AIDS: The Burdens of History*. Berkeley: University of California Press, 1988.

52. Fee, Elizabeth, and Daniel M. Fox, eds. *AIDS: The Making of a Chronic Disease*. Berkeley: University of California Press, 1992.

53. Gostin, Lawrence O. *The AIDS Pandemic: Complacency, Injustice, and Unfulfilled Expectations*. Chapel Hill: University of North Carolina Press, 2004.

54. Gostin, Lawrence O., and Zita Lazzarini. *Human Rights and Public Health in the AIDS Pandemic*. Oxford: Oxford University Press, 1997.

55. Gould, Deborah. *Moving Politics: Emotion and ACT UP's Fight against AIDS*. Chicago: University of Chicago Press, 2009.

56. Grady, Christine. *The Search for an AIDS Vaccine: Ethical Issues in the Development and Testing of a Preventive HIV Vaccine*. Bloomington: Indiana University Press, 1995.

57. Grmek, Mirko D. *History of AIDS: Emergence and Origin of a Modern Pandemic*. Princeton, NJ: Princeton University Press, 1990.

58. Holmberg, Scott. *Scientific Errors and Controversies in the U.S. HIV/AIDS Epidemic: How They Slowed Advances and Were Resolved*. Westport, CT: Praeger, 2008.

59. Inrig, Stephen. *North Carolina & the Problem of AIDS: Advocacy, Politics, & Race in the South*. Chapel Hill: University of North Carolina Press, 2011.

60. Kirp, David L., and Ronald Bayer, eds. *AIDS in the Industrialized Democracies: Passions, Politics, and Policies*. New Brunswick, NJ: Rutgers University Press, 1992.

61. Lord, Alexandra. *Condom Nation: The U.S. Government's Sex Education Campaign from World War I to the Internet*. Baltimore: Johns Hopkins University Press, 2010.

62. Mack, Arien, ed. *In Time of Plague: The History and Social Consequences of Lethal Epidemic Disease*. New York: New York University Press, 1991.

63. Mott, Frank. *Dangerous Sexualities: Medico-Moral Politics in England since 1830*. London: New York: Routledge, 2000.

64. Nguyen, Vinh-Kim. *The Republic of Therapy: Triage and Sovereignty in West Africa's Time of AIDS*. Durham, NC: Duke University Press, 2010.

65. Powell, Mary, and Della Cook. *The Myth of Syphilis: The Natural History of Treponematosis in North America*. Gainesville: University Press of Florida, 2005.

66. Quetel, Claude. *History of Syphilis*. Baltimore: Johns Hopkins University Press, 1990.

Anthrax (see also 403)

67. Jones, Susan D. *Death in a Small Package: A Short History of Anthrax*. Baltimore: Johns Hopkins University Press, 2010.

Beriberi (see "East and Southeast Asia")
Bilharzia; Schistosomiasis

68. Crichton-Harris, Ann. *Poison in Small Measure: Dr. Christopherson and the Cure for Bilharzia*. Boston: Brill, 2009.

69. Farley, John. *Bilharzia: A History of Imperial Tropical Medicine*. New York: Cambridge University Press, 1991.

Cancer (see also "Tobacco Use and Control"; and 631)

70. Aronowitz, Robert. *Unnatural History: Breast Cancer and American Society*. New York: Cambridge University Press, 2007.

71. Ball, Howard. *Cancer Factories: America's Tragic Quest for Uranium Self-Sufficiency*. Westport, CT: Greenwood Press, 1993.

72. Cairns, John. *Matters of Life and Death: Perspectives on Public Health, Molecular Biology, Cancer and Prospects for the Human Race*. Princeton, NJ: Princeton University Press, 1997.

73. Cantor, David, ed. *Cancer in the Twentieth Century*. Baltimore: Johns Hopkins University Press, 2008.

74. Clow, Barbara. *Negotiating Disease: Power and Cancer Care, 1900–1950*. Montreal: McGill-Queen's University Press.

75. Davis, Devra. *The Secret History of the War on Cancer*. New York: Basic Books, 2007.

76. Gardner, Kirsten. *Early Detection: Women, Cancer, & Awareness Campaigns in the Twentieth-Century United States*. Chapel Hill: University of North Carolina Press, 2006.

77. Hayter, Charles. *An Element of Hope: Radium and the Response to Cancer in Canada, 1900–1940*. Montreal: McGill-Queen's University Press, 2005.

78. Kaartinen, Marjo. *Breast Cancer in the Eighteenth Century*. London: Pickering & Chatto, 2013.

79. Kutcher, Gerald. *Contested Medicine: Cancer Research and the Military*. Chicago: University of Chicago Press, 2009.

80. Lerner, Barron. *The Breast Cancer Wars: Hope, Fear and the Pursuit of a Cure in Twentieth-Century America*. New York: Oxford University Press, 2001.

81. Ley, Barbara L. *From Pink to Green: Disease Prevention and the Environmental Breast Cancer Movement*. New Brunswick, NJ: Rutgers University Press, 2009.

82. Leopold, Ellen. *Under the Radar: Cancer and the Cold War*. New Brunswick, NJ: Rutgers University Press, 2009.

83. Löwy, Ilana. *A Woman's Disease: The History of Cervical Cancer.* Oxford: Oxford University Press, 2011.

84. Marcus, Alan. *Cancer from Beef: DES, Federal Food Regulation, and Consumer Confidence.* Baltimore: Johns Hopkins University Press, 1994.

85. Mukherjee, Siddhartha. *The Emperor of All Maladies: A Biography of Cancer.* New York: Scribner, 2010.

86. Olson, James S. *Bathsheba's Breast: Women, Cancer, and History.* Baltimore: Johns Hopkins University Press, 2002.

87. Patterson, James T. *The Dread Disease: Cancer and Modern American Culture.* Cambridge, MA: Harvard University Press, 1987.

88. Proctor, Robert. *The Nazi War on Cancer.* Princeton, NJ: Princeton University Press, 1999.

89. Rettig, Richard A. 1977. *Cancer Crusade: The Story of the National Cancer Act of 1971.* Princeton, NJ: Princeton University Press, 1977.

90. Wailoo, Keith. *How Cancer Crossed the Color Line.* Oxford: Oxford University Press, 2011.

Cholera (see also 401, 486, and 608)

91. Bilson, Geoffrey. *A Darkened House: Cholera in Nineteenth-Century Canada.* Toronto: University of Toronto Press, 1980.

92. Briggs, Charles L., and Clara Mantini-Briggs. *Stories in the Time of Cholera: Racial Profiling during a Medical Nightmare.* Berkeley: University of California Press, 2003.

93. Chambers, John Sharpe. *The Conquest of Cholera.* New York: Macmillan, 1938.

94. Delaporte, François. *Disease and Civilization: The Cholera in Paris, 1832.* Cambridge, MA: MIT Press, 1986.

95. Longmate, Norman. *King Cholera: The Biography of a Disease.* London: Hamish Hamilton, 1966.

96. McGrew, Roderick E. *Russia and the Cholera, 1823–1832.* Madison: University of Wisconsin Press, 1965.

97. McLean, David. *Public Health and Politics in the Age of Reform: Cholera, the State, and the Royal Navy in Victorian Britain.* New York: Palgrave Macmillan, 2006.

98. Pelling, Margaret. *Cholera, Fever and English Medicine, 1825–1865.* New York: Oxford University Press, 1978.

99. Rosenberg, Charles E. *The Cholera Years: The United States in 1832, 1849, and 1866.* Chicago: University of Chicago Press, 1962. Reprint, with a new afterword by the author. Chicago: University of Chicago Press, 1987.

Diphtheria

100. Caulfield, Ernest. *A True History of the Terrible Epidemic Vulgarly Called the Throat Distemper Which Occurred in His Majesty's New England Colonies between the Years 1735 and 1740.* New Haven, CT: Yale Journal of Biology & Medicine, 1939.

101. Hammonds, Evelynn. *Childhood's Deadly Scourge: The Campaign to Control Diphtheria in New York City, 1880–1930.* Baltimore: Johns Hopkins University Press, 1999.

Hookworm

102. Ettling, John. *The Germ of Laziness: Rockefeller Philanthropy and Public Health in the New South.* Cambridge, MA: Harvard University Press, 1981.

Influenza (see also 621)

103. Blakely, Debra. *Mass Mediated Disease: A Case Study Analysis of Three Flu Pandemics and Public Health Policy.* Lanham, MD: Lexington Books, 2006.

104. Bristow, Nancy. *American Pandemic: The Lost Worlds of the 1918 Influenza Epidemic.* New York: Oxford University Press, 2012.

105. Crosby, Alfred W. *America's Forgotten Pandemic: The Influenza of 1918.* 2nd ed. New York: Cambridge University Press, 2003.

106. Davis, Ryan. *The Spanish Flu: Narrative and Cultural Identity in Spain, 1918.* New York: Palgrave Macmillan, 2013.

107. Dehner, George. *Influenza: A Century of Science and Public Health Response.* Pittsburgh, PA: University of Pittsburgh Press, 2012.

108. Farni, Magda, and Esyllt W. Jones, eds. *Epidemic Encounters: Influenza, Society and Culture in Canada, 1918–1920.* Vancouver: University of British Columbia Press, 2012.

109. Giles-Vernick, Tamara, Susan Craddock, and Jennifer Lee Gunn, eds. *Influenza and Public Health: Learning from Past Pandemics.* London: Earthscan, 2010.

110. Honigsbaum, Mark. *Living with Enza: The Forgotten Story of Britain and the Great Flu Epidemic of 1918.* New York: Macmillan, 2009.

111. Humphries, Mark Osborne. *The Last Plague: Spanish Influenza and the Politics of Public Health in Canada.* Toronto: University of Toronto Press, 2013.

112. Johnson, Niall. *Britain and the 1918–19 Influenza Pandemic: A Dark Epilogue.* New York: Routledge, 2006.

113. Patterson, K. David. *Pandemic Influenza, 1700–1900: A Study in Historical Epidemiology.* Totowa, NJ: Rowman & Littlefield, 1986.

114. Rice, Geoffrey. *Black November, the 1918 Influenza Epidemic in New Zealand.* Wellington, NZ: Allen & Unwin, 1988.

115. Silverstein, Arthur M. *Pure Politics and Impure Science: The Swine Flu Affair.* Baltimore: Johns Hopkins University Press, 1981.

Leprosy

116. Demaitre, Luke. *Leprosy in Premodern Medicine: A Malady of the Whole Body.* Baltimore: Johns Hopkins University Press, 2007.

117. Gussow, Zachary. *Leprosy, Racism, and Public Health: Social Policy in Chronic Disease Control.* Boulder, CO: Westview, 1989.

Malaria (see also 258, 364, 379, 519, and 521)

118. Akhtar, Rais, Ashok K. Dutt, and Vandana Wadhwa, eds. *Malaria in South Asia: Eradication and Resurgence during the Second Half of the Twentieth Century.* New York: Springer, 2010.

119. Bell, Andrew M. *Mosquito Soldiers: Malaria, Yellow Fever, and the Course of the American Civil War.* Baton Rouge: Louisiana State University Press, 2010.

120. Bruce-Chwatt, Leonard Jan, and Julian de Zulueta. *The Rise and Fall of Malaria in Europe: A Historico-Epidemiological Study.* New York: Oxford University Press, 1981.

121. Carter, Eric. *Enemy in the Blood: Malaria, Environment, and Development in Argentina.* Tuscaloosa: University of Alabama Press, 2012.

122. Cueto, Marcos. *Cold War, Deadly Fevers: Malaria Eradication in Mexico, 1955–1975.* Baltimore: Johns Hopkins University Press, 2007.

123. Humphreys, Margaret. *Malaria: Poverty, Race, and Public Health in the United States.* Baltimore: Johns Hopkins University Press, 2001.

124. Kazi, Ihtesham. *A Historical Study of Malaria in Bengal.* Dhaka, Bangladesh: Pip, 2004.

125. Packard, Randall. *The Making of a Tropical Disease: A Short History of Malaria.* Baltimore: Johns Hopkins University Press, 2007.

126. Slater, Leo. *War and Disease: Biomedical Research on Malaria in the Twentieth Century.* New Brunswick, NJ: Rutgers University Press, 2009.

127. Snowden, Frank N. *The Conquest of Malaria: Italy, 1900–1962.* New Haven, CT: Yale University Press, 2006.

128. Webb, James. *Humanity's Burden: A Global History of Malaria.* New York, NJ: Cambridge University Press, 2009.

129. Webb, James. *The Long Struggle against Malaria in Africa.* New York: Cambridge University Press, 2014.

Measles (see 605)

Pellagra

130. Etheridge, Elizabeth W. *The Butterfly Caste: A Social History of Pellagra in the South.* Westport, CT: Greenwood Press, 1972.

131. Kraut, Alan. *Goldberger's War: The Life and Work of a Public Health Crusader.* New York: Hill and Wang, 2003.

132. Roe, Daphne A. *A Plague of Corn: The Social History of Pellagra.* Ithaca, NY: Cornell University Press, 1973.

Plague (see also "European Middle Ages"; and 277, 285, 287, and 511)

133. Alexander, J. T. *Bubonic Plague in Early Modern Russia: Public Health and Urban Disaster.* Baltimore: Johns Hopkins University Press, 1980.

134. Benedict, Carol. *Bubonic Plague in Nineteenth-Century China.* Stanford, CA: Stanford University Press, 1996.

135. Benedictow, Ole. *What Disease Was Plague? On the Controversy over the Microbiological Identity of Plague Epidemics of the Past.* Boston: Brill, 2010.

136. Borsch, Stuart. *The Black Death in Egypt and England: A Comparative Study.* Austin: University of Texas Press, 2005.

137. Bowers, Kristy Wilson. *Plague and Public Health in Early Modern Seville.* Rochester, NY: University of Rochester Press, 2013.

138. Bulmus, Birsen. *Plague, Quarantines, and Geopolitics in the Ottoman Empire.* Edinburgh: Edinburgh University Press, 2012.

139. Byrne, Joseph. *Encyclopedia of the Black Death.* Santa Barbara, CA: ABC-CLIO, 2012.

140. Calvi, Giulia. *Histories of a Plague Year: The Social and the Imaginary in Baroque Florence.* Berkeley: University of California Press, 1989.

141. Campbell, Anna Montgomery. *The Black Death and Men of Learning.* New York: Columbia University Press, 1931. Reprint. New York: AMS Press, 1966.

142. Cantor, Norman. *In the Wake of the Plague: The Black Death and the World It Made.* New York: Free Press, 2001.

143. Carmichael, Ann G. *Plague and the Poor in Early Renaissance Florence.* New York: Cambridge University Press, 1986.

144. Chase, Marilyn. *The Barbary Plague: The Black Death in Victorian San Francisco.* New York: Random House, 2003.

145. Christakos, George. *Interdisciplinary Public Health Reasoning and Epidemic Modeling: The Case of Black Death.* New York: Springer, 2005.

146. Cipolla, Carlo M. *Cristofano and the Plague: A Study in the History of Public Health in the Age of Galileo.* Berkeley: University of California Press, 1973.

147. Cipolla, Carlo M. *Faith, Reason, and the Plague in Seventeenth-Century Tuscany.* Ithaca, NY: Cornell University Press, 1979.

148. Cipolla, Carlo M. *Fighting the Plague in Seventeenth-Century Italy.* Madison: University of Wisconsin Press, 1981.

149. Cohn, Samuel. *Cultures of Plague: Medical Thinking at the End of the Renaissance.* New York: Oxford University Press, 2010.

150. Cook, Alexandra, and Noble Cook. *The Plague Files: Crisis Management in Sixteenth-Century Seville.* Baton Rouge: Louisiana State University Press, 2009.

151. Echenberg, Myron. *Plague Ports: The Global Urban Impact of Bubonic Plague, 1894–1901.* New York: New York University Press, 2007.

152. Echenberg, Myron. *Black Death, White Medicine: Bubonic Plague and the Politics of Public Health in Colonial Senegal, 1914–1945.* Portsmouth, NH: Heinemann, 2002.

153. Frandsen, Karl-Erik. *The Last Plague in the Baltic Region 1709–1713.* Copenhagen: Museum Tusculanum Press, 2010.

154. Herlihy, David. *The Black Death and the Transformation of the West.* Cambridge, MA: Harvard University Press, 1997.

155. Hirst, L. Fabian. *The Conquest of Plague: A Study of the Evolution of Epidemiology.* Oxford: Clarendon Press, 1953.

156. Mohr, James. *Plague and Fire: Battling Black Death and the 1900 Burning of Honolulu's Chinatown.* New York: Oxford University Press, 2005.

157. Moote, A. Lloyd, and Dorothy Moote. *The Great Plague: The Story of London's Most Deadly Year.* Baltimore: Johns Hopkins University Press, 2004.

158. Nutton, Vivian, ed. *Pestilential Complexities: Understanding Medieval Plague.* London: Wellcome Trust Centre for the History of Medicine at UCL, 2008.

159. Shrewsbury, J. F. D. *A History of Bubonic Plague in the British Isles.* London: Cambridge University Press, 1970.

160. Slack, Paul. *The Impact of the Plague in Tudor and Stuart England.* London: Routledge & Kegan Paul, 1985.

161. Slack, Paul. *Plague: A Very Short Introduction.* New York: Oxford University Press, 2012.

162. Summers, William C. *The Great Manchurian Plague of 1910–1911: The Geopolitics of an Epidemic Disease.* New Haven, CT: Yale University Press, 2012.

163. Wilson, F. P. *The Plague in Shakespeare's London.* Oxford: Clarendon Press, 1927.

Polio

164. Daniel, Thomas, and Frederick Robbins, eds. *Polio.* Rochester, NY: University of Rochester Press, 1997.

165. Gould, Tony. *A Summer Plague: Polio and Its Survivors.* New Haven, CT: Yale University Press, 1995.

166. Kluger, Jeffrey. *Splendid Solution: Jonas Salk and the Conquest of Polio.* New York: Putnam's, 2004.

167. Offit, Paul. *The Cutter Incident: How America's First Polio Vaccine Led to the Growing Vaccine Crisis.* New Haven, CT: Yale University Press, 2005.

168. Oshinsky, Peter. *Polio: An American Story.* New York: Oxford University Press, 2005.

169. Rogers, Naomi. *Dirt and Disease: Polio before FDR.* New Brunswick, NJ: Rutgers University Press, 1992.

170. Seytrem, Bernard, and Mary Shaffer. *The Death of a Disease: A History of the Eradication of Poliomyelitis.* New Brunswick, NJ: Rutgers University Press, 2005.

171. Smallman-Raynor, Matthew, et al. *Poliomyelitis: Emergence to Eradication.* New York: Oxford University Press, 2006.

172. Wilson, Daniel. *Polio.* Santa Barbara, CA: Greenwood Press / ABC-CLIO, 2009.

Rabies

173. Brown, Karen. *Mad Dogs and Meerkats: A History of Resurgent Rabies in Southern Africa.* Athens: Ohio University Press, 2011.

Rheumatic Fever

174. English, Peter. *Rheumatic Fever in America and Britain: A Biological, Epidemiological, and Medical History.* New Brunswick, NJ: Rutgers University Press, 1999.

SARS

175. Abraham, Thomas. *Twenty-First Century Plague: The Story of SARS.* Baltimore: Johns Hopkins University Press, 2005.

176. Brookes, Tim. *How the World Survived SARS: The First Epidemic of the 21st Century.* Washington, DC: American Public Health Association, 2005.

177. Duffin, Jaclyn, and Arthur Sweetman, eds. *SARS in Context: Memory, History, Policy.* Montreal: McGill-Queen's University Press, 2006.

178. Starling, Arthur. *Plague, SARS, and the Story of Medicine in Hong Kong.* Hong Kong: Hong Kong University Press, 2006.

Scurvy

179. Carpenter, Kenneth J. *The History of Scurvy and Vitamin C.* New York: Cambridge University Press, 1986.

180. Cuppage, Francis. *James Cook and the Conquest of Scurvy.* Westport, CT: Greenwood Press, 1994.

181. Foxhall, Katherine. *Health, Medicine, and the Sea: Australian Voyages, c. 1815–1860.* New York: Palgrave Macmillan, 2012.

182. Torck, Mathieu. *Avoiding the Dire Straits: An Inquiry into Food Provisions and Scurvy in the Maritime and Military History of China and Wider East Asia.* Wiesbaden, Germany: Harrassowitz, 2009.

Sickle-Cell Anemia

183. Nelson, Alondra. *Body and Soul: The Black Panther Party and the Fight against Medical Discrimination.* Minneapolis: University of Minnesota Press, 2011.

184. Tapper, Melbourne. *In the Blood: Sickle Cell Anemia and the Politics of Race.* Philadelphia: University of Pennsylvania Press, 1999.

185. Wailoo, Keith. *Dying in the City of the Blues: Sickle Cell Anemia and the Politics of Race and Health.* Chapel Hill: University of North Carolina Press, 2001.

Smallpox (see also 462, 523, and 551)

186. Blake, John B. *Benjamin Waterhouse and the Introduction of Vaccination: A Reappraisal.* Philadelphia: University of Pennsylvania Press, 1957.

187. Fenner, Frank, et al. *Smallpox and Its Eradication.* Geneva: World Health Organization, 1988.

188. Foege, William. *House on Fire: The Fight to Eradicate Smallpox.* Berkeley: University of California Press, 2011.

189. Henderson, Donald A. *Smallpox: The Death of a Disease; The Inside Story of Eradicating a Worldwide Killer.* Amherst, NY: Prometheus Books, 2009.

190. Hopkins, Donald. *The Greatest Killer: Smallpox in History.* Chicago: University of Chicago Press, 2002.

191. Koplow, David, ed. *Smallpox: The Fight to Eradicate a Global Scourge.* Berkeley: University of California Press, 2003.

192. Miller, Genevieve. *The Adoption of Inoculation for Smallpox in England and France.* Philadelphia: University of Pennsylvania Press, 1957.

193. Naono, Atsuko. *State of Vaccination: The Fight against Smallpox in Colonial Burma.* London: Wellcome Trust Centre for the History of Medicine at University College London, 2009.

194. Razzell, Peter. *The Conquest of Smallpox: The Impact of Inoculation on Smallpox Mortality in Eighteenth Century Britain.* 2nd ed. Firle, UK: Caliban Books, 2003.

195. Sköld, Peter. *The Two Faces of Smallpox: A Disease and Its Prevention in Eighteenth- and Nineteenth-Century Sweden.* Umeå: Demographic Data Base, Umeå University, 1996.

196. Smith, J. R. *The Speckled Monster: Smallpox in England, 1670–1970, with Particular Reference to Essex.* Chelmsford, England: Essex Record Office, 1987.

197. Tucker, Jonathan, and Raymond A. Zilinskas. *The 1971 Smallpox Epidemic in Aralsk, Kazakhstan, and the Soviet Biological Warfare Program.* Monterey, CA: Center for Nonproliferation Studies, Monterey Institute of International Studies, 2002.

198. Williamson, Stanley. *The Vaccination Controversy: The Rise, Reign, and Fall of Compulsory Vaccination for Smallpox.* Liverpool: Liverpool University Press, 2007.

Trypanosomiasis

199. Lyons, Maryinez. *The Colonial Disease: A Social History of Sleeping Sickness in Northern Zaire, 1900–1940.* New York: Cambridge University Press, 1992.

200. Hoppe, Kirk. *Lords of the Fly: Sleeping Sickness Control in British East Africa, 1900–1960.* Westport, CT: Praeger, 2003.

201. McKelvey, John J. *Man against Tsetse: Struggle for Africa.* Ithaca, NY: Cornell University Press, 1973.

202. Perleth, Matthias. *Historical Aspects of American Trypanosomiasis (Chagas' Disease).* Frankfurt am Main, Germany: P. Lang, 1997.

Tuberculosis (see also 347, 505, 680, and 930)

203. Abel, Emily. *Tuberculosis and the Politics of Exclusion: A History of Public Health and Migration to Los Angeles.* New Brunswick, NJ: Rutgers University Press, 2007.

204. Armus, Diego. *The Ailing City: Health, Tuberculosis and Culture in Buenos Aires, 1870–1950.* Durham, NC: Duke University Press, 2011.

205. Barnes, David. *The Making of a Social Disease: Tuberculosis in Nineteenth-Century France.* Berkeley: University of California Press, 1995.

206. Bates, Barbara. *Bargaining for Life: A Social History of Tuberculosis, 1876–1938.* Philadelphia: University of Pennsylvania Press, 1992.

207. Bryder, Linda. *Below the Magic Mountain: A Social History of Tuberculosis in Twentieth-Century Britain.* New York: Oxford University Press, 1988.

208. Bynum, Helen. *Spitting Blood: The History of Tuberculosis.* Oxford: Oxford University Press, 2012.

209. Caldwell, Mark. *The Last Crusade: The War on Consumption, 1862–1954.* New York: Atheneum, 1988.

210. Coker, Richard. *From Chaos to Coercion: Detention and the Control of Tuberculosis.* New York: St. Martin's Press, 2000.

211. Condrau, Flurin, and Michael Worboys. *Tuberculosis Then and Now: Perspectives on the History of an Infectious Disease.* Montreal: McGill-Queen's University Press, 2010.

212. Connolly, Cynthia. *Saving Sickly Children: The Tuberculosis Preventorium in American Life, 1909–1970.* New Brunswick, NJ: Rutgers University Press, 2008.

213. Craddock, Susan. *City of Plagues: Disease, Poverty, and Deviance in San Francisco.* Minneapolis: University of Minnesota Press, 2000.

214. Daniel, Thomas M. *Captain of Death: The Story of Tuberculosis.* Rochester, NY: University of Rochester Press, 1997.

215. Dubos, Rene J., and Dubos, Jean. *The White Plague: Tuberculosis, Man and Society.* Boston: Little, Brown, 1952. Reprint, with additional material. New Brunswick, NJ: Rutgers University Press, 1987.

216. Feldberg, Georgina. *Disease and Class: Tuberculosis and the Shaping of Modern North American Society.* New Brunswick, NJ: Rutgers University Press, 1995.

217. Fortuine, Robert. *"Must We All Die?": Alaska's Enduring Struggle with Tuberculosis.* Fairbanks: University of Alaska Press, 2005.

218. Grygier, Pat S. *A Long Way from Home: The Tuberculosis Epidemic among the Inuit.* Montreal: McGill-Queen's University Press, 1994.

219. Johnston, William. *The Modern Epidemic: A History of Tuberculosis in Japan.* Cambridge, MA: Harvard University Press, 1995.

220. Jones, Greta. *"Captain of All These Men of Death": The History of Tuberculosis in Nineteenth and Twentieth Century Ireland.* Amsterdam: Rodopi, 2001.

221. Kayne, G. Gregory. *The Control of Tuberculosis in England, Past and Present.* London: Oxford University Press, 1937.

222. Lerner, Barron. *Contagion and Confinement: Controlling Tuberculosis along the Skid Road.* Baltimore: Johns Hopkins University Press, 1998.

223. McCuiag, Katherine. *The Weariness, the Fever, and the Fret: The Campaign against Tuberculosis in Canada, 1900–1950.* Montreal: McGill-Queen's University Press, 1999.

224. Nagelkerke, Nico J. D. *Courtesans and Consumption: How Sexually Transmitted Infections Drive Tuberculosis Epidemics.* Delft, Netherlands: Eburon, 2012.

225. Ott, Katherine. *Fevered Lives: Tuberculosis in American Culture since 1870.* Cambridge, MA: Harvard University Press, 1996.

226. Roberts, Charlotte A., and Jane E. Buikstra. *The Bioarchaeology of Tuberculosis: A Global View on a Reemerging Disease.* Gainesville: University Press of Florida, 2003.

227. Smith, F. B. *The Retreat of Tuberculosis, 1850–1950.* New York: Croom Helm, 1988.

228. Waksman, Selman A. *The Conquest of Tuberculosis.* Berkeley: University of California Press, 1964.

Typhoid Fever (see also "Water Supply" and "Food and Drug Regulation")

229. Leavitt, Judith Walzer. *Typhoid Mary: Captive to the Public's Health.* Boston: Beacon Press, 1996.

230. McCarthy, Michael P. *Typhoid and the Politics of Public Health in Nineteenth-Century Philadelphia.* Philadelphia: American Philosophical Society, 1987.

231. Smith, David F., and H. Leslie Diack. *Food Poisoning, Policy, and Politics: Corned Beef and Typhoid in Britain in the 1960s.* Rochester, NY: Boydell Press, 2005.

Typhus (see also "Housing" and "Military")

232. Baumslag, Naomi. *Murderous Medicine: Nazi Doctors, Human Experimentation, and Typhus.* Westport, CT: Praeger, 2005.

233. Pelis, Kim. *Charles Nicolle, Pasteur's Imperial Missionary: Typhus and Tunisia.* Rochester, NY: University of Rochester Press, 2006.

234. Talty, Stephan. *The Illustrious Dead: The Terrifying Story of How Typhus Killed Napoleon's Greatest Army.* New York: Crown, 2009.

235. Weindling, Paul. *Epidemics and Genocide in Eastern Europe, 1890–1945.* New York: Oxford University Press, 2000.

236. Zinsser, Hans. *Rats, Lice and History: Being a Study in Biography, Which, after Twelve Preliminary Chapters Indispensable for the Preparation of the Lay Reader, Deals with the Life History of Typhus Fever.* Boston: Atlantic Monthly Press, 1935.

Yellow Fever (see also 379 and 400)

237. Delaporte, François. *The History of Yellow Fever: An Essay on the Birth of Tropical Medicine.* Cambridge, MA: MIT Press, 1991.

238. Duffy, John. *Sword of Pestilence: The New Orleans Yellow Fever Epidemic of 1853.* Baton Rouge: Louisiana State University Press, 1966.

239. Ellis, John H. *Yellow Fever and Public Health in the New South.* Lexington: University Press of Kentucky, 1992.

240. Espinosa, Mariola. *Epidemic Invasions: Yellow Fever and the Limits of Cuban Independence, 1878–1930.* Chicago: University of Chicago Press, 2009.

241. Estes, J. Worth, and Billy G. Smith, eds. *A Melancholy Scene of Devastation: The Public Response to the 1793 Philadelphia Yellow Fever Epidemic.* Canton, MA: Science History Publications, 1997.

242. Humphreys, Margaret. *Yellow Fever and the South*. Baltimore: Johns Hopkins University Press, 1999.

243. Nuwer, Deanne. *Plague among the Magnolias: The 1878 Yellow Fever Epidemic in Mississippi*. Tuscaloosa: University of Alabama Press, 2009.

244. Powell, John. *Bring Out Your Dead: The Great Plague of Yellow Fever in Philadelphia in 1793*. Philadelphia: University of Pennsylvania Press, 1993.

245. Smith, Billy G. *Ship of Death: A Voyage That Changed the Atlantic World*. New Haven, CT: Yale University Press, 2013.

246. Trask, Benjamin H. *Fearful Ravages: Yellow Fever in New Orleans, 1796–1905*. Lafayette: Center for Louisiana Studies, University of Louisiana at Lafayette, 2005.

III. HISTORICAL PERIODS BEFORE 1801
Ancient; before 500 CE (see also 116, 265, and 936)

247. Abbott, Frank Frost, and Allan Chester Johnson. *Municipal Administration in the Roman Empire*. Princeton, NJ: Princeton University Press, 1926.

248. Bagnall, Roger S., and Bruce W. Frier. *The Demography of Roman Egypt*. New York: Cambridge University Press, 1994.

249. Cohn-Haft, Louis. *The Public Physicians of Ancient Greece*. Northampton, MA: Department of History of Smith College, 1956.

250. Grmek, Mirko D. *Diseases in the Ancient Greek World*. Baltimore: Johns Hopkins University Press, 1989.

251. Hope, Valerie, and Eireann Marshall. *Death and Disease in the Ancient City*. New York: Routledge, 2000.

252. Jackson, Ralph. *Doctors and Diseases in the Roman Empire*. Norman: University of Oklahoma Press, 1988.

253. Kottek, Samuel. *Medicine and Hygiene in the Works of Flavius Josephus*. New York: Brill, 1994.

254. Lambert, Patricia. *Bioarchaeological Studies of Life in the Age of Agriculture: A View from the Southeast*. Tuscaloosa: University of Alabama Press, 2000.

255. Nriagu, Jerome O. *Lead and Lead Poisoning in Antiquity*. New York: Wiley, 1983.

256. Parker, Robert. *Miasma: Pollution and Purification in Early Greek Religion*. Oxford: Clarendon Press, 1983.

257. Pechenkina, Kate, and Marc Oxenham, eds. *Bioarchaeology of East Asia: Movement, Contact, Health*. Gainesville: University Press of Florida, 2013.

258. Sallares, Robert. *Malaria and Rome: A History of Malaria in Ancient Italy*. New York: Oxford University Press, 2002.

259. Scheidel, Walter. *Death on the Nile: Disease and the Demography of Roman Egypt*. Boston: Brill, 2001.

260. Yegül, Fikret. *Baths and Bathing in Classical Antiquity*. Cambridge, MA: MIT Press, 1992.

European Middle Ages; Other Parts of the World: 500 to 1450
(see also "Plague"; and 116, 166, 418, 511, 593, and 936)

261. Eckert, Edward. *The Structure of Plagues and Pestilences in Early Modern Europe: Central Europe, 1560–1640*. New York: Karger, 1996.

262. Little, Lester. *Plague and the End of Antiquity: The Pandemic of 541–750.* New York: Cambridge University Press, 2007.

263. Mormando, Franco, and Thomas Worcester, eds. *Piety and Plague: From Byzantium to the Baroque.* Kirksville, MO: Truman State University Press, 2007.

264. Paravicini Bagliani, Agostino, and Francesco Santi. *The Regulation of Evil: Social and Cultural Attitudes to Epidemics in the Late Middle Ages.* Florence: Sismel, 1998.

265. Pormann, Peter. *Epidemics in Context: Greek Commentaries on Hippocrates in the Arabic Tradition.* Boston: De Gruyter, 2011.

266. Rawcliffe, Carole. *Urban Bodies: Communal Health in Late Medieval English Towns and Cities.* Woodbridge, Suffolk: Boydell, 2013.

267. Russell, Andrew W., ed. *The Town and State Physician in Europe from the Middle Ages to the Enlightenment.* Wolfenbuttel: Herzog August Bibliothek, 1981.

268. Scott, Susan, and Christopher Duncan. *Biology of Plagues: Evidence from Historical Populations.* New York: Cambridge University Press, 2001.

269. Stathakopoulos, Dionysios. *Famine and Pestilence in the Late Roman and Early Byzantine Empire: A Systematic Survey of Subsistence Crises and Epidemics.* Burlington, VT: Ashgate, 2004.

270. Stearns, Justin K. *Infectious Ideas: Contagion in Premodern Islamic and Christian Thought in the Western Mediterranean.* Baltimore: Johns Hopkins University Press, 2011.

271. Woolgar, C. M., D. Serjeantson, and T. Waldron, eds. *Food in Medieval England: Diet and Nutrition.* New York: Oxford University Press, 2006.

European Renaissance; Early Modern Europe; Other Parts of the World: 1450 to 1800 (see also "Plague"; and 78, 100, 180, 192, 194, 195, 241, 244, 263, 267, 268, 371, 418, and 936)

272. Andrew, Donna T. *Philanthropy and Police: London Charity in the Eighteenth Century.* Princeton, NJ: Princeton University Press, 1989.

273. Caulfield, Ernest. *The Infant Welfare Movement in the Eighteenth Century.* New York: Hoeber, 1931.

274. Cipolla, Carlo. *Public Health and the Medical Profession in the Renaissance.* New York: Cambridge University Press, 1976.

275. Clouse, Michele. *Medicine, Government, and Public Health in Philip II's Spain: Shared Interests, Competing Authorities.* Burlington, VT: Ashgate, 2011.

276. Cockayne, Emily. *Hubbub: Filth, Noise & Stench in England, 1600–1770.* New Haven, CT: Yale University Press, 2007.

277. Crawshaw, Jane. *Plague Hospitals: Public Health for the City in Early Modern Venice.* Farnham, Surrey, UK: Ashgate, 2012.

278. Dobson, Mary J. *Contours of Death and Disease in Early Modern England.* Cambridge: New York: Cambridge University Press, 1997.

279. Fissell, Mary E. *Patients, Power, and the Poor in Eighteenth-Century Bristol.* New York: Cambridge University Press, 1991.

280. Grell, Ole Peter, and Andrew Cunningham, eds. *Health Care and Poor Relief in Protestant Europe, 1500–1700.* New York: Routledge, 1997.

281. Jones, Colin. *Charity and Bienfaisance: The Treatment of the Poor in the Montpellier Region, 1740–1815.* New York: Cambridge University Press, 1982.

282. Lederer, David. *Madness, Religion and the State in Early Modern Europe: A Bavarian Beacon.* New York: Cambridge University Press, 2006.

283. Lindemann, Mary. *Medicine and Society in Early Modern Europe.* 2nd ed. New York: Cambridge University Press, 2010.

284. McGough, Laura J. *Gender, Sexuality, and Syphilis in Early Modern Venice: The Disease That Came to Stay.* New York: Palgrave Macmillan, 2011.

285. Martin, A. Lynn. *Plague? Jesuit Accounts of Epidemic Disease in the 16th Century.* Kirksville, MO: Sixteenth Century Journal Publishers, 1996.

286. Mikkeli, Heikki. *Hygiene in the Early Modern Medical Tradition.* Helsinki: The Finnish Academy of Science and Letters, 1999.

287. Naphy, William G. *Plagues, Poisons, and Potions: Plague-Spreading Conspiracies in the Western Alps, c. 1530–1640.* New York: Palgrave, 2002.

288. Park, Katherine. *Doctors and Medicine in Early Renaissance Florence.* Princeton, NJ: Princeton University Press, 1985.

289. Pelling, Margaret. *The Common Lot: Sickness, Medical Occupations, and the Urban Poor in Early Modern England: Essays.* New York: Longman, 1998.

290. Pullan, Brian S. *Rich and Poor in Renaissance Venice: The Social Institutions of a Catholic State.* Cambridge, MA: Harvard University Press, 1971.

291. Riley, James C. *The Eighteenth-Century Campaign to Avoid Disease.* New York: St. Martin's Press, 1987.

292. Rusnock, Andrea. *Vital Accounts: Quantifying Health and Population in Eighteenth-Century England and France.* New York: Cambridge University Press, 2002.

293. Schwartz, Robert M. *Policing the Poor in Eighteenth-Century France.* Chapel Hill: University of North Carolina Press, 1988.

294. Siena, Kevin. *Venereal Disease, Hospitals, and the Urban Poor: London's "Foul Wards," 1600–1800.* Rochester, NY: University of Rochester Press, 2004.

295. Stein, Claudia. *Negotiating the French Pox in Early Modern Germany.* Burlington, VT: Ashgate, 2009.

296. Steinbicker, Carl R. *Poor Relief in the Sixteenth Century.* Washington, DC: Catholic University of America, 1937.

IV. GEOGRAPHICAL DIVISIONS
United States

297. Blake, John B. *Public Health in the Town of Boston, 1630–1822.* Cambridge, MA: Harvard University Press, 1959.

298. Blumenthal, David, and James A. Morone. *The Heart of Power: Health and Politics in the Oval Office.* Berkeley: University of California Press, 2009.

299. Cassedy, James H. *Charles V. Chapin and the Public Health Movement.* Cambridge, MA: Harvard University Press, 1962.

300. Colgrove, James, Gerald E. Markowitz, and David Rosner, eds. *The Contested Boundaries of American Public Health.* New Brunswick, NJ: Rutgers University Press, 2008.

301. Colgrove, James. *Epidemic City: The Politics of Public Health in New York.* New York: Russell Sage Foundation, 2011.

302. Duffy, John. *A History of Public Health in New York City.* 2 vols. New York: Russell Sage Foundation, 1968–74.

303. Duffy, John. *Epidemics in Colonial America*. Baton Rouge: Louisiana State University Press, 1953.

304. Duffy, John. *The Sanitarians: A History of American Public Health*. Urbana: University of Illinois Press, 1990.

305. Estes, J. Worth, and David M. Goodman. *The Changing Humors of Portsmouth: The Medical Biography of an American Town, 1623–1983*. Boston: Countway Library, 1986.

306. Fairchild, Amy, Ronald Bayer, James Keith Colgrove, and Daniel Wolfe. *Searching Eyes: Privacy, the State, and Disease Surveillance in America*. New York: Milbank Memorial Fund, 2007.

307. Finger, Simon. *The Contagious City: The Politics of Public Health in Early Philadelphia*. Ithaca, NY: Cornell University Press, 2012.

308. Fortuine, Robert. *Chills and Fever: Health and Disease in the Early History of Alaska*. Fairbanks: University of Alaska Press, 1989.

309. Galishoff, Stuart. *Newark, the Nation's Unhealthiest City, 1832–1895*. New Brunswick, NJ: Rutgers University Press, 1988.

310. Galishoff, Stuart. *Safeguarding the Public Health, Newark, 1895–1918*. Westport, CT: Greenwood Press, 1975.

311. Howard, William Travis, Jr. *Public Health Administration and the Natural History of Disease in Baltimore, Maryland, 1797–1920*. Washington, DC: Carnegie Institution, 1924.

312. Jordan, Philip D. *The People's Health: A History of Public Health in Minnesota to 1948*. St. Paul: Minnesota Historical Society, 1953.

313. Leavitt, Judith Walzer. *The Healthiest City: Milwaukee and the Politics of Health Reform*. With a new preface. Madison: University of Wisconsin Press, 1996.

314. Leavitt, Judith Walzer, and Ronald Numbers, eds. *Sickness and Health in America: Readings in the History of Medicine and Public Health*. 3rd ed. rev. Madison: University of Wisconsin Press, 1997.

315. Mullan, Fitzhugh. *Plagues and Politics: The Story of the United States Public Health Service*. New York: Basic Books, 1989.

316. Rosen, George. *Preventive Medicine in the United States 1900–1975: Trends and Interpretations*. New York: Science History Publications, 1975.

317. Rosenberg, Charles E. *The Care of Strangers: The Rise of America's Hospital System*. New York: Basic Books, 1987.

318. Rosenkrantz, Barbara G. *Public Health and the State: Changing Views in Massachusetts, 1842–1936*. Cambridge, MA: Harvard University Press, 1972.

319. Rosner, David, ed. *Hives of Sickness: Public Health and Epidemics in New York City*. New Brunswick, NJ: Rutgers University Press, 1995.

320. Smillie, Wilson G. *Public Health: Its Promise for the Future; A Chronicle of the Development of Public Health in the United States, 1607–1914*. New York: Macmillan, 1955.

321. Stange, Marion. *Vital Negotiations: Protecting Settlers' Health in Colonial Louisiana and South Carolina, 1720–1763*. Göttingen: V&R unipress, 2012.

322. Stevens, Rosemary. *In Sickness and in Wealth: American Hospitals in the Twentieth Century*. New York: Basic Books, 1989.

323. Tomes, Nancy. *The Gospel of Germs: Men, Women, and the Microbe in American Life*. Cambridge, MA: Harvard University Press, 1998.

324. Ward, John, and Christian Warren, eds. *Silent Victories: The History and Practice of Public Health in Twentieth-Century America*. New York: Oxford University Press, 2007.

325. Warner, John Harley, and Janet Tighe, eds. *Major Problems in the History of American Medicine and Public Health: Documents and Essays.* Boston: Houghton Mifflin, 2001.

326. Williams, Ralph C. *The United States Public Health Service, 1798–1950.* Washington, DC: Government Printing Office, 1951.

327. Wright, Russell. *Chronology of Public Health in the United States.* Jefferson, NC: McFarland, 2005.

Canada (see also "SARS"; and 91, 108, 111, 223, and 586)

328. MacDougall, Heather A. *Activists and Advocates: Toronto's Health Department, 1883–1983.* Toronto: Dundurn Press, 1990.

329. Naylor, C. David. *Private Practice, Public Payment: Canadian Medicine and the Politics of Health Insurance, 1911–1966.* Montreal: McGill-Queen's University Press, 1986.

330. Taylor, Malcolm G. *Health Insurance and Canadian Public Policy: The Seven Decisions that Created the Canadian Health Insurance System.* Montreal: McGill-Queen's University Press, 1978. Abridged edition published as *Insuring National Health Care: The Canadian Experience.* Chapel Hill: University of North Carolina Press, 1990.

Minorities, Immigration, Race, and Health in North America (see also "Sickle-Cell Anemia"; and 90, 117, 123, 156, 213, 217, 218, 575, 577, 770, and 878)

331. Bard, Robert. *Immigration at the Golden Gate: Passenger Ships, Exclusion, and Angel Island.* Westport, CT: Praeger, 2008.

332. Boyd, Robert. *The Coming of the Spirit of Pestilence: Introduced Infectious Diseases and Population Decline among Northwest Coast Indians, 1774–1874.* Seattle: University of Washington Press, 1999.

333. Bushnell, O. A. *The Gifts of Civilization: Germs and Genocide in Hawai'i.* Honolulu: University of Hawaii Press, 1993.

334. DeJong, David H. *"If You Knew the Conditions": A Chronicle of the Indian Medical Service and American Indian Health Care, 1908–1955.* Lanham, MD: Lexington Books, 2008.

335. Downs, Jim. *Sick from Freedom: African-American Illness and Suffering during the Civil War and Reconstruction.* New York: Oxford University Press, 2012.

336. Fairchild, Amy. *Science at the Borders: Immigrant Medical Inspection and the Shaping of the Modern Industrial Labor Force, 1891 to 1930.* Baltimore: Johns Hopkins University Press, 2003.

337. Fortuine, Robert. *A Century of Adventure in Northern Health: The Public Health Service Commissioned Corps in Alaska 1879–1978.* Landover, MD: PHS Commissioned Officers Foundation for the Advancement of Public Health, 2006.

338. Hull, Kathleen, *Pestilence and Persistence: Yosemite Indian Demography and Culture in Colonial California.* Berkeley: University of California Press, 2009.

339. Gamble, Vanessa Northington. *Making a Place for Ourselves: The Black Hospital Movement, 1920–1945.* New York: Oxford University Press, 1995.

340. Hackett, Paul. *"A Very Remarkable Sickness": Epidemics in the Petit Nord, 1670–1846.* Winnipeg: University of Manitoba Press, 2002.

341. Hutchinson, Dale L. *Tatham Mound and the Bioarchaeology of European Contact: Disease and Depopulation in Central Gulf Coast Florida*. Gainesville: University Press of Florida, 2006.

342. Jones, David S. *Rationalizing Epidemics: Meanings and Uses of American Indian Mortality since 1600*. Cambridge, MA: Harvard University Press, 2004.

343. Jones, James. *Bad Blood: The Tuskegee Syphilis Experiment*. New and expanded ed. New York: Free Press, 1993.

344. Kalton, Paul. *Epidemics and Enslavement: Biological Catastrophe in the Native Southeast, 1492–1715*. Lincoln: University of Nebraska Press, 2007.

345. Kiple, Kenneth F., and Virginia Himmelsteib King. *Another Dimension to the Black Diaspora: Diet, Disease and Racism*. New York: Cambridge University Press, 1981.

346. Kunitz, Stephen J. *Disease Change and the Role of Medicine: The Navajo Experience*. Berkeley: University of California Press, 1983.

347. McBride, David. *From TB to AIDS: Epidemics among Urban Blacks since 1900*. Albany: SUNY Press, 1991.

348. McCandless, Peter. *Slavery, Disease, and Suffering on the Southern Lowcountry*. New York: Cambridge University Press, 2011.

349. McKiernan-González, John. *Fevered Measures: Public Health and Race at the Texas-Mexico Border, 1848–1942*. Durham, NC: Duke University Press, 2012.

350. Mann, Barbara Alice. *The Tainted Gift: The Disease Method of Frontier Expansion*. Santa Barbara, CA: Praeger, 2009.

351. Markel, Howard. *Quarantine: East European Jewish Immigrants and the New York City Epidemics of 1892*. Baltimore: Johns Hopkins University Press, 1997.

352. Molina, Natalia. *Fit to Be Citizens? Public Health and Race in Los Angeles, 1879–1939*. Berkeley: University of California Press, 2006.

353. Reverby, Susan. *Examining Tuskegee: The Infamous Syphilis Study and Its Legacy*. Chapel Hill: University of North Carolina Press, 2009.

354. Roberts, Samuel. *Infectious Fear: Politics, Disease, and the Health Effects of Segregation*. Chapel Hill: University of North Carolina Press, 2009.

355. Savitt, Todd L. *Medicine and Slavery: The Diseases and Health Care of Blacks in Antebellum Virginia*. Urbana: University of Illinois Press, 1978.

356. Savitt, Todd. *Race and Medicine in Nineteenth- and Early-Twentieth-Century America*. Kent, OH: Kent State University Press, 2007.

357. Shah, Nayan. *Contagious Divides: Epidemics and Race in San Francisco's Chinatown*. Berkeley: University of California Press, 2001.

358. Thornton, Russell. *American Indian Holocaust and Survival: A Population History since 1492*. Norman: University of Oklahoma Press, 1987.

359. Trennert, Robert A. *White Man's Medicine: Government Doctors and the Navajo, 1863–1955*. Albuquerque: University of New Mexico Press, 1998.

360. Wilson, Jamie J. *Building a Healthy Black Harlem: Health Politics in Harlem, New York, from the Jazz Age to the Great Depression*. Amherst, NY: Cambria Press, 2009.

361. Young, T. Kue. *Health Care and Cultural Change: The Indian Experience in the Central Subarctic*. Toronto: University of Toronto Press, 1988.

Latin America and the Caribbean
(see also 92, 121, 122, 202, 204, 240, 349, 714, and 801)

362. Agostoni, Claudia. *Monuments of Progress: Modernization and Public Health in Mexico City, 1876–1910.* Boulder: University Press of Colorado, 2003.

363. Armus, Diego. *The Ailing City: Health, Tuberculosis and Culture in Buenos Aires, 1870–1950.* Durham, NC: Duke University Press, 2011.

364. Armus, Diego, ed. *Disease in the History of Modern Latin America: From Malaria to AIDS.* Durham, NC: Duke University Press, 2003.

365. Birn, Anne-Emanuelle. *Marriage of Convenience: The Rockefeller International Health and Revolutionary Mexico.* Rochester, NY: University of Rochester Press, 2006.

366. Chevalier, Jacques, and Andrés Sánchez Bain. *The Hot and the Cold: Ills of Humans and Maize in Native Mexico.* Toronto: University of Toronto Press, 2003.

367. Danielson, Ross. *Cuban Medicine.* New Brunswick, NJ: Transaction Books, 1979.

368. De Barros, Juanita, Steven Palmer, and David Wright, eds. *Health and Medicine in the Circum-Caribbean, 1800–1968.* New York: Routledge, 2009.

369. Diaz-Briquets, Sergio. *The Health Revolution in Cuba.* Austin: University of Texas Press, 1983.

370. Donahue, John M. *The Nicaraguan Revolution in Health: From Somoza to the Sandinistas.* South Hadley, MA: Bergin & Garvey, 1986.

371. Fields, Sherry. *Pestilence and Headcolds: Encountering Illness in Colonial Mexico.* New York: Columbia University Press, 2008.

372. Fisher, Lawrence E. *Colonial Madness: Mental Health in the Barbadian Social Order.* New Brunswick, NJ: Rutgers University Press, 1985.

373. Gragnolati, Michele, Magnus Lindelöw, and Bernard Couttolenc. *Twenty Years of Health System Reform in Brazil: An Assessment of The Sistema Único De Saúde.* Washington, DC: World Bank, [2013].

374. Hirschfield, Katherine. *Health, Politics, and Revolution in Cuba since 1898.* New Brunswick, NJ: Transaction Publishers, 2007.

375. Jenson, Niklas. *For the Health of the Enslaved: Slaves, Medicine and Power in the Danish West Indies, 1803–1848.* Copenhagen: Museum Tusculanum Press, 2012.

376. Jones, Margaret. *Public Health in Jamaica, 1850–1940: Neglect, Philanthropy and Development.* Kingston, Jamaica: University of West Indies Press, 2013.

377. Lopez-Alonso, Moramay. *Measuring Up: A History of Living Standards in Mexico, 1850–1950.* Stanford, CA: Stanford University Press, 2012.

378. McCrae, Heather. *Diseased Relations: Epidemics, Public Health, and State-Building in Yucatán, Mexico, 1847–1924.* Albuquerque: University of New Mexico Press, 2010.

379. McNeill, John Robert. *Mosquito Empires: Ecology and War in the Greater Caribbean, 1620–1914.* New York: Cambridge University Press, 2010.

380. Palmer, Steven. *From Popular Medicine to Medical Populism: Doctors, Healers and Public Power in Costa Rica, 1900–1940.* Durham, NC: Duke University Press, 2003.

381. Palmer, Steven. *Launching Global Health: The Caribbean Odyssey of the Rockefeller Foundation.* Ann Arbor: University of Michigan Press, 2010.

382. Peard, Julian. *Race, Place, and Medicine: The Idea of the Tropics in Nineteenth-Century Brazilian Medicine.* Durham, NC: Duke University Press, 1999.

383. Riley, James C. *Poverty and Life Expectancy: The Jamaica Paradox.* New York: Cambridge University Press, 2005.

384. Stepan, Nancy Leys. *Beginnings of Brazilian Science: Oswaldo Cruz, Medical Research and Policy, 1890–1920.* New York: Science History, 1976.

385. Stepan, Nancy Leys. *The Hour of Eugenics: Race, Gender, and Nation in Latin America.* Ithaca, NY: Cornell University Press, 1991.

386. Zulawski, Ann. *Unequal Cures: Public Health and Political Change in Bolivia, 1900–1950.* Durham, NC: Duke University Press, 2007.

Europe: General (see also 120, 908, and 929)

387. Baldwin, Peter. *Contagion and the State in Europe, 1830–1930.* New York: Cambridge University Press, 1999.

388. Barona, Josep. *The Problem of Nutrition: Experimental Science, Public Health, and Economy in Europe, 1914–1945.* New York: Peter Lang, 2010.

389. Bourdelais, Patrice. *Epidemics Laid Low: A History of What Happened in Rich Countries.* Baltimore: Johns Hopkins University Press, 2006.

390. Brunton, Deborah, ed. *Medicine Transformed: Health, Disease, and Society in Europe, 1800–1930.* Manchester, UK: Manchester University Press, 2004.

391. Solomon, Susan Gross, Lion Murard, and Patrick Zylberman, eds. *Shifting Boundaries of Public Health: Europe in the Twentieth Century.* Rochester, NY: University of Rochester Press, 2008.

Continental Europe (see also 41, 88, 94, 96, 106, 127, 133, 205, 232, 235, 740, 744, 750, 783, 806, 811, 817, 875, and 909)

392. Ackerknecht, Erwin H. *Rudolph Virchow: Doctor, Statesman, Anthropologist.* Madison: University of Wisconsin Press, 1953.

393. Ackerman, Evelyn B. *Health Care in the Parisian Countryside, 1800–1914.* New Brunswick, NJ: Rutgers University Press, 1990.

394. Baloutzova, Svetla. *Demography and Nation: Social Legislation and Population Policy in Bulgaria, 1918–1944.* Budapest, Hungary: Central European University Press, 2011.

395. Barnes, David. *The Great Stink of Paris and the Nineteenth-Century Struggle against Filth and Germs.* Baltimore: Johns Hopkins University Press, 2006.

396. Bernstein, Frances L., Christopher Burton, and Dan Healey, eds. *Soviet Medicine: Culture, Practice, and Science.* DeKalb: Northern Illinois University Press, 2010.

397. Bucur, Maria. *Eugenics and Modernization in Interwar Romania.* Pittsburgh, PA: University of Pittsburgh Press, 2002.

398. Coleman, William. *Death Is a Social Disease: Public Health and Political Economy in Early Industrial France.* Madison: University of Wisconsin Press, 1982.

399. Coleman, William. *Yellow Fever in the North: The Methods of Early Epidemiology.* Madison: University of Wisconsin Press, 1987.

400. Ellis, Jack D. *The Physician-Legislators of France: Medicine and Politics in the Early Third Republic, 1870–1914.* New York: Cambridge University Press, 1990.

401. Evans, Richard J. *Death in Hamburg: Society and Politics in the Cholera Years, 1830–1910.* New York: Oxford University Press, 1987.

402. Filtzer, Donald A. *The Hazards of Urban Life in Late Stalinist Russia: Health, Hygiene, and Living Standards, 1943–1953.* New York: Cambridge University Press, 2010.

403. Guilleman, Jeanne. *Anthrax: The Investigation of a Deadly Outbreak.* Berkeley: University of California Press, 1999.

404. Heidenheimer, Arnold J., and Nils Elvander, eds. *The Shaping of the Swedish Health System.* New York: St. Martin's Press, 1980.

405. Henze, Charlotte. *Disease, Health Care, and Government in Late Imperial Russia: Life and Death on the Volga, 1823–1914.* New York: Routledge, 2011.

406. Hildreth, Martha L. *Doctors, Bureaucrats, and Public Health in France, 1888–1902.* New York: Garland, 1987.

407. Hutchinson, John F. *Politics and Public Health in Revolutionary Russia, 1890–1918.* Baltimore: Johns Hopkins University Press, 1990.

408. Larsen, Øivind. *Epidemic Diseases in Norway in a Period of Change: An Atlas of Some Selected Infectious Diseases and the Attitudes towards Them 1868–1900.* Oslo: Unipub, 2000.

409. McNeely, Ian. *"Medicine on a Grand Scale": Rudolf Virchow, Liberalism, and the Public Health.* London: Wellcome Trust, 2002.

410. Navarro, Vicente. *Social Security and Medicine in the USSR: A Marxist Critique.* Lexington, MA: Lexington Books, 1977.

411. Niemi, Marjaana. *Public Health and Municipal Policy Making: Britain and Sweden, 1900–1940.* Burlington, VT: Ashgate, 2007.

412. Proctor, Robert. *The Nazi War on Cancer.* Princeton, NJ: Princeton University Press, 1999.

413. Promitzer, Christian, Sevastē Troumpeta, and Marius Turda, eds. *Health, Hygiene, and Eugenics in Southeastern Europe to 1945.* Budapest, Hungary: Central European University Press, 2011.

414. Solomon, Susan Gross, and John F. Hutchinson, eds. *Health and Society in Revolutionary Russia.* Bloomington: Indiana University Press, 1990.

415. Spree, Reinhard. *Health and Social Class in Imperial Germany: A Social History of Mortality, Morbidity, and Inequality.* New York: Berg, 1988.

416. Stark, Tricia. *The Body Soviet: Propaganda, Hygiene, and the Revolutionary State.* Madison: University of Wisconsin Press, 2008.

417. Sundin, Jan, and Sam Willner. *Social Change and Health in Sweden: 250 Years of Politics and Practice.* Stockholm: Swedish National Institute of Public Health, 2007.

418. Vigarello, Georges. *Concepts of Cleanliness: Changing Attitudes in France since the Middle Ages.* New York: Cambridge University Press, 1988.

419. Weindling, Paul. *Health, Race, and German Politics between National Unification and Nazism, 1870–1945.* New York: Cambridge University Press, 1989.

420. Wilsford, David. *Doctors and the State: The Politics of Health Care in France and the United States.* Durham, NC: Duke University Press, 1991.

Ireland and Great Britain

421. Barrington, Ruth. *Health, Medicine and Politics in Ireland, 1900–1970.* Dublin: Institute of Public Administration, 1987.

422. Barry, Jonathan, and Colin Jones, eds. *Medicine and Charity before the Welfare State.* New York: Routledge, 1991.

423. Berridge, Virginia. *Health and Society in Britain since 1939.* New York: Cambridge University Press, 1999.

424. Brand, Jeanne L. *Doctors and the State: The British Medical Profession and Government Action in Public Health, 1810–1912.* Baltimore: Johns Hopkins Press, 1965.

425. Brundage, Anthony. *England's "Prussian Minister": Edwin Chadwick and the Politics of Government Growth, 1832–1854*. University Park: Pennsylvania State University Press, 1988.

426. Carpenter, Mary. *Health, Medicine, and Society in Victorian England*. Santa Barbara, CA: Praeger, 2010.

427. Connell, K. H. *The Population of Ireland*. Oxford: Clarendon Press, 1950. Reprint. Westport, CT: Greenwood Press, 1975.

428. Crossman, Virginia, and Peter Gray, eds. *Poverty and Welfare in Ireland, 1838–1948*. Dublin: Irish Academic Press, 2011.

429. Delmege, J. A. *Toward National Health: Or, Health and Hygiene in England from Roman to Victorian Times*. New York: Macmillan, 1932.

430. Eyler, John. *Sir Arthur Newsholme and State Medicine, 1885–1935*. New York: Cambridge University Press, 1997.

431. Eyler, John M. *Victorian Social Medicine: The Ideas and Methods of William Farr*. Baltimore: Johns Hopkins University Press, 1979.

432. Finer, S. E. *The Life and Times of Sir Edwin Chadwick*. London: Methuen, 1952.

433. Fox, Daniel M. *Health Policies, Health Politics: The British and American Experience, 1911–1965*. Princeton, NJ: Princeton University Press, 1986.

434. Frazer, William M. *A History of English Public Health, 1834–1939*. London: Balliere, Tindall & Cox, 1950.

435. Freeman, Mark, Eleanor Gordon, Krista Maglen, and M. A. Crowther, eds. *Medicine, Law, and Public Policy in Scotland, c. 1850–1990*. Dundee, Scotland: Dundee University Press, 2011.

436. Gray, B. Kirkman. *A History of English Philanthropy from the Dissolution of the Monasteries to the Taking of the First Census*. London: King, 1905.

437. Hamlin, Christopher. *Public Health and Social Justice in the Age of Chadwick: Britain, 1800–1854*. New York: Cambridge University Press, 1998.

438. Hardy, Anne. *Health and Medicine in Britain since 1860*. New York: Palgrave, 2001.

439. Honigsbaum, Frank. *The Struggle for the Ministry of Health (1914–1919)*. London: Bell, 1971.

440. Jenkinson, Jacqueline. *Scotland's Health, 1919–1948*. New York: Peter Lang, 2002.

441. Jones, Greta. *Social Hygiene in Twentieth-Century Britain*. Wolfeboro, NH: Croom Helm, 1986.

442. Jones, Greta, and Elizabeth Malcolm, eds. *Medicine, Disease and the State in Ireland, 1650–1940*. Cork, Ireland: Cork University Press, 1999.

443. Lambert, Royston. *Sir John Simon, 1816–1904, and English Social Administration*. London: McKibbon & Kee, 1963.

444. Lewis, Jane. *What Price Community Medicine? The Philosophy, Practice, and Politics of Public Health since 1919*. Brighton, UK: Wheatsheaf, 1986.

445. Lewis, R. A. *Edwin Chadwick and the Public Health Movement, 1832–1854*. London: Longmans, Green, 1952.

446. Marland, Hilary. *Medicine and Society in Wakefield and Huddersfield, 1780–1870*. New York: Cambridge University Press, 1987.

447. Midwinter, Eric C. *Social Administration in Lancashire, 1830–1860: Poor Law, Public Health and Police*. Manchester, UK: Manchester University Press, 1969.

448. Navarro, Vicente. *Class Struggle, the State, and Medicine: An Historical and Contemporary Analysis of the Medical Sector in Great Britain.* New York: Prodist, 1978.

449. Newman, George. *The Building of a Nation's Health.* London: Macmillan, 1939.

450. Parfit, Jessie. *The Health of a City: Oxford 1770–1974.* Oxford: Amate Press, 1987.

451. Pickstone, John V. *Medicine and Industrial Society: A History of Hospital Development in Manchester and Its Region, 1752–1946.* Dover, NH: Manchester University Press, 1985.

452. Sheard, Sally, and Liam Donaldson. *The Nation's Doctor: The Role of the Chief Medical Officer 1855–1998.* Seattle, WA: Radcliffe, 2006.

453. Smith, F. B. *The People's Health 1830 to 1910.* New York: Holmes & Meier, 1979.

454. Smith, George, Daniel Dorling, and Mary Shaw, eds. *Poverty, Inequality, and Health in Britain, 1800–2000: A Reader.* Bristol, UK: Policy Press, 2001.

455. Watson, Roger. *Edwin Chadwick, Poor Law, and Public Health.* London: Longman, 1969.

456. Welshman, John. *Municipal Medicine: Public Health in Twentieth-Century Britain.* New York: Peter Lang, 2000.

457. Wohl, Anthony S. *Endangered Lives: Public Health in Victorian Britain.* Cambridge, MA: Harvard University Press, 1983.

458. Woods, Robert, and John Woodward, eds. *Urban Disease and Mortality in Nineteenth-Century England.* New York: St. Martin's Press, 1984.

459. Worboys, Michael. *Spreading Germs: Diseases, Theories, and Medical Practice in Britain, 1865–1900.* New York: Cambridge University Press, 2000.

Oceania, Australia, and New Zealand (see also 114 and 568)

460. Anderson, Warwick. *The Collectors of Lost Souls: Turning Kuru Scientists into Whitemen.* Baltimore: Johns Hopkins University Press, 2008.

461. Bryder, Linda, ed. *A Healthy Country: Essays on the Social History of Medicine in New Zealand.* Wellington, NZ: Bridget Williams, 1991.

462. Campbell, Judith. *Invisible Invaders: Smallpox and Other Diseases in Aboriginal Australia, 1780–1880.* Carlton, South Australia: Melbourne University Press, 2002.

463. Cumpston, J. H. L. *Health and Disease in Australia: A History.* Canberra: Australian Government Publishing Service, 1989.

464. Curson, P. H. *Times of Crisis: Epidemics in Sydney, 1788–1900.* Sydney: Sydney University Press, 1985.

465. Davies, Margrit. *Public Health and Colonialism: The Case of German New Guinea 1884–1914.* Wiesbaden, Germany: Harrassowitz, 2002.

466. Denoon, Donald. *Public Health in Papua New Guinea: Medical Possibility and Social Constraint, 1884–1984.* New York: Cambridge University Press, 1989.

467. Dow, Derek. *Maori Health and Government Policy, 1840–1940.* Wellington, NZ: Victoria University Press, 1999.

468. Durie, Mason. *Whaiora: Māori Health Development.* New York: Oxford University Press, 1994.

469. Foley, Jean. *In Quarantine: A History of Sydney's Quarantine Station, 1828–1984.* Kenthurst, NSW, Australia: Kangaroo Press, 1995.

470. Kampf, Antje. *Mapping Out the Venereal Wilderness: Public Health and STD in New Zealand, 1920–1980.* Berlin: LIT, 2007.

471. Lange, Raeburn. *May the People Live: A History of Maori Health Development 1900–1920.* Auckland, NZ: Auckland University Press, 1999.

472. Lewis, Milton J. *The People's Health: Public Health in Australia,* 1788–1950. Westport, CT: Praeger, 2003.

473. Lewis, Milton, and Kerrie L. MacPherson, eds. *Public Health in Asia and the Pacific: Historical and Comparative Perspectives.* New York: Routledge, 2008.

474. Mayne, A. J. C. *Fever, Squalor and Vice: Sanitation and Social Policy in Victorian Sydney.* St. Lucia: University of Queensland Press, 1982.

475. Miles, John. *Infectious Diseases: Colonising the Pacific?* Dunedin, NZ: University of Otago Press, 1997.

476. Petrow, Stefan, *Sanatorium of the South? Public Health and Politics in Hobart and Launceston, 1875–1914.* Hobart: Tasmanian Historical Research Association, 1995.

477. Spencer, Margaret. *Public Health in Papua New Guinea 1870–1939.* Brisbane: Australian Centre for International & Tropical Health & Nutrition, 1999.

478. Wood, Pamela. *Dirt: Filth and Decay in a New World Arcadia.* Auckland, NZ: Auckland University Press, 2005.

Sub-Saharan Africa (see also "Tripanosomiasis" and "Bilharzia"; and 64, 129, 152, 173, 563, 824, and 828)

479. Addae, Stephen, *History of Western Medicine in Ghana, 1880–1960.* Edinburgh: Durham Academic Press, 1997.

480. Ashitey, Gilfrod A. *An Epidemiology of Disease Control in Ghana, 1901–1990.* Accra: Ghana Universities Press, 1994.

481. Beck, Ann. *Medicine, Tradition and Development in Kenya and Tanzania, 1920–1970.* Waltham, MA: Crossroads Press, 1981.

482. Carlson, Dennis G. *African Fever: A Study of British Science, Technology and Politics in West Africa, 1787–1864.* New York: Science History, 1984.

483. Cranefield, Paul F. *Science and Empire: East Coast Fever in Rhodesia and the Transvaal.* New York: Cambridge University Press, 1991.

484. Crombé, Xavier, and Jean-Hervé Jézéquel. *A Not-So Natural Disaster: Niger 2005.* New York: Columbia University Press, 2009.

485. Curtin, Philip D. *Death by Migration: Europe's Encounter with the Tropical World in the Nineteenth Century.* New York: Cambridge University Press, 1989.

486. Echenberg, Myron. *Africa in the Time of Cholera: A History of Pandemics from 1815 to the Present.* Cambridge, UK: Cambridge University Press, 2011.

487. Geissler, Wenzel, and Catherine Molyneux, eds. *Evidence, Ethos and Experiment: The Anthropology and History of Medical Research in Africa.* New York: Berghahn, 2011.

488. Gelfand, Michael. *A Service to the Sick: A History of the Health Services for Africans in Southern Rhodesia (1890–1953).* Gwelo, Zimbabwe: Mambo Press, 1976.

489. Hartwig, Gerald W., and K. David Patterson, eds. *Disease in African History: An Introductory Survey and Case Studies.* Durham, NC: Duke University Press, 1978.

490. Headrick, Rita. *Colonialism, Health and Illness in French Equatorial Africa, 1885–1935.* Atlanta, GA: African Studies Association Press, 1994.

491. King, Michael, and Elspeth King. *The Story of Medicine and Disease in Malawi: The 150 Years since Livingstone.* Blantyre, Malawi: Montfort, 1992.

492. Jong, Joop T. V M. de. *A Descent into African Psychiatry.* Amsterdam: Royal Tropical Institute, 1987.

493. Kinsman, John. *AIDS Policy in Uganda: Evidence, Ideology, and the Making of an African Success Story.* New York: Macmillan, 2010.

494. Kitaw, Yayehyirad, et al. *The Evolution of Public Health in Ethiopia 1941–2010.* Addis Ababa, Ethiopia: Ethiopian Public Health Association (EPHA), 2012.

495. Laidler, Percy Ward, and Michael Gelfand. *South Africa: Its Medical History, 1652–1898: A Medical and Social Study.* Cape Town, South Africa: Struik, 1971.

496. McCulloch, Jock. *South Africa's Gold Mines & the Politics of Silicosis.* Suffolk, UK: James Currey, 2012.

497. Maynard, Kent. *Making Kedjom Medicine: A History of Public Health and Well-Being in Cameroon.* Westport, CT: Praeger, 2004.

498. Molefi, Rodgers. *A Medical History of Botswana, 1885–1966.* Gaborone, Botswana: Botswana Society, 1996.

499. Ndege, George. *Health, State and Society in Kenya: Faces of Contact and Change.* Rochester, NY: University of Rochester Press, 2001.

500. Ngalamulume, Kalala. *Colonial Pathologies, Environment, and Western Medicine in Saint-Louis-Du-Senegal, 1867–1920.* New York: Peter Lang, 2012.

501. Packard, Randall M. *White Plague, Black Labor: Tuberculosis and the Political Economy of Health and Disease in South Africa.* Berkeley: University of California Press, 1989.

502. Patterson, K. David. *Health in Colonial Ghana: Disease, Medicine, and Socio-Economic Change, 1900–1955.* Waltham, MA: Crossroads Press, 1981.

503. Prince, Ruth J., and Rebecca Marsland, eds. *Making Public and Unmaking Health an Africa: Ethnographic and Historical Perspectives.* Athens: Ohio University Press, 2013.

504. Schram, R. *A History of the Nigerian Health Services.* Ibadan, Nigeria: Ibadan University Press, 1971.

505. Scott, David. *Epidemic Disease in Ghana, 1901–1961.* New York: Oxford University Press, 1965.

506. Tsikoane, Tumelo. *A History of Tuberculosis in Lesotho (1900–80) with Special Reference to Control Policy and Practice.* Roma: National University of Lesotho, 1998.

507. Turshen, M. *The Political Ecology of Disease in Tanzania.* New Brunswick, NJ: Rutgers University Press, 1984.

508. Wallace, Marion. *Health, Power and Politics in Windhoek, Namibia, 1915–1945.* Basel, Switzerland: Schlettwein, 2002.

North Africa and the Middle East (see also 136, 138, 233, and 845)

509. Barnea, Tamara, and Rafiq Husseini, eds. *Separate and Cooperate, Cooperate and Separate: The Disengagement of the Palestine Health Care System from Israel and Its Emergence as an Independent System.* Westport, CT: Praeger, 2002.

510. Dağlar, Oya. *War, Epidemics, and Medicine in the Late Ottoman Empire (1912–1918).* Haarlem, Netherlands: Sota, 2008.

511. Dols, Michael W. *The Black Death in the Middle East.* Princeton, NJ: Princeton University Press, 1977.

512. Ebrahimnejad, Hormoz. *Medicine, Public Health, and the Qājār State: Patterns of Medical Modernization in Nineteenth-Century Iran.* Boston: Brill, 2004.

513. Floor, Willem. *Public Health in Qajar Iran.* Washington, DC: Mage Publishers, 2004.

514. Gallagher, Nancy Elizabeth. *Egypt's Other Wars: Epidemics and the Politics of Public Health.* Syracuse, NY: Syracuse University Press, 1990.

515. Gallagher, Nancy Elizabeth. *Medicine and Power in Tunisia, 1780–1900.* New York: Cambridge University Press, 1983.

516. Kottek, Samuel, ed. *Infectious Diseases and Epidemics in the Land of Israel.* Jerusalem: The Hebrew University Magnes Press, 2013.

517. Kuhnke, LaVerne. *Lives at Risk: Public Health in Nineteenth-Century Egypt.* Berkeley: University of California Press, 1990.

518. Shvarts, Shifra. *The Workers' Health Fund in Eretz Israel: Kupat Holim, 1911–1937.* Rochester, NY: University of Rochester Press, 2002.

519. Sufian, Sandra M. *Healing the Land and the Nation: Malaria and the Zionist Project in Palestine, 1920–1947.* Chicago: University of Chicago Press, 2007.

520. Yildirm, Nuran. *A History of Healthcare in Istanbul: Health Organizations, Epidemics, Infections and Disease Control, Preventive Health Institutions, Hospitals, Medical Education.* Istanbul, Turkey: İstanbul Üniversitesi: Istanbul 2010 European Capital of Culture, 2010.

South Asia (see also 118, 124, 816, and 881)

521. Akhtar, Rais, Ashok K. Dutt, and Vandana Wadha, eds. *Malaria in South Asia: Eradication and Resurgence during the Second Half of the Twentieth Century.* New York: Springer, 2010.

522. Amrith, Sunil. *Decolonizing International Health: India and Southeast Asia, 1930–65.* New York: Palgrave Macmillan, 2006.

523. Arnold, David. *Colonizing the Body: State Medicine and Epidemic Disease in Nineteenth-Century India.* Berkeley: University of California Press, 1993.

524. Bhattacharya, Sanjoy. *Expunging Variola: The Control and Eradication of Smallpox in India, 1947–1977.* New Delhi: Orient Longman, 2006.

525. Bhattacharya, Sanjoy, Mark Harrison, and Michael Worboys. *Fractured States: Small Pox, Public Health and Vaccination Policy in British India, 1800–1947.* New Delhi: Orient Longman, 2005.

526. Chakrabarti, Pratik. *Bacteriology in British India: Laboratory Medicine and the Tropics.* Rochester, NY: University of Rochester Press, 2012.

527. Dyson, Tim. *India's Historical Demography: Studies in Famine, Disease and Society.* London: Curzon, 1989.

528. Goswami, Tinmi. *Sanitising Society: Public Health and Sanitation in Colonial Bengal, 1880–1947.* New Delhi: B.R., 2011.

529. Gracia, Fatima de Silva. *Health and Hygiene in Colonial Goa (1510–1961).* New Delhi: Concept, 1994.

530. Guha, Sumit. *Health and Population in South Asia: From Earliest Times to the Present.* London: Hurst, 2001.

531. Harrison, Mark. *Public Health in British India: Anglo-Indian Preventive Medicine 1859–1914.* New York: Cambridge University Press, 1994.

532. Hewa, Soma. *Colonialism, Tropical Disease, and Imperial Medicine: Rockefeller Philanthropy in Sri Lanka.* Lanham, MD: University Press of America, 1995.

533. Jeffery, Roger. *The Politics of Health in India.* Berkeley: University of California Press, 1988.

534. Jones, Margaret. *Health Policy in Britain's Model Colony: Ceylon, 1900–1948.* New Delhi: Wellcome Trust Centre for the History of Medicine, 2004.

535. Pati, Biswamy, and Mark Harrison. *The Social History of Health and Medicine in Colonial India.* New York: Routledge, 2009.

536. Pati, Biswamoy, and Mark Harrison, eds. *Health, Medicine, and Empire: Perspectives on Colonial India.* Hyderabad, India: Orient Longman, 2001.

537. Ramanna, Mridula. *Western Medicine and Public Health in Colonial Bombay, 1845–1895.* London: Sangam, 2002.

538. Ratna, Kalpish. *Uncertain Life and Sure Death: Medicine and Mahamaari in Maritime Mumbai.* Mumbai: Maritime History Society, 2008.

539. Samanta, Arabinda. *Malarial Fever in Colonial Bengal, 1820–1939: Social History of an Epidemic.* Kolkata: Firma KLM, 2002.

540. Satya, Laxman. *Medicine, Disease, and Ecology in Colonial India: The Deccan Plateau in the Nineteenth Century.* New Delhi: Manohar, 2008.

541. Winther, Paul C. *Anglo-European Science and the Rhetoric of Empire: Malaria, Opium and British Rule in India, 1756–1895.* Lanham, MD: Lexington, 2005.

East and Southeast Asia (see also "Beriberi" and "SARS"; and 118, 134, 162, 182, 219, 193, 473, 824, 826, and 911)

542. Aldous, Christopher, and Akihito Suzuki. *Reforming Public Health in Occupied Japan, 1945–52: Alien Prescriptions?* New York: Routledge, 2012.

543. Au, Sokhieng. *Mixed Medicines: Health and Culture in French Colonial Cambodia.* Chicago: University of Chicago Press, 2011.

544. Bay, Alexander R. *Beriberi in Modern Japan: The Making of a National Disease.* Rochester, NY: University of Rochester Press, 2012.

545. Borowy, Iris, ed. *Uneasy Encounters: the Politics of Medicine and Health in China, 1900–1937.* New York: Peter Lang, 2009.

546. De Bevoise, Ken. *Agents of Apocalypse: Epidemic Disease in the Colonial Philippines.* Princeton, NJ: Princeton University Press, 1995.

547. DiMoia, John. *Reconstructing Bodies: Biomedicine, Health, and Nation Building in South Korea since 1945.* Stanford, CA: Stanford University Press, 2013.

548. Hanson, Marta. *Speaking of Epidemics in Chinese Medicine: Disease and the Geographic Imagination in Late Imperial China.* New York: Routledge, 2011.

549. Hillier, S. M., and J. A. Jewell. *Health Care and Traditional Medicine in China, 1800–1982.* Boston: Routledge & Kegan Paul, 1983.

550. Jannetta, Ann. *Epidemics and Mortality in Early Modern Japan.* Princeton, NJ: Princeton University Press, 1987.

551. Jannetta, Ann. *The Vaccinators: Smallpox, Medical Knowledge, and the "Opening" of Japan.* Stanford, CA: Stanford University Press, 2007.

552. Leung, Angela, and Charlotte Furth. *Health and Hygiene in Chinese East Asia: Policies and Publics in the Long Twentieth Century.* Durham, NC: Duke University Press, 2010.

553. Lucas, AnElissa. *Chinese Medical Modernization: Comparative Policy Continuities, 1930s–1980s.* New York: Praeger, 1982.

554. Macpherson, Kerrie L. *A Wilderness of Marshes: The Origins of Public Health in Shanghai, 1843–1893.* New York: Oxford University Press, 1987.

555. Manderson, Lenore. *Sickness and the State: Health and Illness in Colonial Malaya, 1870–1940*. New York: Cambridge University Press, 1996.

556. Monnaie, Lawrence, and Harold Cook. *Global Movements, Local Concerns: Medicine and Health in Southeast Asia*. Singapore: NUS Press, 2012.

557. Peckham, Robert, and David Pomfret. *Imperial Contagions: Medicine, Hygiene, and Cultures of Planning in Asia*. Hong Kong: Hong Kong University Press, 2013.

558. Richaell, Judith. *Disease and Demography in Colonial Burma*. Singapore: NUS, 2006.

559. Rogaski, Ruth. *Hygienic Modernity: Meanings of Health and Disease in Treaty-Port China*. Berkeley: University of California Press, 2004.

560. Ryan, Jennifer, Lincoln C. Chen, and Tony Saich, eds. *Philanthropy for Health in China*. Bloomington: Indiana University Press, 2014.

561. Williams, Robert R. *Toward the Conquest of Beriberi*. Cambridge, MA: Harvard University Press, 1961.

V. AREAS OF CONCERN IN PUBLIC HEALTH
Alcoholism; Drug Addiction (see also "Tobacco Use"; and 541 and 746)

562. Acker, Carolyn. *Creating the American Junkie: Addiction Research in the Classic Era of Narcotic Control*. Baltimore: Johns Hopkins University Press, 2002.

563. Akyeampong, Emmanuel K. *Drink, Power, and Cultural Change: A Social History of Alcohol in Ghana, c. 1800 to Recent Times*. Oxford: James Currey, 1996.

564. Burnham, John. *Bad Habits: Drinking, Smoking, Taking Drugs, Gambling, Sexual Misbehavior, and Swearing in American History*. New York: New York University Press, 1993.

565. Burns, Eric. *The Spirits of America: A Social History of Alcohol*. Philadelphia: Temple University Press, 2004.

566. Courtwright, David. *Forces of Habit: Drugs and the Making of the Modern World*. Cambridge, MA: Harvard University Press, 2001.

567. Courtwright, David. *Dark Paradise: A History of Opiate Addiction in America*. Enl. ed. Cambridge, MA: Harvard University Press, 2001.

568. Fitzgerald, Ross, and Trevor Jordan. *Under the Influence: A History of Alcohol in Australia*. New York: ABC Books / HarperCollins, 2009.

569. Foxcroft, Louise. *The Making of Addiction: The "Use and Abuse" of Opium in Nineteenth-Century Britain*. Burlington, VT: Ashgate, 2007.

570. Gerritsen, Jan-Willem. *The Control of Fuddle and Flash: A Sociological History of the Regulation of Alcohol and Opiates*. Boston: Brill, 2000.

571. Gootenberg, Paul, ed. *Cocaine: Global Histories*. New York: Routledge, 1999.

572. Hickman, Timothy. *The Secret Leprosy of Modern Days: Narcotic Addiction and Cultural Crisis in the United States, 1870–1920*. Amherst: University of Massachusetts Press, 2007.

573. Holt, Mack P. *Alcohol: A Social and Cultural History*. New York: Berg, 2006.

574. Kandall, Stephen R. *Substance and Shadow: Women and Addiction in the United States*. Cambridge, MA: Harvard University Press, 1996.

575. Lerner, Barron H. *One for the Road: Drunk Driving Since 1900*. Baltimore: Johns Hopkins University Press, 2011.

576. McGregor, J. E. *Drink and the City: Alcohol and Alcohol Problems in Urban UK since the 1950s*. Nottingham, UK: Nottingham University Press, 2012.

577. Mancall, Peter. *Deadly Medicine: Indians and Alcohol in Early America*. Ithaca, NY: Cornell University Press, 1995.

578. Mars, Sarah G. *The Politics of Addiction: Medical Conflict and Drug Dependence in England since the 1960s*. Basingstoke, UK: Palgrave Macmillan, 2012.

579. Mold, Alex. *Heroin: The Treatment of Addiction in Twentieth-Century Britain*. DeKalb: Northern Illinois University Press, 2008.

580. Mold, Alex, and Virginia Berridge. *Voluntary Action and Illegal Drugs: Health and Society in Britain since the 1960s*. New York: Palgrave Macmillan, 2010.

581. Murdock, Catherine. *Domesticating Drink: Women, Men, and Alcohol in America, 1870–1940*. Baltimore: Johns Hopkins University Press, 1998.

582. Musto, David. *The American Disease: Origins of Narcotics Control*. 3rd ed. New York: Oxford University Press, 1999.

583. Musto, David, and Pamela Korsmeyer. *The Quest for Drug Control: Politics and Federal Policy in a Period of Increasing Substance Abuse, 1963–1981*. New Haven, CT: Yale University Press, 2002.

584. Nichols, James. *The Politics of Alcohol: A History of the Drink Question in England*. New York: Palgrave, 2011.

585. Seddon, Toby. *A History of Drugs: Drugs and Freedom in the Liberal Age*. New York: Routledge, 2010.

586. Smart, Reginald G., and Alan C. Ogborne, *Northern Spirits: A Social History of Alcohol in Canada*. Toronto: ARF, 1996.

587. Strang, John, and Michael Gossop, eds. *Heroin Addiction and the British System*. New York: Routledge, 2005.

588. Spear, H. B. *Heroin Addiction Care and Control: The British System, 1916–1984*. London: DrugScope, 2002.

589. Tracy, Sarah. *Alcoholism in America: From Reconstruction to Prohibition*. Baltimore: Johns Hopkins University Press, 2005.

590. Tracy, Sarah, and Carolyn Acker, eds. *Altering American Consciousness: The History of Alcohol and Drug Use in the United States, 1800–2000*. Amherst: University of Massachusetts Press, 2004.

591. Warsh, Cheryl, ed. *Drink in Canada: Historical Essays*. Montreal: McGill-Queen's University Press, 1993.

Communicable Disease Control; Vaccination and Anti-Vaccination (see also "General")

592. Cliff, Andrew, and Matthew Smallman-Raynor. *Oxford Textbook of Infectious Disease Control: A Geographical Analysis from Medieval Quarantine to Global Eradication*. Oxford: Oxford University Press, 2013.

593. Conrad, Lawrence, and Dominik Wujastyk. *Contagion: Perspectives from Pre-modern Societies*. Burlington, VT: Ashgate, 2000.

594. Colgrove, James. *State of Immunity: The Politics of Vaccination in Twentieth-Century America*. Berkeley: University of California Press, 2006.

595. Dowling, Harry. *Fighting Infection: Conquests of the Twentieth Century*. Cambridge, MA: Harvard University Press, 1977.

596. Durbach, Nadja. *Bodily Matters: The Anti-vaccination Movement in England, 1853–1907*. Durham, NC: Duke University Press, 2005.

597. Greenwood, David. *Antimicrobial Drugs: Chronicle of a Twentieth Century Medical Triumph.* New York: Oxford University Press, 2008.

598. Heller, Jacob. *The Vaccine Narrative.* Nashville, TN: Vanderbilt University Press, 2008.

599. Kitta, Andrea. *Vaccinations and Public Concern in History: Legend, Rumor, and Risk Perception.* New York: Routledge, 2012.

600. Magner, Lois. *A History of Infectious Diseases and the Microbial World.* Westport, CT: Praeger, 2009.

601. Pollock, George. *An Epidemiological Odyssey: The Evolution of Communicable Disease Control.* Dordrecht, Netherlands: Springer, 2012.

602. Stepan, Nancy. *Eradication: Ridding the World of Diseases Forever?* London: Reaktion Books, 2011.

Demography, Statistics, and Epidemiology (see also "General"; and 113, 120, 131, 145, 155, 174, 338, 377, 383, 394, 399, 408, 415, 480, 527, 592, 806, and 846)

603. Cassedy, James H. *American Medicine and Statistical Thinking, 1800–1860.* Cambridge, MA: Harvard University Press, 1984.

604. Cassedy, James H. *Demography in Early America: Beginnings of the Statistical Mind, 1600–1800.* Cambridge, MA: Harvard University Press, 1969.

605. Cliff, Andrew, Peter Haggett, and Matthew Smallman-Raynor. *Measles: An Historical Geography of a Major Human Viral Disease from Global Expansion to Local Retreat, 1840–1990.* Cambridge, MA: Blackwell, 1993.

606. Coleman, William. *Yellow Fever in the North: The Methods of Early Epidemiology.* Madison: University of Wisconsin Press, 1987.

607. Daston, Lorraine. *Classical Probability in the Enlightenment.* Princeton, NJ: Princeton University Press, 1988.

608. Hempel, Sandra. *The Strange Case of the Broad Street Pump: John Snow and the Mystery of Cholera.* Berkeley: University of California Press, 2007.

609. Kawakita, Yoshio, Shizu Sakai, and Yasuo Ōtsuka, eds. *History of Epidemiology: Proceedings of the 13th International Symposium on the Comparative History of Medicine— East and West.* St. Louis, MO: Ishiyaku EuroAmerica, 1993.

610. Koch, Tom. *Disease Maps: Epidemics on the Ground.* Chicago: University of Chicago Press, 2011.

611. Keating, Conrad. *Smoking Kills: The Revolutionary Life of Richard Doll.* Oxford: Signal Books, 2009.

612. Lancaster, H. O. *Expectations of Life: A Study in the Demography, Statistics and History of World Mortality.* New York: Springer, 1990.

613. Levy, Daniel, and Susan Brink. *A Change of Heart: How the Framingham Heart Study Helped Unravel the Mysteries of Cardiovascular Disease.* New York: Knopf, 2005.

614. Lilienfeld, Abraham M., ed. *Times, Places, and Persons: Aspects of the History of Epidemiology.* Baltimore: Johns Hopkins University Press, 1980.

615. Livi Bacci, Massimo. *Population and Nutrition: An Essay on European Demographic History.* New York: Cambridge University Press, 1991.

616. Morabia, Alfredo. *A History of Epidemiologic Methods and Concepts.* Boston: Birkhäuser, 2004.

617. Porter, Theodore. *The Rise of Statistical Thinking, 1820–1900.* Princeton, NJ: Princeton University Press, 1986.

618. Scott, Susan, and Christopher Duncan. *Human Demography and Disease.* New York: Cambridge University Press, 1998.

619. Susser, Mervyn, and Zena Stein. *Eras in Epidemiology: The Evolution of Ideas.* New York: Oxford University Press, 2009.

620. Top, Franklin H., ed. *The History of American Epidemiology.* St. Louis, MO: Mosby, 1952.

621. Vilensky, Joel A. *Encephalitis Lethargica: During and after the Epidemic.* New York: Oxford University Press, 2011.

Dental Public Health

622. Freeze, R. Allan, and Jay H. Lehr. *The Fluoride Wars: How a Modest Public Health Measure Became America's Longest-Running Political Melodrama.* Hoboken, NJ: Wiley, 2009.

623. Martin, Brian. *Scientific Knowledge in Controversy: The Social Dynamics of the Fluoridation Debate.* Albany: SUNY Press, 1991.

624. Picard, Alyssa. *Making the American Mouth: Dentists and Public Health in the Twentieth Century.* New Brunswick, NJ: Rutgers University Press, 2009.

Emergency Management (see also 924 and 928)

625. Brennan, Virginia, ed. *Natural Disasters and Public Health: Hurricanes Katrina, Rita, and Wilma.* Baltimore: Johns Hopkins University Press, 2009.

626. Wall, Barbra Mann, and Arlene W. Keeling, eds. *Nurses on the Front Line: When Disaster Strikes, 1878–2010.* New York: Springer, 2011.

Environmental Health; Sanitation (see also "Water Supply and Purification"; and 81, 195, 256, 379, 395, 418, 474, 478, 528, 255, and 910)

627. Allen, Michelle. *Cleansing the City: Sanitary Geographies in Victorian London.* Athens: Ohio University Press, 2008.

628. Berridge, Virginia, and Martin Gorsky, eds. *Environment, Health, and History.* New York: Palgrave Macmillan, 2012.

629. Black, Maggie, and Ben Fawcett. *The Last Taboo: Opening the Door on the Global Sanitation Crisis.* Sterling, VA: Earthscan, 2008.

630. Brimblecombe, Peter. *The Big Smoke: A History of Air Pollution in London since Medieval Times.* New York: Methuen, 1987.

631. Brown, Phil, and Edwin J. Mikkelsen. *No Safe Place: Toxic Waste, Leukemia, and Community Action.* Berkeley: University of California Press, 1990.

632. Caufield, Catherine. *Multiple Exposures, Chronicles of the Radiation Age.* London: Seeker & Warburg, 1989.

633. Cohen, William A., and Ryan Johnson, eds. *Filth: Dirt, Disgust, and Modern Life.* Minneapolis: University of Minnesota Press, 2005.

634. Davies, Kate. *The Rise of the U.S. Environmental Health Movement.* Lanham, MD: Rowman & Littlefield, 2013.

635. Dunlap, T. R. *DDT: Scientists, Citizens, and Public Policy.* Princeton, NJ: Princeton University Press, 1981.

636. Dyck, Erika, and Christopher Fletcher, eds. *Locating Health: Historical Investigations of Health and Place.* London: Pickering and Chatto, 2005.

637. English, Peter. *Old Paint: A Medical History of Childhood Lead Poisoning in the United States to 1980.* New Brunswick, NJ: Rutgers University Press, 2001.

638. Fee, Elizabeth. *Garbage: The History and Politics of Trash in New York City.* New York: New York Public Library, 1994.

639. Fletcher, Thomas H. *From Love Canal to Environmental Justice: The Politics of Hazardous Waste on the Canada-U.S Border.* Toronto: University of Toronto Press, 2003.

640. Gottlieb, Robert. *Forcing the Spring: The Transformation of the American Environmental Movement.* Washington, DC: Island Press, 1993.

641. Grieco, Antonio, Sergio Iavicoli, and Giovanni Berlinguer, eds. *Contributions to the History of Occupational and Environmental Prevention: 1st International Conference on the History of Occupational and Environmental Prevention.* New York: Elsevier, 1999.

642. Halliday, Stephen. *The Great Filth: The War against Disease in Victorian England.* Stroud, Gloucestershire: Sutton, 2007.

643. Hays, Samuel P. *Beauty, Health, and Permanence: Environmental Health and Politics in the United States, 1955–1985.* New York: Cambridge University Press, 1987.

644. Kessel, Anthony. *Air, the Environment, and Public Health.* Cambridge, UK: Cambridge University Press, 2006.

645. Markowitz, Gerald, and David Rosner. *Deceit and Denial: The Deadly Politics of Industrial Pollution.* Berkeley: University of California Press, 2012.

646. Markowitz, Gerald, and David Rosner. *Lead Wars: The Politics of Science and the Fate of America's Children.* Berkeley: University of California Press; New York: Milbank Memorial Fund, 2013.

647. Medvedev, Grigori. *The Truth about Chernobyl.* New York: Basic Books, 1991.

648. Medvedev, Zhores. *The Legacy of Chernobyl.* New York: Norton, 1990.

649. Melosi, Martin V. *Garbage in the Cities: Refuse, Reform, and the Environment: 1880–1980.* College Station: Texas A&M University Press, 1981.

650. Melosi, Martin V., ed. *Pollution and Reform in American Cities, 1870–1930.* Austin: University of Texas Press, 1980.

651. Melosi, Martin V. *The Sanitary City: Environmental Services in Urban America from Colonial Times to the Present.* Pittsburgh, PA: University of Pittsburgh Press, 2008.

652. Nash, Linda. *Inescapable Ecologies: A History of Environment, Disease, and Knowledge.* Berkeley: University of California Press, 2006.

653. Price-Smith, Andrew. *The Health of Nations: Infectious Disease, Environmental Change, and Their Effects on National Security and Development.* Cambridge MA: MIT Press, 2002.

654. Sellers, Christopher. *Crabgrass Crucible: Suburban Nature and the Rise of Environmentalism in Twentieth Century.* Chapel Hill: University of North Carolina Press, 2012.

655. Sellers, Christopher. *Hazards of the Job: From Industrial Disease to Environmental Health Science.* Chapel Hill: University of North Carolina Press, 1997.

656. Smith, Derek R. *Creating Environmental and Occupational Health.* Sydney: Sydney University Press, 2010.

657. Stephens, Martha. *The Treatment: The Story of Those Who Died in the Cincinnati Radiation Test.* Durham, NC: Duke University Press, 2002.

658. Sternglass, Ernest J. *Secret Fallout: Low-Level Radiation from Hiroshima to Three-Mile Island.* New York: McGraw-Hill, 1981.

659. Sullivan, Marianne. *Tainted Earth: Smelters, Public Health, and the Environment.* New Brunswick, NJ: Rutgers University Press, 2014.

660. Tarr, Joel A. *The Search for the Ultimate Sink: Urban Pollution in Historical Perspective.* Akron, OH: University of Akron Press, 2011.

661. Walker, J. Samuel. *Three Mile Island: A Nuclear Crisis in Historical Perspective.* Berkeley: University of California.

662. Tone, Andrea. *Devices and Desires: A History of Contraception in America.* New York: Hill &Wang, 2001.

663. Warren, Christian. *Brush with Death: A Social History of Lead Poisoning.* Baltimore: Johns Hopkins University Press, 2000.

664. Wedeen, Richard P. *Poison in the Pot: The Legacy of Lead.* Carbondale: Southern Illinois Press, 1984.

665. Whorton, J. *Before Silent Spring: Pesticides and Public Health in Pre-DDT America.* Princeton, NJ: Princeton University Press, 1974.

666. Williams, Marilyn Thornton. *Washing "The Great Unwashed": Public Baths in Urban America, 1840–1920.* Columbus: Ohio State University Press, 1991.

Food and Drug Regulation (see also "Typhoid," and "Veterinary")

667. Bewley-Taylor, David. *The United States and International Drug Control, 1909–1997.* New York: Continuum, 2001.

668. Boyle, Eric. *Quack Medicine: A History of Combating Health Fraud in Twentieth-Century America.* Santa Barbara, CA: Praeger, 2013.

669. Carpenter, Daniel. *Reputation and Power: Organizational Image and Pharmaceutical Regulation at the FDA.* Princeton, NJ: Princeton University Press, 2010.

670. Gaudillière, Jean-Paul, ed. *Ways of Regulating Drugs in the 19th and 20th Centuries.* New York: Palgrave Macmillan, 2013.

671. Gradman, Christoph, and Jonathan Simon, eds. *Evaluating and Standardizing Therapeutic Agents, 1890–1950.* New York: Palgrave Macmillan, 2010.

672. Hilts, Philip J. *Protecting America's Health: The FDA, Business, and One Hundred Years of Regulation.* New York: Knopf, 2003.

673. Jackson, Charles O. *Food and Drug Legislation in the New Deal.* Princeton, NJ: Princeton University Press, 1970.

674. Kat, Gwen. *Dying to be Beautiful: The Fight for Safe Cosmetics.* Columbus: Ohio State University Press, 2005.

675. Okun, Mitchell. *Fair Play in the Marketplace: The First Battle for Pure Food and Drugs.* DeKalb: Northern Illinois University Press, 1986.

676. Paulus, Ingeborg. *The Search for Pure Food: A Sociology of Legislation in Britain.* London: Robertson, 1974.

677. Parrish, Richard. *Defining Drugs: How Government Became the Arbiter of Pharmaceutical Fact.* New Brunswick, NJ: Transaction, 2003.

678. Pray, W. Steven. *A History of Nonprescription Product Regulation.* Binghamton, NY: Pharmaceutical Products Press, 2003.

679. Stieb, Ernst W. *Drug Adulteration: Detection and Control in Nineteenth Century Britain.* Madison: University of Wisconsin Press, 1966.

680. Young, James Harvey. *Pure Food: Securing the Federal Food and Drugs Act of 1906*. Princeton, NJ: Princeton University Press, 1989.

681. Young, James Harvey. *The Toadstool Millionaires: A Social History of Patent Medicines in America before Federal Regulation*. Princeton, NJ: Princeton University Press, 1961.

682. Waddington, Keir. *The Bovine Scourge: Meat, Tuberculosis and Public Health, 1850–1914*. Rochester, NY: Boydell, 2006.

Health Education (see also 61 and 416)

683. Beier, Lucinda. *For Their Own Good: The Transformation of English Working-Class Health Culture, 1880–1970*. Columbus: Ohio State University Press, 2008.

684. Berridge, Virginia, and Kelly Loughlin, eds. *Medicine, the Market and Mass Media: Producing Health in the Twentieth Century*. New York: Routledge, 2005.

685. Davis, Allen. *Spearheads for Reform: The Social Settlements and the Progressive Movement, 1890 to 1914*. New Brunswick, NJ: Rutgers University Press, 1985.

686. Green, Harvey. *Fit for America: Health, Fitness, Sport, and American Society*. New York: Pantheon Books, 1986.

687. Hansen, Bert. *Picturing Medical Progress from Pasteur to Polio: A History of Mass Media Images and Popular Attitudes in America*. New Brunswick, NJ: Rutgers University Press, 2009.

688. McLendon, William W., Floyd W. Denny, and William B. Blythe. *Bettering the Health of the People: W. Reece Berryhill, the UNC School of Medicine, and the North Carolina Good Health Movement*. Chapel Hill: University of North Carolina at Chapel Hill Library, 2007.

689. Pernick, Martin S. *The Black Stork: Eugenics and the Death of "Defective" Babies in American Medicine and Motion Pictures since 1915*. New York: Oxford University Press, 1996.

690. Poirier, Suzanne. *Chicago's War on Syphilis, 1937–1940: The Times, the* Trib *and the Clap Doctor*. Urbana: University of Illinois Press, 1995.

691. Reagan, Leslie J., Nancy Tomes, and Paula A. Treichler, eds. *Medicine's Moving Pictures: Medicine, Health and Bodies in American Movies and Television*. Rochester, NY: University of Rochester Press, 2007.

692. Serlin, David, ed. *Imagining Illness: Public Health and Visual Culture*. Minneapolis: University of Minnesota Press, 2010.

693. Warsh, Cheryl Krasnick, ed. *Gender, Health, and Popular Culture: Historical Perspectives*. Waterloo, Ontario: Wilfrid Laurier University Press, 2011.

694. Whorton, James C. *Crusaders for Fitness: The History of American Health Reformers*. Princeton, NJ: Princeton University Press, 1982.

Housing; Urban Health (see also 251, 638, 649, and 666)

695. Burnett, John. *A Social History of Housing, 1815–1985*. 2d ed. New York: Methuen, 1986.

696. Carroll, Lydia. *In The Fever King's Preserves: Sir Charles Cameron and the Dublin Slums*. Dublin: Farmar, 2011.

697. Daunton, M. J., ed. *Housing the Workers, 1850–1914: A Comparative Perspective*. London: Leicester University Press, 1990.

698. Burton, Linda. *Communities, Neighborhoods, and Health: Expanding the Boundaries of Place*. New York: Springer, 2011.

699. Freund, Daniel. *American Sunshine: Diseases of Darkness and the Quest for Natural Light.* Chicago: University of Chicago Press, 2012.

700. Gauldie, Enid. *Cruel Habitations: A History of Working-Class Housing 1780–1918.* New York: Harper & Row, 1974.

701. Jackson, Mark. *Health and the Modern Home.* New York: Routledge, 2007.

702. Melosi, Martin. *The Sanitary City: Urban Infrastructure in America from Colonial Times to the Present.* Baltimore: Johns Hopkins University Press, 2000.

703. Morgan, Nigel. *Deadly Dwellings: Housing & Health in a Lancashire Cotton Town: Preston from 1840 to 1914.* Preston, UK: Mullion Books, 1993.

704. Shapiro, Ann-Louise. *Housing the Poor of Paris, 1850–1902.* Madison: University of Wisconsin Press, 1985.

705. Sheard, Sally, and Helen Power, eds. *Body and City: Histories of Urban Public Health.* Burlington, VT: Ashgate, 2000.

706. Wohl, Anthony S. *The Eternal Slum: Housing and Social Policy in Victorian London.* Montreal: McGill-Queen's University Press, 1977.

International Health; Tropical Medicine; Port Quarantine (see also "Bilharzia," "Malaria," "Smallpox," "Tripanosomiasis," "Yellow Fever" and all tropical and developing countries; and 151, 233, 351, 365, 381, and 469)

707. Arnold, David. *Warm Climates and Western Medicine: The Emergence of Tropical Medicine, 1500–1900.* Atlanta, GA: Rodopi, 1996.

708. Bala, Poonam. *Biomedicine as a Contested Site: Some Revelations in Imperial Contexts.* Lanham, MD: Lexington Books, 2009.

709. Bashford, Alison. *Medicine at the Border: Disease, Globalization and Security, 1850 to the Present.* New York: Palgrave Macmillan, 2006.

710. Birn, Anne-Emanuelle, and Theodore Brown, eds. *Comrades in Health: U.S. Health Internationalists, Abroad and at Home.* New Brunswick, NJ: Rutgers University Press, 2013.

711. Booker, John. *Maritime Quarantine: The British Experience, c. 1650–1900.* Burlington VT: Ashgate, 2007.

712. Borowy, Iris. *Coming to Terms with World Health: The League of Nations Health Organisation, 1921–1946.* New York: Peter Lang, 2009.

713. Bruyn, George, and Charles Poser. *The History of Tropical Neurology: Nutritional Disorders.* Canton, MA: Science History Publications, 2003.

714. Cueto, Marcos. *The Value of Health: A History of the Pan American Health Organization.* Rochester, NY: University of Rochester Press, 2007.

715. Eager, J. M. *The Early History of Quarantine: Origin of Sanitary Measures Directed against Yellow Fever.* Washington, DC: Government Printing Office, 1903.

716. Farley, John. *Brock Chisholm, the World Health Organization, and the Cold War.* Vancouver: UBC Press, 2008.

717. Farley, John. *To Cast Out Disease: A History of the International Health Division of the Rockefeller Foundation (1913–1951).* New York: Oxford University Press, 2004.

718. Haynes, Douglas. *Imperial Medicine: Patrick Manson and the Conquest of Tropical Disease.* Philadelphia: University of Pennsylvania Press, 2001.

719. Howard-Jones, Norman. *The Scientific Background of the International Sanitary Conferences, 1851–1938.* Geneva: World Health Organization, 1975.

720. Johnson, Ryan, and Amna Khalid. *Public Health in the British Empire: Intermediaries, Subordinates, and the Practice of Public Health, 1850–1960.* New York: Routledge, 2012.

721. Kantner, John, and Andrew Kantner. *The Struggle for International Consensus on Population and Development.* New York: Palgrave Macmillan, 2006.

722. Moran, Michelle, *Colonizing Leprosy: Imperialism and the Politics of Public Health in the United States.* Chapel Hill: University of North Carolina Press, 2007.

723. Neill, Deborah. *Networks in Tropical Medicine: Internationalism, Colonialism, and the Rise of a Medical Specialty, 1890–1930.* Stanford, CA: Stanford University Press, 2012.

724. Page, Benjamin, and Davis Malone, eds. *Philanthropic Foundations and the Globalization of Scientific Medicine and Public Health: Proceedings of a Conference Jointly Sponsored by Quinnipiac University and the Rockefeller Archive Center.* Lanham, MD: University Press of America, 2007.

725. Price-Smith, Andrew. *Contagion and Chaos: Disease, Ecology, and National Security in the Era of Globalization.* Cambridge, MA: MIT Press, 2009.

726. Rhodes, John. *The End of Plagues: The Global Battle against Infectious Diseases.* New York City: Palgrave Macmillan, 2013.

727. Shchepin, Oleg P., and Waldermar V. Yermakov. *International Quarantine.* Madison, CT: International Universities Press, 1991.

Laboratories

728. Etheridge, Elizabeth W. *Sentinel for Health: A History of the Centers for Disease Control.* Berkeley: University of California Press, 1991.

729. Harden, Victoria A. *Inventing the NIH: Federal Biomedical Research Policy, 1887–1937.* Baltimore: Johns Hopkins University Press, 1986.

730. Smith, George Winston. *Medicines for the Union Army: The United States Army Laboratories during the Civil War.* New York: Pharmaceutical Products Press, 2001.

731. Williams, R. E. O. *Microbiology for the Public Health: The Evolution of the Public Health Laboratory Service, 1939–1980.* London: Public Health Laboratory Service, 1985.

Maternal and Child Health; Women's Health Issues; Gender and Health; Reproductive Health (see also 70, 76, 78, 80, 81, 86, 100, 212, 637, 646, 663, 689, 693, 874, 879, and 880)

732. Apple, Rima. *Mothers and Medicine: A Social History of Infant Feeding.* Madison: University of Wisconsin Press, 1987.

733. Apple, Rima. *Women, Health, and Medicine in America: A Historical Handbook.* New York: Garland, 1990.

734. Baird, Karen L. *Beyond Reproduction: Women's Health, Activism, and Public Policy.* Madison, NJ: Fairleigh Dickinson University Press, 2009.

735. Borsay, Anne, and Pamela Dale, eds. *Disabled Children: Contested Caring, 1850–1979* London: Pickering & Chatto, 2012.

736. Bradbury, Dorothy Edith. *Four Decades of Action for Children: A History of the Children's Bureau.* Washington, DC: Government Printing Office, 1962.

737. Comacchio, Cynthia. *Nations Are Built of Babies: Saving Ontario's Mothers and Children, 1900–1940.* Montreal: McGill-Queen's University Press, 1993.

738. Comacchio, Cynthia, Janet Golden, and George Weisz, eds. *Healing the World's Children: Interdisciplinary Perspectives on Child Health in the Twentieth Century*. Montreal: McGill-Queen's University Press, 2008.

739. Crocker, Ruth. *Cultivating Health: Los Angeles Women and Public Health Reform*. New Brunswick, NJ: Rutgers University Press, 2009.

740. David, Henry P., ed. *From Abortion to Contraception: A Resource to Public Policies and Reproductive Behavior in Central and Eastern Europe from 1917 to the Present*. Westport, CT: Greenwood Press, 1999.

741. Davis, Tom. *Sacred Work: Planned Parenthood and Its Clergy Alliances*. New Brunswick, NJ: Rutgers University Press, 2005.

742. Dwork, Deborah. *War is Good for Babies and Other Young Children: A History of the Infant and Child Welfare Movement in England, 1898–1918*. New York: Tavistock, 1987.

743. Garcia, Jo, Robert Kilpatrick, and Martin Richards, eds. *The Politics of Maternity Care: Services for Childbearing Women in Twentieth-Century Britain*. Oxford: Clarendon Press, 1990.

744. Gijswijt-Hofstra, Marijke, and Hilary Marland. *Cultures of Child Health in Britain and the Netherlands in the Twentieth Century*. New York: Rodopi, 2003.

745. Golden, Janet, Richard A. Meckel, and Heather Munro Prescott, eds. *Children and Youth in Sickness and in Health: A Historical Handbook and Guide*. Westport, CT: Greenwood Press, 2004.

746. Golden, Janet. *Message in a Bottle: The Making of Fetal Alcohol Syndrome*. Cambridge, MA: Harvard University Press, 2005.

747. Gordon, Linda. *Heroes of Their Own Lives: The Politics and History of Family Violence—Boston, 1880–1960*. Urbana: University of Illinois Press, 2002.

748. Gordon, Linda. *Women's Body, Women's Right: A Social History of Birth Control in America*. Rev. ed. New York: Penguin, 1990.

749. Greenlees, Janet, and Linda Bryder, eds. *Western Maternity and Medicine, 1880–1990*. London: Pickering & Chatto, 2013.

750. Heywood, Colin. *Childhood in Nineteenth-Century France: Work, Health, and Education among the "Classes Populaires."* New York: Cambridge University Press, 1988.

751. Holz, Rose. *The Birth Control Clinic in a Marketplace World*. Rochester, NY: University of Rochester Press, 2012.

752. Klaus, Alisa. *Every Child a Lion: The Origins of Maternal and Infant Health Policy in the United States and France, 1890–1920*. Ithaca, NY: Cornell University Press, 1993.

753. Koslow, Jennifer. *Cultivating Health: Los Angeles Women and Public Health Reform*. New Brunswick, NJ: Rutgers University Press, 2009.

754. Jones, Kathleen. *Taming the Troublesome Child: American Families, Child Guidance, and the Limits of Psychiatric Authority*. Cambridge, MA: Harvard University Press, 1999.

755. Ladd-Taylor, Molly, ed. *Raising a Baby the Government Way: Mothers' Letters to the Children's Bureau, 1915–1932*. New Brunswick, NJ: Rutgers University Press, 1986.

756. Leavitt, Judith W., ed. *Women and Health in America: Historical Readings*. Madison: University of Wisconsin Press, 1984.

757. Leavitt, Judith W. 1986. *Brought to Bed: Childbearing in America, 1750–1950*. New York: Oxford University Press.

758. Lewis, Jane. *The Politics of Motherhood: Child and Maternal Welfare in England, 1900–1939*. Montreal: McGill-Queen's University Press, 1980.

759. Mac Lellan, Anne, and Alice Mauger, eds. *Growing Pains: Childhood Illness in Ireland, 1750–1950*. Dublin: Irish Academic Press, 2013.

760. Marks, Lara V. *Metropolitan Maternity: Maternal and Infant Welfare Services in Early Twentieth Century London*. Atlanta, GA: Rodopi, 1996.

761. Meckel, Richard A. *Save the Babies: American Public Health Reform and the Prevention of Infant Mortality, 1850–1920*. Baltimore: Johns Hopkins University Press, 1990.

762. Mohr, James C. *Abortion in America: The Origins and Evolution of National Policy, 1800–1900*. New York: Oxford University Press, 1978.

763. Newton, Hannah. *The Sick Child in Early Modern England*. Oxford: Oxford University Press, 2012.

764. Perkins, Barbara P. *The Medical Delivery Business: Health Reform, Childbirth, and the Economic Order*. New Brunswick, NJ: Rutgers University Press, 2004.

765. Preston, Samuel H., and Michael R Haines. *Fatal Years: Child Mortality in Late Nineteenth-Century America*. Princeton, NJ: Princeton University Press, 1991.

766. Quiroga, Virginia A. Metaxas. *Poor Mothers and Babies: A Social History of Childbirth and Child Care Institutions in Nineteenth-Century New York City*. New York: Garland, 1989.

767. Reagan Leslie J. *When Abortion Was a Crime Women, Medicine, and Law, 1867–1963*. Berkeley: University of California Press, 1997.

768. Reed, James. *From Private Vice to Public Virtue: The Birth Control Movement and American Society since 1830*. New York: Basic Books, 1978.

769. Reed, Laurie, and Paula Saukko. *Governing the Female Body: Gender, Health, and Networks of Power*. Albany: SUNY Press, 2010.

770. Smith, Susan. *Sick and Tired of Being Sick and Tired: Black Women's Health Activism, 1890–1950*. Philadelphia: University of Pennsylvania Press, 1995.

771. Sussman, George D. *Selling Mother's Milk: The Wet-Nursing Business in France, 1715–1914*. Urbana: University of Illinois Press, 1982.

772. Verbrugge, Martha H. *Able-Bodied Womanhood: Personal Health and Social Change in Nineteenth Century Boston*. New York: Oxford University Press, 1998.

773. Watkins, Elizabeth S. *On the Pill: A Social History of Oral Contraception*. Baltimore: Johns Hopkins University Press, 1998.

774. Watkins, Elizabeth S. *The Estrogen Elixir: A History of Hormone Replacement in America*. Baltimore: Johns Hopkins University Press, 2007.

Medical Care Organization and Delivery
(see also 329, 330, 373, 404, 417, and 420)

775. Berridge, Virginia, ed. *Making Health Policy: Networks in Research and Policy after 1945*. New York: Rodopi, 2005.

776. Derickson, Alan. *Health Security for All: Dreams of Universal Health Care in America*. Baltimore: Johns Hopkins University Press, 2005.

777. Engel, Jonathan. *Poor People's Medicine: Medicaid and American Charity Care since 1965*. Durham, NC: Duke University Press, 2006.

778. Freeman, Mark, Eleanor Gordon, Krista Maglen, and M. A. Crowther, eds. *Medicine, Law, and Public Policy in Scotland, c. 1850–1990*. Dundee, Scotland: Dundee University Press, 2011.

779. Gordon, Colin. *Dead on Arrival: The Politics of Health Care in Twentieth-Century America*. Princeton, NJ: Princeton University Press, 2003.

780. Hodgkinson, Ruth G. *The Origins of the National Health Service: The Medical Services of the New Poor Law, 1834–1871*. Berkeley: University of California Press, 1967.

781. Hoffman, Beatrix. *Health Care for Some: Rights and Rationing in the United States since 1930*. Chicago: University of Chicago Press, 2012.

782. Hoffman, Beatrix. *The Wages of Sickness: The Politics of Health Insurance in Progressive America*. Chapel Hill: University of North Carolina Press, 2001.

783. Hollingsworth, J. Rogers, Jerald Hage, and Robert Hanneman. *State Intervention in Medical Care: Consequences for Britain, France, Sweden, and the United States, 1890–1970*. Ithaca, NY: Cornell University Press, 1990.

784. Honigsbaum, Frank. *The Division in British Medicine: A History of the Separation of General Practice from Hospital Care, 1911–1968*. New York: St. Martin's Press, 1979.

785. Honigsbaum, Frank. *Health, Happiness, and Security: The Creation of the National Health Service*. London: Routledge, 1989.

786. Navarro, Vicente. *Medicine under Capitalism*. New York: Prodist, 1976.

787. Numbers, Ronald L. *Almost Persuaded: American Physicians and Compulsory Health Insurance, 1912–1920*. Baltimore: Johns Hopkins University Press, 1978.

788. Numbers, Ronald L., ed. *Compulsory Health Insurance: The Continuing American Debate*. Westport, CT: Greenwood Press, 1982.

789. Opdycke, Sandra. *No One Was Turned Away: The Role of Public Hospitals in New York City since 1900*. New York: Oxford University Press, 1999.

790. Sardell, A. *The U.S. Experiment in Social Medicine: The Community Health Center Program, 1965–1986*. Pittsburgh, PA: University of Pittsburgh Press, 1988.

791. Shryock, Richard Harrison. *Medical Licensing in America, 1650–1965*. Baltimore: Johns Hopkins Press, 1967.

792. Starr, Paul. *Remedy and Reaction: The Peculiar American Struggle over Health Care Reform*. New Haven, CT: Yale University Press, 2011.

793. Starr, Paul. *The Social Transformation of American Medicine*. New York: Basic Books, 1982.

794. Stevens, Robert Bocking, and Rosemary Stevens. *Welfare Medicine in America: A Case Study of Medicaid*. New York: Free Press, 1974.

795. Stevens, Rosemary. *American Medicine and the Public Interest*. New Haven, CT: Yale University Press, 1971.

796. Stevens, Rosemary. *Medical Practice in Modern England: The Impact of Specialization and State Medicine*. New Haven, CT: Yale University Press, 1966.

797. Stevens, Rosemary. *The Public-Private Health Care State: Essays on the History of American Health Care Policy*. New Brunswick, NJ: Transaction Publishers, 2007.

798. Webster, Charles. *Problems of Health Care: The National Health Service before 1957*. London: HMSO, 1988.

799. Weiss, Lawrence D. *Private Medicine and Public Health: Profit, Politics and Prejudice in the American Health Care Enterprise*. Boulder, CO: Westview, 1997.

800. Weisz, George. *Chronic Disease in the Twentieth Century*. Baltimore: Johns Hopkins University Press, 2014.

Mental Health (see also 282, 372, and 492)

801. Ablard, Jonathan. *Madness in Buenos Aires: Patients, Psychiatrists, and the Argentine State, 1880–1983*. Athens: Ohio University Press, 2008.

802. Andrews, Jonathan. *"They're in the Trade . . . of Lunacy, They 'Cannot Interfere'—They Say": The Scottish Lunacy Commissioners and Lunacy Reform in Nineteenth-Century Scotland*. London: Wellcome Trust, 1998.

803. Barham, Peter. *Forgotten Lunatics of the Great War*. New Haven, CT: Yale University Press, 2004.

804. Bartlett, Peter. *The Poor Law of Lunacy: The Administration of Pauper Lunatics in Mid-Nineteenth-Century England*. London: Leicester University Press, 1999.

805. Bartlett, Peter, and David Wright. *Outside the Walls of the Asylum: The History of Care in the Community, 1750–2000*. New Brunswick, NJ: Transaction, 1999.

806. Blackshaw, Gemma, and Sabine Wieber. *Journeys into Madness: Mapping Mental Illness in the Austro-Hungary Empire*. New York: Berghahn, 2012.

807. Brown, Phil. *The Transfer of Care: Psychiatric Deinstitutionalization and Its Aftermath*. Boston: Routledge & Kegan Paul, 1985.

808. Cox, Catherine. *Negotiating Insanity in the Southeast of Ireland, 1820–1900*. New York: Palgrave Macmillan, 2012.

809. Crossley, Nick. *Contesting Psychiatry: Social Movements in Mental Health*. New York: Routledge, 2006.

810. Dain, Norman. *Concepts of Insanity in the United States, 1789–1865*. New Brunswick, NJ: Rutgers University Press, 1964.

811. Danto, Elizabeth. *Freud's Free Clinics: Psychoanalysis & Social Justice, 1918–1938*. New York: Columbia University Press, 2005.

812. Deutsch, Albert. *The Mentally Ill in America*. 2nd ed. New York: Columbia University Press, 1948.

813. Dowbiggin, Ian. *Keeping America Sane: Psychiatry and Eugenics in the United States and Canada, 1880–1940*. Ithaca, NY: Cornell University Press, 2003.

814. Dowdall, George. *The Eclipse of the State Mental Hospital: Policy, Stigma, and Organization*. Albany: SUNY Press, 1996.

815. Eghigian, Greg. *From Madness to Mental Health: Psychiatric Disorder and Its Treatment in Western Civilization*. New Brunswick, NJ: Rutgers University Press, 2010.

816. Ernst, Waltraud. *Mad Tales from the Raj: The European Insane in British India, 1800–1858*. New York: Routledge, 1991.

817. Gijswijt-Hofstra, Marijke, and Roy Porter, eds. *Cultures of Psychiatry and Mental Health Care in Postwar Britain and the Netherlands*. Atlanta, GA: Rodopi, 1998.

818. Gijswijt-Hofstra, Marijke, et al, eds. *Psychiatric Cultures Compared: Psychiatry and Mental Health care in the Twentieth Century: Comparisons and Approaches*. Amsterdam: Amsterdam University Press, 2005.

819. Grob, Gerald N. *From Asylum to Community: Mental Health Policy in Modern America*. Princeton, NJ: Princeton University Press, 1991.

820. Grob, Gerald N. *The Mad among Us: A History of the Care of America's Mentally Ill*. New York: Free Press, 1994.

821. Grob, Gerald N. *Mental Illness and American Society, 1875–1940*. Princeton, NJ: Princeton University Press, 1983.

822. Grob, Gerald N. *Mental Institutions in America: Social Policy to 1875.* New York: Free Press, 1973.

823. Jones, Kathleen. *Asylums and After: A Revised History of the Mental Health Services: From the Early 18th Century to the 1990s.* Atlantic Highlands, NJ: Athlone, 1993.

824. Jones, Tiffany. *Psychiatry, Mental Institutions, and the Mad in Apartheid South Africa.* New York: Routledge, 2012.

825. Moran, James E. *Committed to the State Asylum: Insanity and Society in Nineteenth-Century Quebec and Ontario.* Montreal: McGill-Queen's University Press, 2000.

826. Ng, Beng Yeong. *Till the Break of Day: A History of Mental Health Services in Singapore, 1841–1993.* Singapore: Singapore University Press, 2001.

827. Ng, Vivien W. *Madness in Late Imperial China.* Norman: University of Oklahoma Press, 1991.

828. Parle, Julie. *States of Mind: Searching for Mental Health in Natal and Zululand, 1868–1918.* Scottsville, South Africa: University of KwaZulu-Natal Press, 2007.

829. Prior, Pauline. *Mental Health and Politics in Northern Ireland: A History of Service Development.* Brookfield, VT: Avebury, 1993.

830. Prior, Pauline, ed. *Asylums, Mental Health Care, and the Irish: Historical Studies, 1800–2010.* Dublin: Irish Academic Press, 2012.

831. Paulson, George. *Closing the Asylums: Causes and Consequences of the Deinstitutionalization Movement.* Jefferson, NC: McFarland & Co., 2012.

832. Raz, Mical. *What's Wrong with the Poor? Psychiatry, Race, and the War on Poverty.* Chapel Hill: University of North Carolina Press, 2013.

833. Reid, Fiona. *Broken Men: Shell Shock, Treatment and Recovery in Britain, 1914–1930.* New York: Continuum, 2010.

834. Rothman, David. *The Discovery of the Asylum: Social Order and Disorder in the New Republic.* Rev. ed. Boston: Little, Brown, 1990.

835. Torrey, E. Fuller. *How the Federal Government Destroyed the Mental Illness Treatment System.* Oxford: Oxford University Press, 2014.

836. Torrey, E. Fuller. *Out of the Shadows: Confronting America's Mental Illness Crisis.* New York: John Wiley, 1997.

837. Torrey, E. Fuller, and Judy Miller. *The Invisible Plague: The Rise of Mental Illness from 1750 to the Present.* New Brunswick, NJ: Rutgers University Press, 2001.

**Military; Naval; War and Health (see also "Influenza," and "Scurvy";
and 79, 82, 97, 119, 197, 234, 335, 403, 510, 803, 833, 870, and 928)**

838. Allison, R. S. *Sea Diseases: The Story of a Great Natural Experiment in Preventive Medicine in the Royal Navy.* London: John Bale, 1943.

839. Byerly, Carol R. *Fever of War: The Influenza Epidemic in the U.S. Army during World War I.* New York: New York University Press, 2005.

840. Bayne-Jones, Stanhope. *The Evolution of Preventive Medicine in the United States Army, 1607–1939.* Washington, DC: Office of the Surgeon General, 1968.

841. Cirillo, Vincent. *Bullets and Bacilli: The Spanish-American War and Military Medicine.* New Brunswick, NJ: Rutgers University Press, 2004.

842. Gillett, Mary C. *The Army Medical Department, 1917–1941.* Washington: U.S. Army Center for Military History, 2009.

843. Harrison, Mark. *Medicine and Victory: British Military Medicine in the Second World War*. New York: Oxford University Press, 2004.

844. Lindee, M. Susan. *Suffering Made Real: American Science and the Survivors at Hiroshima*. Chicago: University of Chicago Press, 1994.

845. Özdemir, Hikmet. *The Ottoman Army, 1914–1918: Disease and Death on the Battlefield*. Salt Lake City: University of Utah Press, 2008.

846. Smallman-Raynor, Matthew, and Andrew Cliff. *War Epidemics: An Historical Geography of Infectious Diseases in Military Conflict and Civil Strife, 1850–2000*. New York: Oxford University Press, 2004.

847. Wintermute, Bobby. *Public Health and the U.S. Military: A History of the Army Medical Department, 1818–1917*. New York: Routledge, 2011.

Nursing (see also 626)

848. Breckenridge, Mary. *Wide Neighborhoods: A Story of the Frontier Nursing Service*. New York: Harper, 1952. Reprint. Lexington: University Press of Kentucky, 1981.

849. Bartlett, Marie. *The Frontier Nursing Service: America's First Rural Nurse-Midwife Service and School*. Jefferson, NC: McFarland, 2008.

850. Buhler-Wilkerson, Karen. *False Dawn: The Rise and Decline of Public Health Nursing, 1900–1930*. New York: Garland, 1989.

851. Yrjälä, Ann. *Public Health and Rockefeller Wealth: Alliance Strategies in the Early Formation of Finnish Public Health Nursing*. Åbo: Åbo Akademi University Press, 2005.

Nutrition (see also "Beriberi" and "Scurvy"; and 269, 271, 388, 402, 484, 615, 711, and 838)

852. Akiyama, Yuriko. *Feeding the Nation: Nutrition and Health in Britain before World War One*. New York: Tauris, 2008.

853. Atkins, Peter, Peter Lummel, and Derek J. Oddy, eds. *Food and the City in Europe since 1800*. Burlington, VT: Ashgate, 2007.

854. Cain, Louis P., and Donald G. Paterson. *The Children of Eve: Population and Well-Being in History*. Malden, MA: Wiley-Blackwell, 2012.

855. Cantor, David, Christian Bonah, and Matthias Dörries, eds. *Meat, Medicine, and Human Health in the Twentieth Century*. London: Pickering & Chatto, 2010.

856. Clarkson, Leslie, and E. Margaret Crawford. *Feast and Famine: Food and Nutrition in Ireland, 1500–1920*. New York: Oxford University Press, 2001.

857. Clay, Karen, and Werner Troesken. *Deprivation and Disease in Early Twentieth-Century America*. Cambridge, MA: National Bureau of Economic Research, 2006.

858. Drummond, J. C., and Anne Wilbraham. *The Englishman's Food: Five Centuries of English Diet*. Rev. ed. London: Jonathan Cape, 1958.

859. Floud, Roderick, Kenneth W. Wachter, and Annabel Gregory. *Height, Health, and History: Nutritional Status in the United Kingdom, 1750–1980*. New York: Cambridge University Press, 1990.

860. Floud, Roderick, et al. *The Changing Body: Health, Nutrition, and Human Development in the Western World since 1700*. New York: Cambridge University Press, 2011.

861. Kamminga, Harmke, and Andrew Cunningham, eds. *The Science and Culture of Nutrition, 1840–1940*. Atlanta, GA: Rodopi, 1995.

862. Newman, Lucile F., et al., eds. *Hunger in History: Food Shortage, Poverty and Deprivation.* Cambridge, MA: Basil Blackwell, 1990.

863. Scott, Susan, and Christopher Duncan. *Demography and Nutrition: Evidence from Historical and Contemporary Populations.* Malden, MA: Blackwell Science, 2002.

864. Semba, Richard. *The Vitamin A Story: Lifting the Shadow of Death.* Basel: Karger, 2012.

865. Smith, David F., ed. *Nutrition in Britain: Science, Scientists, and Politics in the Twentieth Century.* New York: Routledge, 1997.

866. Vernon, James. *Hunger: A Modern History.* Cambridge, MA: Belknap Press of Harvard University Press, 2007.

867. Steckel, Richard H., and Jerome C. Rose. *The Backbone of History: Health and Nutrition in the Western Hemisphere.* New York: Cambridge University Press, 2002.

868. Ulijaszek, Stanley, Neil Mann, and Sarah Elton. *Evolving Human Nutrition: Implications for Public Health.* New York: Cambridge University Press, 2012.

869. Veit, Helen, *Modern Food, Moral Food: Self-Control, Science, and the Rise of Modern American Eating in the Early Twentieth Century.* Chapel Hill: University of North Carolina Press, 2013.

870. Watt, J., et al., eds. *Starving Sailors: The Influence of Nutrition upon Naval and Maritime History.* Greenwich, UK: National Maritime Museum, 1981.

Occupational Health (see also 71, 496, 501, 641, 655, 656, 752, and 927)

871. Bartrip, Peter. *The Home Office and the Dangerous Trades: Regulating Occupational Disease in Victorian and Edwardian Britain.* New York: Rodopi, 2002.

872. Bayer, Ronald, ed. *The Health and Safety of Workers: Case Studies in the Politics of Professional Responsibility.* New York: Oxford University Press, 1988.

873. Beardsley, Edward H. *A History of Neglect: Health Care for Blacks and Mill Workers in the Twentieth-Century South.* Knoxville: University of Tennessee Press, 1987.

874. Clark, Claudia. *Radium Girls, Women and Industrial Health Reform: 1910–1935.* Chapel Hill: University of North Carolina Press, 1997.

875. Derickson, Alan. *Black Lung: Anatomy of a Public Health Disaster.* Ithaca, NY: Cornell University Press, 1998.

876. Derickson, Alan. *Workers' Health, Workers' Democracy: The Western Miners' Struggle, 1891–1925.* Ithaca, NY: Cornell University Press, 1989.

877. Gordon, Bonnie. *Phossy-Jaw and the French Match Workers: Occupational Health and Women in the Third Republic.* New York: Garland, 1989.

878. Hahamovitch, Cindy. *The Fruits of Their Labor: Atlantic Coast Farmworkers and the Making of Migrant Poverty, 1870–1945.* Chapel Hill: University of North Carolina Press, 1997.

879. Harrison, Barbara. *Not Only the "Dangerous Trades": Women's Work and Health in Britain, 1880–1914.* Bristol, PA: Taylor & Francis, 1996.

880. Hepler, Alison. *Women in Labor: Mothers, Medicine, and Occupational Health in the United States, 1890–1980.* Columbus: Ohio State University Press, 2000.

881. Jones, Tara. *Corporate Killing: Bhopals Will Happen.* London: Free Association, 1988.

882. Judkins, Bennett M. *We Offer Ourselves as Evidence: Toward Workers' Control of Occupational Health.* New York: Greenwood Press, 1986.

883. Long, Vicky. *The Rise and Fall of the Healthy Factory: The Politics of Industrial Health in Britain, 1914–60.* Houndmills, UK: Palgrave Macmillan, 2011.

884. Mulcahy, Richard. *A Social Contract for the Coal Fields: The Rise and Fall of the United Mine Workers of America Welfare and Retirement Fund*. Knoxville: University of Tennessee Press, 2000.

885. Murphy, Michelle. *Sick Building Syndrome and the Problem of Uncertainty: Environmental Politics, Technoscience, and Women Workers*. Durham, NC: Duke University Press, 2006.

886. Oliver, Thomas. *Dangerous Trades: History of Health and Safety at Work*. Bristol: Thoemmes Continuum, 2004.

887. Riley, James. *Sick, Not Dead: The Health of British Workingmen during the Mortality Decline*. Baltimore: Johns Hopkins University Press, 1997.

888. Rosen, George. *The History of Miners' Diseases: A Medical and Social Interpretation*. New York: Schuman's, 1943.

889. Rosner, David, and Markowitz, Gerald E. *Deadly Dust: Silicosis and the Politics of Occupational Disease in Twentieth-Century America*. Princeton, NJ: Princeton University Press, 1991.

890. Rosner, David, and Markowitz, Gerald, eds. *Dying for Work: Workers' Safety and Health in Twentieth-Century America*. Bloomington: Indiana University Press, 1987.

891. Sellers, Christopher, and Joseph Mellings, eds. *Dangerous Trade: Histories of Industrial Hazards across a Globalizing World*. Philadelphia: Temple University Press, 2011.

892. Sicherman, Barbara. *Alice Hamilton: A Life in Letters*. Cambridge, MA: Harvard University Press, 1984.

893. Smith, Barbara Ellen. *Digging Our Own Graves: Coal Miners and the Struggle over Black Lung Disease*. Philadelphia: Temple University Press, 1987.

894. Teleky, Ludwig. *History of Factory and Mine Hygiene*. New York: Columbia University Press, 1948.

895. Weindling, Paul, ed. *The Social History of Occupational Health*. Dover, NH: Croom Helm, 1985.

896. Whiteside, James. *Regulating Danger: The Struggle for Mine Safety in the Rocky Mountain Coal Industry*. Lincoln: University of Nebraska Press, 1990.

Prison Medicine

897. Sim, Joe. *Medical Power in Prisons: The Prison Medical Service in England, 1774–1989*. Philadelphia: Open University Press, 1990.

Professional Education; Schools of Public Health (see also 688)

898. Bator, Paul Adolphus. *Within Reach of Everyone: A History of the University of Toronto School of Hygiene and the Connaught Laboratories*. Ottawa: Canadian Public Health Association, 1990.

899. Bhopal, Raj, and John Last. *Public Health: Past, Present, and Future; Celebrating Academic Public Health in Edinburgh, 1902–2002*. Norwich, UK: TSO, 2004.

900. Fee, Elizabeth. *Disease and Discovery: A History of the Johns Hopkins School of Hygiene and Public Health, 1916–1939*. Baltimore: Johns Hopkins University Press, 1987.

901. Fee, Elizabeth, and Roy M. Acheson, eds. *A History of Education in Public Health: Health That Mocks the Doctor's Rules*. New York: Oxford University Press, 1990.

902. Korstad, Robert Rodgers. *Dreaming of a Time: The School of Public Health, the University of North Carolina at Chapel Hill, 1939–1989*. Chapel Hill: University of North Carolina Press, 1990.

903. Power, Helen J. *Tropical Medicine in the Twentieth Century: A History of the Liverpool School of Tropical Medicine 1898–1990*. New York: Columbia University Press, 1999.

904. *Saving Lives Millions at a Time*. Baltimore: Johns Hopkins Bloomberg School, 2004.

905. Schneider, Donna, and David E. Lilienfeld. *Public Health: The Development of a Discipline*. 2 vols. New Brunswick, NJ: Rutgers University Press, 2008–2011.

906. Wilkinson, Lisa, and Anne Hardy. *Prevention and Cure: The London School of Hygiene & Tropical Medicine; A 20th Century Quest for Global Public Health*. New York: Kegan Paul, 2001.

Rural Health

907. Barney, Sandra. *Authorized to Heal: Gender, Class, and the Transformation of Medicine in Appalachia, 1880–1930*. Chapel Hill: University of North Carolina Press, 2000.

908. Barona, Josep, and Steven Cherry, eds. *Health and Medicine in Rural Europe (1850–1945)*. València, Spain: Seminari d'Estudis sobre la Ciència, 2005.

909. Ransel, David. *Village Mothers: Three Generations of Change in Russia and Tataria*. Bloomington: Indiana University Press, 2000.

910. Valenčius, Conovery Bolton. *The Health of the Country: How American Settlers Understood Themselves and Their Land*. New York: Basic Books, 2002.

Tobacco Use and Control (see also 611)

911. Benedict, Carol. *Golden-Silk Smoke: A History of Tobacco in China, 1550–2010*. Berkeley: University of California Press, 2011.

912. Berridge, Virginia. *Marketing Health: Smoking and the Discourse of Public Health in Britain, 1945–2000*. Oxford : New York: Oxford University Press, 2007.

913. Brandt, Allan. *The Cigarette Century: The Rise, Fall, and Deadly Persistence of the Product That Defined American*. New York: Basic Books, 2007.

914. Cordry, Harold V. *Tobacco: A Reference Handbook*. Santa Barbara, CA: ABC-Clio, 2001.

915. Gately, Ian. *Tobacco: The Story of How Tobacco Seduced the World*. New York: Grove Press, 2001.

916. Gilman, Sandor, and Zhou Xun, eds. *Smoke: A Global History of Smoking*. London: Reaktion, 2004.

917. Givel, Michael, and Andrew Spivak. *Heartland Tobacco War*. Lanham, MD: Lexington, 2013.

918. Hughes, Jason. *Learning to Smoke: Tobacco Use in the West*. Chicago: University of Chicago Press, 2003.

919. Proctor, Robert N. *Golden Holocaust: Origins of the Cigarette Catastrophe and the Case for Abolition*. Berkeley: University of California Press, 2012.

920. Winter, Joseph. C. *Tobacco Use by Native North American: Sacred Smoke and Silent Killer*. Norman: University of Oklahoma Press, 2000.

921. Wolfson, Mark. *The Fight against Big Tobacco: The Movement, the State and the Public's Health*. New York: Aldine de Gruyter, 2001.

Veterinary Public Health (see also 84 and 483)

922. Brown, Karen, and Daniel Gilfoyle. *Healing the Herds: Disease, Livestock Economies, and the Globalization of Veterinary Medicine*. Athens: Ohio University Press, 2010.

923. Smith, Gary, and Alan Kelly, eds. *Food Security in a Global Economy: Veterinary Medicine and Public Health.* Philadelphia: University of Pennsylvania Press, 2008.

Voluntary and Professional Organizations

924. Bennett, Angela. *The Geneva Convention: The Hidden Origins of the Red Cross.* Stroud UK: Sutton, 2005.

925. Bernstein, Nancy R. *The First One Hundred Years: Essays on the History of the American Public Health Association.* Washington, DC: American Public Health Association, 1972.

926. Dittmer, John. *The Good Doctors: The Medical Committee for Human Rights and the Struggle for Social Justice in Health Care.* New York: Bloomsbury Press, 2009.

927. Grieco, Antonio. *Origins of Occupational Health Associations in the World.* Boston: Elsevier, 2003.

928. Hutchinson, John. *Champions of Charity: War and the Rise of the Red Cross.* Boulder, CO: Westview: 1996.

929. Leon Sanz, Pilar. *Health Institutions at the Origin of the Welfare Systems in Europe.* Pamplona: Ediciones Universidad de Navarra, 2010.

930. Shryock, Richard Harrison. *National Tuberculosis Association, 1904–1954: A Study of the Voluntary Health Movement in the United States.* New York: National Tuberculosis Association, 1957.

Water Supply and Purification
(see also "Cholera," "Typhoid Fever," and "Dental")

931. Ashby, Thomas. *The Aqueducts of Ancient Rome.* Oxford: Clarendon Press, 1935.

932. Blake, Nelson. *Water for the Cities: A History of the Urban Water Supply Problem in the United States.* Syracuse, NY: Syracuse University Press, 1956.

933. Cain, Louis. *Sanitary Strategy for a Lakefront Metropolis: The Case of Chicago.* DeKalb: Northern Illinois University Press, 1978.

934. Goubert, Jean-Pierre. *The Conquest of Water: The Advent of Health in the Industrial Age.* Princeton, NJ: Princeton University Press, 1989.

935. Hamlin, Christopher. *A Science of Impurity: Water Analysis in Nineteenth Century Britain.* Berkeley: University of California Press, 1990.

936. Kosso, Cynthia, and Anne Scott. *The Nature and Function of Water, Baths, Bathing, and Hygiene from Antiquity through the Renaissance.* Boston: Brill, 2009.

937. Luckin, Bill. *Pollution and Control: A Social History of the Thames in the Nineteenth Century.* Boston: Adam Hilger, 1986.

938. McGuire, Michael J. *The Chlorine Revolution: Water Disinfection and the Fight to Save Lives.* Denver, CO: American Water Works Association, 2013.

939. Reid, Donald. *Paris Sewers and Sewermen: Realities and Representations.* Cambridge, MA: Harvard University Press, 1991.

940. Robins, F. W. *The Story of Water Supply.* New York: Oxford University Press, 1946.

941. Smith, Denis, ed. *Water Supply and Public Health Engineering.* Brookfield, VT: Ashgate, 1999.

942. Troesken, Werner. *The Great Lead Water Pipe Disaster.* Cambridge, MA: MIT Press, 2006.